On Call
Surgery

Other Titles in the ON CALL Series

Adams & Bresnick: **On Call Procedures,** *2nd Edition, 2006*

Bernstein, Levin, Poag & Rubinstein: **On Call Psychiatry,** *3rd edition, 2006*

Chin: **On Call Obstetrics and Gynecology,** *3rd Edition, 2006*

Henry & Mathur: **On Call Laboratory Medicine and Pathology,** *2000*

Khan: **On Call Cardiology,** *3rd Edition, 2006*

Marshall & Mayer: **On Call Neurology,** *3rd Edition, 2006*

Marshall & Ruedy: **On Call Principles and Protocols,** *4th Edition, 2004*

Nocton & Gedeit: **On Call Pediatrics,** *3rd Edition, 2006*

On Call Surgery

GREGG A. ADAMS, MD, FACS

Acting Chair, Department of Surgery
Director of Surgical Education
Santa Clara Valley Medical Center
San Jose, California
Clinical Instructor
Department of General Surgery
Stanford University Medical Center
Stanford, California

STEPHEN D. BRESNICK, MD, DDS

Clinical Assistant Professor of Surgery
Division of Plastic and Reconstructive
  Surgery
University of Southern California School
  of Medicine
Los Angeles, California

3 rd edition

SAUNDERS
ELSEVIER

1600 John E Kennedy Blvd.
Ste 1800
Philadelphia, PA 19103-2899

ON CALL SURGERY

ISBN-13: 978-1-4160-2441-5
ISBN-10: 1-4160-2441-7

Notice

Knowledge and best practice in this field are constantly changing. As new research and experience broaden our knowledge, changes in practice treatment and drug therapy may become necessary or appropriate. Readers are advised to check the most current information provided (i) on procedures featured or (ii) by the manufacturer of each product to be administered, to verify the recommended dose or formula, the method and duration of administration, and contraindications. It is the responsibility of the practitioner, relying on his or her own experience and knowledge of the patient, to make diagnoses, to determine dosages and the best treatment for each individual patient, and to take all appropriate safety precautions. To the fullest extent of the law, neither the Publisher nor the Authors assume any liability for any injury and/or damage to persons or property arising out of or related to any use of the material contained in this book.

The Publisher

Library of Congress Cataloging-in-Publication Data

Adams, Gregg A.
    On call: surgery / Gregg A. Adams, Stephen D. Bresnick.–3rd ed.
      p. ; cm.
    Includes index.
    ISBN 1-4160-2441-7
    1. Surgical emergencies–Handbooks, manuals, etc. I. Title: Surgery. II. Bresnick, Stephen D. III. Title.
    [DNLM: 1. Emergencies–Handbooks. 2. Surgical Procedures, Operative–Handbooks. WO 39 A213o 2006]
RD93.A32 2006
617'.026–dc22

2005057525

Acquisitions Editor: Jim Merritt
Developmental Editor: Nicole DiCicco
Designer: Ellen Zanolle

Printed in the United States of America

Working together to grow
libraries in developing countries
www.elsevier.com | www.bookaid.org | www.sabre.org

ELSEVIER   BOOK AID International   Sabre Foundation

Last digit is the print number: 9   8   7   6   5   4   3   2   1

Dedicated to Maria Allo, MD—surgeon, teacher, mentor, friend.

Preface

Medicine changes daily. In particular, residency training is evolving to address new challenges such as decreased work hours and new regulatory and privacy guidelines. "Best practices" and clinical guidelines are becoming prominent, and computerized health records make vast amounts of information available without actually saving any time. Despite these changes in the infrastructure of how medical care is delivered, patients still have very high expectations of your time and abilities. With fewer hours to meet patients' needs and more information available at your fingertips, it is imperative that an organized approach be used to diagnose and treat clinical syndromes. In addition, limiting work hours has created a situation where patients must routinely be "checked-out" to an on-call resident, placing new emphasis on communication between colleagues and consultants.

Many educational situations occur during nights spent "on call." Although this is a time of learning, it is also a time of stress, owing to fatigue, heavy workloads, and decreased availability of staff support. In addition, the on-call team may have responsibility for patients about whom limited information is available. *On Call Surgery* is designed to meet the needs of today's surgeon. In a very concise and organized fashion, the text will lead medical students, residents, and practitioners of all levels through a safe and relevant evaluation of clinical on-call problems.

Gregg A. Adams

Stephen D. Bresnick

Acknowledgments

We acknowledge all of our teachers, including our parents, instructors, fellow residents and students, and especially our patients.

Thank you also to those who tolerated many late nights of typing and those many others who contributed, directly and indirectly, to this work.

Structure of the Book

Most medical didactic education starts with a disease process, explaining first the pathophysiology and then revealing the clinical findings. The training at the bedside, however, starts with a physical complaint or a finding, and the underlying disease is only revealed through careful listening, observation, and deduction. A wide differential diagnosis is then created, recognizing that in order to *make* a diagnosis, you must first *think* of a diagnosis. Then the differential diagnosis is pared down using history, physical examination, and the judicious use of laboratory and radiographic studies.

In order to more fully follow the line of thinking at the bedside, the structure of *On Call Surgery* starts with the initial phone call from a bedside care provider, describing a patient problem. A list of likely diagnoses is generated and a plan for assessment and management of the patient is outlined. Particular emphasis is placed on those diseases that pose the greatest risk to a patient and the special needs of the preoperative and postoperative patient.

PHONE CALL

The initial phone call from the bedside care provider describes the patient symptoms and signs.

Questions

Pertinent questions are listed that help clarify the nature and severity of the problem.

Orders

Orders or instructions that will increase the safety of the patient or help rapidly diagnosis the patient are listed.

Not all of these orders need be used in each scenario.

Inform RN

Let the bedside care provider (often an RN) know when to expect you at the bedside to evaluate the patient.

ELEVATOR THOUGHTS

These are the Differential Diagnoses lists. The phrase "Elevator Thoughts" was coined by Shane Marshall and John Ruedy in the first edition of *On Call: Principles and Protocols*, in recognition that an elevator ride often stands between you and your patient. They encourage you to use that time wisely by thinking about the possible causes of a specific symptom or complaint.

MAJOR THREAT TO LIFE

These are those disease processes that pose the most serious risk to the patient and must be ruled out first.

BEDSIDE

The evaluation at the bedside is divided into various steps, starting from the moment you walk into the room.

Quick Look Test

This is a rapid visual assessment of the patient. It should be practiced with every patient encounter. Quickly divide your patient into one of three categories: well, sick, or critical. This will help focus your next steps and give you a guide as to how rapidly the remainder of the assessment needs to be made.

Airway and Vital Signs

The next evaluation of any patient is a quick assessment of the patient's breathing, vital signs, and fluid status. Special note is made of any recent changes or instability. Breathing or circulatory difficulties are dealt with immediately as life-threatening conditions.

Selective History, Chart Review, and Physical Examination

Next is a limited and directed history and physical examination, which is generally problem directed. This departs from the standard 30- to 60-minute interview practiced in medical school or the unhurried evaluation of a new patient. The motivation is different when the physician is on call. A specific complaint is to be addressed, and although that often expands into an assessment of several systems, other aspects of the patient's care, unrelated to the current complaint, do not need to be evaluated at this time. Sources of pertinent information are obtained from the bedside caregiver, from the patient, and from the chart. Remember that much information has already been obtained and is organized in the bedside chart, but be careful not to rely completely on this information. Circumstances may dictate further questioning and examination not already documented.

MANAGEMENT

Some management begins before the assessment is complete. In such cases, the steps needed to keep a patient safe should be begun before continuing with other steps.

The text also contains helpful Appendices and a Formulary of commonly used medications. A comprehensive list of necessary Formulae is also included.

The structure and content of *On Call Surgery* will be helpful as points of reference and guides to the management of many of the typical problems encountered while caring for surgical patients. We believe that the reader will find *On Call Surgery* to be one of the most valuable resources available.

Contents

Appendices

Commonly Used Abbreviations

Many hospitals limit some types of abbreviations in clinical notes and in orders so as to avoid ambiguity and to improve patient safety. Check with your institution to confirm that an abbreviation is useable. For example, the Joint Commission for the Accreditation of Hospital Organizations (JCAHO) has recently discouraged the following abbreviations: **qD** (daily), **QOD** (every other day), **U** (units), **IU** (international units), **MS** and **MSO$_4$** (morphine sulfate), and **MgSO$_4$** (magnesium sulfate). In addition, it is generally good policy to avoid adding a trailing zero after a decimal point (e.g., write "2" rather than "2.0") and be sure to include the preceding zero before a decimal point (e.g., write "0.5" rather than ".5").

ABCs	airway, breathing, circulation (first steps of evaluating a critically ill patient)
Abd.	abdomen
ABG	arterial blood gas
ABI	ankle-brachial index*
AC	*ante cibum* (before meals)
ACE	angiotensin-converting enzyme
ACS	acute coronary syndrome
ACTH	adrenocorticotrophic hormone
ADH	antidiuretic hormone
AF	atrial fibrillation
AIDS	acquired immunodeficiency syndrome
ALT	alanine aminotransferase (SGPT)
AMI	acute myocardial infarction (often MI)
ant.	anterior
Ao.	aorta

*Denotes that a formula is listed in Appendix G.

AP	anterior-to-posterior direction (as in path of x-rays)
ARDS	adult respiratory distress syndrome
ASA	acetylsalicylic acid (aspirin)
ASD	atrioseptal defect
AST	aspartate aminotransferase (SGOT)
ATN	acute tubular necrosis
AV	atrioventricular
AZT	zidovudine
B	bilateral
BBB	bundle branch block (usually right or left)
ß-hCG	beta-human chorionic gonadotropin
BID	*bis in die*, twice a day
BP	blood pressure*
BPH	benign prostatic hypertrophy
bpm	beats per minute
BS	breath sounds
BUN	blood urea nitrogen
°C	degrees centigrade, or Celsius
C & S	culture and sensitivity
Ca+	calcium ion
CAD	coronary artery disease
CBC	complete blood count
cc	cubic centimeter (milliliter)
CCU	critical care unit
CHF	congestive heart failure
CI	cardiac index*
Cl−	chloride ion
cm	centimeter
cm H$_2$O	centimeters of water*
CMV	cytomegalovirus
CN	cranial nerve
CNS	central nervous system

---

*Denotes that a formula is listed in Appendix G.

CO	cardiac output*
CO₂	carbon dioxide
COPD	chronic obstructive pulmonary disease
COX-2	cyclo-oxygenase isoenzyme-2
CPB	cardiopulmonary bypass
CPK	creatine phosphokinase
CPP	cerebral perfusion pressure (MAP– ICP)*
CPR	cardiopulmonary resuscitation
CPT	chest physiotherapy
Cr	creatinine
CrCl	creatinine clearance*
CSF	cerebrospinous fluid
CT	computed tomography
CVA	cerebrovascular accident (stroke)
CVP	central venous pressure
CXR	chest x-ray
D5NS	5% dextrose in normal saline
D5W	5% dextrose in sterile water
D10W	10% dextrose in sterile water
D20W	20% dextrose in sterile water
D50W	50% dextrose in sterile water
DBP	diastolic blood pressure
DDAVP	1-desamino-(8-ᴅ-arginine)-vasopressin, desmopressin
DI	diabetes insipidus
DIC	disseminated intravascular coagulation
DKA	diabetic ketoacidosis
dl	deciliter
DM	diabetes mellitus
DT	delirium tremens
DVT	deep venous thrombosis
Dx	diagnosis
ECF	extracellular fluid

*Denotes that a formula is listed in Appendix G.

ECG, EKG	electrocardiogram
EDTA	disodium edentate
EEG	electroencephalogram
EMD	electromechanical dissociation (PEA)
ERCP	endoscopic retrograde cholangiopancreoscopy
ET	endotracheal
Extrem.	extremity examination
°F	degrees Fahrenheit
FFP	fresh frozen plasma
FHx	family history
FiO$_2$	fraction of oxygen in inspired air
Fr	French (diameter in mm)
g	gram
GI	gastrointestinal
GN	glomerulonephritis
gran.	granulocytes, polymorphonucleocytes (PMNs)
GU	genitourinary
H$_2$	histamine receptor type-2
H&P	history and physical examination
HAV	hepatitis A virus
Hb	hemoglobin
HBV	hepatitis B virus
HCl	hydrochloride, hydrochloric acid
HCO$_3^-$	bicarbonate ion*
Hct	hematocrit
HCTZ	hydrochlorothiazide
HCV	hepatitis C virus
HDV	hepatitis D virus
HEENT	head, eyes, ears, nose, throat examination
HEV	hepatitis E virus
HIV	human immunodeficiency virus
HPI	history of present illness

*Denotes that a formula is listed in Appendix G.

HR	heart rate
HS	*hora somni*, at bedtime
HTN	hypertension
Hx	history
IABP	intra-aortic balloon pump
ICF	intracellular fluid
ICP	intracranial pressure
ICU	intensive care unit
IJ	internal jugular vein (or line)
IM	intramuscular
inf.	inferior
INR	international normalizing ratio
I/O	intake and output measurements
IP	intraperitoneal
IV	intravenous
IVC	inferior vena cava
IVF	intravenous fluids
J	joule
JVD	jugular venous distention
K⁺	potassium ion
kg	kilogram
KUB	"kidney, ureter, bladder," a flat-plate radiograph of the abdomen
L	left side
L	liter
lat.	lateral
LDH	lactate dehydrogenase
LFT	liver function tests
LLL	left lower lobe (of the lung)
LLQ	left lower quadrant (of the abdomen)
LMWH	low-molecular-weight heparin
LOC	level of consciousness, loss of consciousness

LP	lumbar puncture
LR	lactated Ringer solution
LUL	left upper lobe (of the lung)
LUQ	left upper quadrant (of the abdomen)
lymph.	lymphocytes
MAO	monoamine oxidase
MAP	mean arterial pressure*
mcg, mgm	microgram
med.	medial
mEq	milliequivalent
mg	milligram
Mg$^+$	magnesium ion
MI	myocardial infarction (often AMI for acute myocardial infarction)
ml	milliliter
mm	millimeter
mm^3	cubic millimeter
mm Hg	millimeters of mercury*
mmol	millimolar concentration
MAOI	monoamine oxidase inhibitor
MOSF	multiorgan system failure
mOsm	milliosmolar concentration*
MRI	magnetic resonance imaging
MS	mental status
MV	mitral valve
N$_2$	nitrogen*
Na$^+$	sodium ion*
NAVELS	nerve artery vein empty space lymphatics symphysis pubis
neuro.	neurological examination
NG	nasogastric
NPH	neutral protamine Hagedorn insulin
NPO	*nil per os*, nothing by mouth

---

*Denotes that a formula is listed in Appendix G.

NS	normal saline
NSAID	nonsteroidal anti-inflammatory drug
O$^-$	O-type, Rh-negative blood
O$_2$	oxygen
O&P	ova and parasite examination
OR	operating room
OT	occupational therapy
P	pulse rate
PA	posterior-to-anterior direction (as in path of x-rays)
P[A-a]O$_2$	alveolar-arterial oxygen gradient*
PAC	premature atrial contraction
PAO$_2$	alveolar partial pressure of oxygen*
PaO$_2$	arterial partial pressure of oxygen
PAR	"procedure, alternatives, risk," used with surgical informed consent
PAT	paroxysmal atrial tachycardia
PC	*post cibum,* after meals
PCO$_2$	partial pressure of carbon dioxide
PCWP	pulmonary capillary wedge pressure
PE	physical examination
PEA	pulseless electrical activity (EMD)
PEEP	positive end expiratory pressure
PFT	pulmonary function test
pH (−)	log of hydrogen ion concentration
PICC	peripherally inserted central catheter
PID	pelvic inflammatory disease
plt	platelet count
PMHx	past medical history
PMN	polymorphonucleocytes, granulocytes
PND	paroxysmal nocturnal dyspnea
PO	*per os,* by mouth
POD	postoperative day

---

*Denotes that a formula is listed in Appendix G.

post.	posterior
PPD	purified protein derivative (for TB testing)
PPN	peripherally delivered parenteral nutrition
PR	per rectum
pRBC	packed red blood cells
PRN	*pro re nata*, as necessary
PSHx	past surgical history
PT	physical therapy
PT	prothrombin time
PTT, aPTT	partial thromboplastin time
PUD	peptic ulcer disease
PVC	premature ventricular contraction
PVR	pulmonary vascular resistance
q	each (as in qHS, or "at each hour of sleep")
QID	*quarter in die*, four times a day
R	right side
RAD	reactive airway disease
RBC	red blood cell, erythrocytes
resp.	respiratory
RLL	right lower lobe (of the lung)
RLQ	right lower quadrant (of the abdomen)
RML	right middle lobe (of the lung)
RN	registered nurse
R/O	rule out
ROS	review of systems
RR	respiratory rate
RUL	right upper lobe (of the lung)
RUQ	right upper quadrant (of the abdomen)
Rx	prescription
SaO$_2$	oxygen saturation of arterial blood
SBE	subacute bacterial endocarditis
SBP	spontaneous bacterial peritonitis

SBP	systolic blood pressure
SC	subcutaneous
SG	specific gravity
SGOT	serum glutamic-oxaloacetic transaminase (AST)
SGPT	serum glutamic-pyruvic transaminase (ALT)
SHx	social history
SIADH	syndrome of inappropriate secretion of antidiuretic hormone
SIRS	systemic inflammatory response syndrome
SL	sublingual
SLE	systemic lupus erythematosus
SOB	short of breath, shortness of breath
sp.	species
S/P	status post
SQ	subcutaneous
SSRI	selective serotonin reuptake inhibitor
SSS	sick sinus syndrome
stat	*statim*, immediately
sup.	superior
SV	stroke volume*
SVC	superior vena cava
SvO$_2$	oxygen saturation of venous blood
SVR	systemic vascular resistance*
SVT	supraventricular tachycardia
Sx	symptom
T	temperature
TB	tuberculosis
TCP	transcutaneous pacing
TFT	thyroid function test
TIA	transient ischemic attack
TID	*ter in die*, three times a day
TKO, TKVO	(IV fluid rate sufficient) to keep (vein) open

---

*Denotes that a formula is listed in Appendix G.

TMP/SFX	trimethoprim/sulfamethoxazole
tPA	tissue plasminogen activator
TPN	total parenteral nutrition
TPVR	total peripheral vascular resistance
Tx	treatment
UA	urinalysis
UO	urine output
URI	upper respiratory infection
US	ultrasound
UTI	urinary tract infection
VC	vena cava
VF	ventricular fibrillation
VMA	vanillylmandelic acid
VP	ventriculoperitoneal
V/Q	ventilation/perfusion
VS	vital signs
VSD	ventriculoseptal defect
VT, V-Tach	ventricular tachycardia
WBC	white blood cell
WPW	Wolff-Parkinson-White syndrome
wt.	weight
ZN	Ziehl-Neelsen stain

Introduction

1

Approach to On-Call Surgical Problems

Why write a book on surgical on-call problems? All surgical training programs require time spent "on call." This is the time, usually overnight or during weekends, during which a physician is responsible for the care of hospitalized patients. It is also the time when new clinical problems arise. These times have extraordinary educational value, but are also the source of great stress. While on call, the physician is typically among the first to encounter significant changes in the condition of a patient and variances in recovery patterns. Hence, it is a unique time to hone clinical skills. However, under current training practices, a significant amount of the time spent "on-call" occurs early in the educational process and the individual may not have encountered a wide range of clinical situations. Being on call often requires many late hours and prioritizing of numerous tasks. In addition, being on call usually requires "cross coverage," or responsibility for patients for whom the on-call physician may have little familiarity or information. Often life-threatening changes in a patient's condition may be hidden under seemingly innocuous symptoms. Knowledge and anticipation of these problems may make a great difference in the patient's outcome. It is useful, therefore, to have a scheme to evaluate and administer care to patients in a rapid but thorough and organized fashion.

This book provides an outline for the organization and implementation of care plans in response to many on-call surgical situations. It is written for the intern and junior resident, but we hope that the information will be useful for persons at all levels of training. Obviously, not all on-call situations could be covered, but emphasis has been placed on the more common and more life-threatening problems.

The structure of this book follows closely the flow of information as it reaches the individual on call. Most chapters are divided into six major headings, as follows:

Phone Call
Elevator Thoughts
Major Threat to Life
Bedside
Management
Special Surgical Considerations

PHONE CALL

The first notification of a change in the status of a patient is often a phone call from the bedside caregiver. During that phone call the status of the patient and the urgency of the response must be assessed immediately. It is also important to determine whether the patient is pre- or postoperative. If necessary, orders for immediate action are given and initial laboratory studies are ordered. The bedside care provider should be given an estimate of when to expect the physician's arrival at the bedside. Rarely, the problem may be handled entirely over the phone, but usually, a bedside evaluation is required to fully assess the situation. If there is any question, always err toward a bedside evaluation.

ELEVATOR THOUGHTS

The travel time to the bedside is wisely spent in consideration of the differential diagnosis of the presenting symptom. These are called "elevator thoughts." This term was coined by Shane A. Marshall, MD, and John Ruedy, MD, in the first edition of On Call: Principles and Protocols, and it refers to the long distances through the hospital that often have to be covered while on call. Elevator thoughts may also be used to organize a plan of action once at the bedside. The differential diagnoses given in this text are not meant to be complete; attention is given to those that are most common and to those that could be life threatening. Always bear in mind that there are many uncommon causes of symptoms, which can be diagnosed or treated with simple measures, and these must also be entertained. Know what the preliminary plan of action will be before arriving at the bedside.

MAJOR THREAT TO LIFE

In many clinical situations there is a potential of serious injury or risk to life, although these outcomes are thankfully uncommon. Many patients are initially hospitalized to anticipate or treat these potential complications. This section will focus on those observations and tests that will best ensure the safety of the patient. The major threat to life is rarely the most common item on the differential diagnosis list.

In clinical practice it is a wise educational tool to imagine what the major threat is to each patient each day, pre- and postoperatively, and to outline the plan of action. Although these threats may not become a reality, the anticipation of a bad outcome leads to appropriate vigilance and avoidance tactics, and to suitable preparation in the face of an unfortunate event.

BEDSIDE

This section deals with the evaluation of the patient at the bedside. This evaluation may be divided into three steps.

Quick Look Test

Once at the bedside, the first look at the patient is often the best assessment of the severity of the complaint. This begins as you enter the patient's room and involves a rapid scan of the patient's general condition. A patient, who is calm and conversant with stable vital signs, may require less speed of action than one who is acutely distressed or unstable. Patients may be divided into the following three broad groups:

1. **Comfortable:** At ease, with stable or normal vital signs
2. **Sick:** Requiring attention; recent changes or abnormalities in signs or symptoms with an indication of patient discomfort
3. **Critical:** Moribund or very unstable; about to die

This "first look" should become second nature. Practice it with every patient contact, such as on rounds in the morning or in the clinic, so that it becomes **automatic**.

Vital Signs

The next evaluation of any patient is a quick assessment of the patient's breathing, vital signs, and fluid status. Special note is made of any recent changes or instability. As with any emergency situation, aberrations to airway breathing, or circulation are dealt with immediately as life-threatening conditions. Follow the **A, B, C's**.

Selective History, Chart Review, and Physical Examination

Next is a limited and directed history and physical examination, which is generally problem directed. This is a departure from the standard 30- to 60-minute interview practiced in medical school, or the unhurried evaluation of a new patient. The motivation is different when the physician is on call. A specific complaint is to be addressed, and although that often expands into an assessment of several systems, other aspects of the patient's care, unrelated to the current complaint, do not need to be evaluated at this time. Sources of pertinent information are obtained from the bedside caregiver, from the patient, and from the chart. Remember that much information has already been obtained and is organized in the bedside chart, but be careful not to rely completely on this information. Circumstances may dictate further questioning and examination not already documented.

MANAGEMENT

Emergency measures and initial laboratory studies are described in an Initial Management section.

Further management issues, based on findings in the history and physical examination, are then discussed in the Definitive Management section.

SPECIAL SURGICAL CONSIDERATIONS

In those situations where special considerations are necessary, specific to a particular surgical technique or patient, they will be addressed in a separate section. Chapter 2 has a complete explanation.

FURTHER INFORMATION

The book also has several helpful appendices which outline reading of chest x-rays, ECGs, and list commonly used formulae and medications. Wherever possible, information is placed in list or table form to assist in quick reference.

Special Considerations for Surgical Patients

Surgical patients are different from other patients in the hospital. Physiologic changes in their condition that become apparent on call may be due to the disease process that prompted their admission or may be due to the surgical procedure that was used to treat them. Often the same symptom will require different considerations in a preoperative patient than in a postoperative patient. Also important is the time elapsed since the day of the operation and the type of procedure performed. This section will be devoted to considerations that are specific to the surgical patient. Problems and considerations specific to individual surgical specialties will also be addressed.

PREOPERATIVE CONSIDERATIONS

Preoperative patients are broadly divided into the following three categories: elective, urgent, and emergent.

The elective patient may not be acutely ill, but may require a surgical procedure. A good example is the patient admitted for bowel preparation before abdominal surgery or the patient admitted for diagnostic procedures. Perturbations in their health, such as fever or chest pain, may be enough to cancel an elective procedure, pending further evaluation of the problem.

The urgent patient may be more ill, and the disease state that was the reason for admission may cause changes in the patient's condition. Knowledge of the pathophysiology of the disease will often make it easier to anticipate and circumvent these problems, but occasionally a patient's condition will deteriorate to the point that urgency becomes emergency.

The emergent patient requires the most immediate attention and thought. Any patient, including an elective patient, can become an emergent patient at any time. In the assessment of the emergent patient, always consider whether it is appropriate to move the patient to an intensive care unit or to the operating room. Also ask yourself whether you need assistance in assessing or dealing with the problem, and call in extra help as needed. Being on call is a learning experience, and there is no reason to avoid consulting with others.

Preoperative patients soon will be in the operating room, where their condition may drastically change. Therefore, preparation of the patient for surgery should be considered when conditions allow (see Chapter 24). Postoperative patients will do best when they have had adequate preoperative hydration, nutrition, and pharmacologic preparation. Specific considerations including preoperative antibiotic therapy and bowel preparation will be addressed in subsequent chapters.

POSTOPERATIVE CONSIDERATIONS

The delivery of anesthetic agents and the performance of major surgical procedures may have profound physiologic effects on a patient. Fluid shifts are common, and the patient may require hemodynamic monitoring, fluid resuscitation, and electrolyte measurement and correction. Specific organ physiology may be permanently altered, as with the transplantation of a kidney or with extensive bowel resection. Various surgical results may need to be protected, such as the integrity of a new anastomosis or the blood flow to a free-flap graft. Many postoperative considerations are specific to the procedure performed and will be addressed in the appropriate chapters.

Hypothermia is a common postoperative finding. Although found mostly after extensive surgical procedures or in trauma patients, it is of general interest because it may occur in a variety of patients, regardless of the procedure performed.

A core temperature of <36°C persisting 1 to 2 hours postoperatively is a significant complication. It is frequent after extensive intra-abdominal procedures and in septic, seriously injured, and very ill patients. Common etiologies include long periods of time with the patient's skin or abdominal contents exposed to subphysiologic temperatures, or massive rehydration with cool replacement fluids.

Expect patients with hypothermia to have vasoconstriction with an associated increase in systemic vascular resistance (SVR). Hypothermia may contribute to tachycardia and to hyperventilation, especially in the setting of shivering. In addition, as the patient is rewarmed, cooler peripheral beds are reperfused, which may slow further rewarming and contribute to postoperative acidosis.

The treatment includes awareness of the potential for hypothermia in the operating room, rapid operative procedures, warm intravenous (IV) solutions, warmed humidified gases in ventilated patients, and warming blankets.

Hypothermia alters mental state, affects blood coagulation, and prolongs the half-lives of many medications. It is also possible to overcorrect in the treatment of hypothermia, and the result should not be confused with postoperative fever (see Chapter 11).

Documentation of On-Call Problems

An important aspect of management of on-call problems is the appropriate documentation of events. This is essential for the continued efficient care of the patient. In addition, the medical chart is a medicolegal document, and it should be as accurate and complete as possible. Documentation is required for every patient evaluated. This may be just a short note for a simple problem, or it may require a complete rendering of a complex intervention.

As shorter work hours continue to shorten and as use of "night float" positions becomes more frequent, adequate communication about patients will become very important. The concept of "sign-out" at the end of a shift is not an unfamiliar one to surgical residents, but the quality of that sign-out needs to be high if the on-call resident is to be able to adequately and efficiently tend to problems in the middle of the night. It is a skill that we could all improve. Likewise, when something happens to a patient that is not in your primary care, the onus is upon you to adequately document the events for the team coming on in the morning.

An example of an on-call note is as follows:

RESIDENT ON-CALL NOTE

(Date and Time)
   Called by RN to evaluate patient because of fever.
   The patient is a 65-year-old man, who is 2 days status post exploratory laparotomy for presumed bowel obstruction; 20 cm of questionably necrotic small bowel was removed, and a primary anastomosis was performed without complication. His postoperative course has been complicated by initial shortness of breath associated with a mild fever (38°C) and an oxygen requirement on postoperative day 1, which resolved with diuretics and ambulation. His course since has been uncomplicated. He has been ambulatory without difficulty but has not yet been ready for oral feedings. His current therapies include IV hydration with 5% dextrose in one-half normal saline (D5½ NS) at 75 mL/hour, nasogastric suction, parenteral antibiotic therapy, ambulation, and incentive spirometry.

(List current medications)
The physical examination is directed toward the evaluation of the problem described.

Vital signs (VS):	Temperature: 38.6°C
	Pulse: 107 beats/minute
	Respiration: 20/minute
	Blood pressure: 136 mm Hg/85 mm Hg
Head, eyes, ears, nose, and throat (HEENT):	Nasogastric tube in place, normally functioning. Output over the last 24 hours: 1550 mL (75 mL in the last hour). Green, nonbloody fluid. No sinus tenderness.
Cardiovascular system (CVS):	Regular rate and rhythm, mild tachycardia. No murmur.
Respiration:	Basilar rales with poor aeration. Incentive spirometer hidden in bottom drawer of personal items. No documented use since last shift.
Abdomen:	Wound clean without discharge. No erythema. Abdomen is soft, with mild incisional tenderness. No peritoneal signs. No organomegaly.
Urinary:	No urinary catheter. Urine output is >800 mL/shift. No dysuria complaints. No tenderness over bladder or flanks.
IV sites:	No erythema. Day 2 of current site (left dorsal hand).
Legs:	No calf tenderness.

Laboratory analysis, as follows, is dictated by the history and physical examination:

Complete blood count (CBC):	
White blood cell (WBC):	6700/mcL
Hemoglobin (Hb):	12 g/dL
Hematocrit (Hct):	42%
Platelet (Plt):	267,000/mcL
Urinalysis:	No WBC, 3 to 5 red blood cells, occasional epithelial cells. Negative for leukocyte esterase, specific gravity: 1.125.
Chest x-ray:	Bibasilar atelectasis without specific infiltrate.

The diagnosis and treatment should be clear; list any further studies that might be useful. Also list who might have been contacted.

Assessment: Probable atelectasis; must also consider pulmonary infection or reaction to antibiotic therapy.

Postoperative day 2.
Day 2 antibiotic therapy *(list agents used)*.

Treatment: 1. Incentive spirometry every hour, the importance of which was reiterated to the patient and his family.
2. Continue antibiotic therapy.
3. Repeat chest x-ray and CBC in A.M.
4. Consider sputum analysis.
5. Plan discussed with RN and chief resident *(time)*.

COMMUNICATION

Complete medical care is a team approach, and adequate communication is vital for consistent and appropriate treatment of patients. It is important to document the chart in a complete and *legible* fashion. Do not forget that many practitioners and others read and rely on the information written in the medical record, for example, the primary care team, the nurses directly involved in the patient's care, the consulting teams, and occasionally the patient or family. Any of these individuals may contribute significantly to the care of the patient.

Often, medical approaches to treating patients on call represent differences in treatment philosophies, and these may be educational. Remember as well that communication should occur in all directions along the hierarchy of caregivers, to interns and to medical students, and to family, bedside caregivers, chief residents, and attending physicians.

If professional disagreements arise, air them privately, not in the chart.

On-Call Hazards

The practice of medicine has inherent risks. The exposure to blood- and secretion-borne diseases is significant and should always be considered. Specifically, the transmission of human immunodeficiency virus (HIV) to a health care provider from an infected patient, although infrequent, is always a risk. Hepatitis B and C are other blood-borne pathogens. Hepatitis is particularly worrisome because only a small viral inoculum can result in disease transmission. Precautions must *always* be taken, especially in those patients about whom you have no firsthand knowledge (Table 4–1).

Before blood contact occurs, find out what the hospital policies are regarding treatment of significant blood-borne exposures. Know where to seek first aid as required, and make sure that your tetanus and hepatitis B vaccinations are up to date (Table 4–2).

TABLE 4–1 **Universal Precautions to Prevent Transmission of HIV**

Universal Precautions

Because a medical history and physical examination cannot reliably identify all patients infected with HIV or other blood-borne pathogens, blood and body fluid precautions should be consistently used for all patients, especially those in emergency care settings in which the risk of blood exposure is increased and the infection status of the patient is usually not known.

1. Use appropriate barrier protection to prevent skin and mucous membrane exposure when exposure to blood, body fluids containing blood, or other body fluids to which universal precautions apply (see below), is anticipated. Wear gloves when touching blood or body fluids, mucous membranes, or nonintact skin of all patients, when handling items or surfaces soiled with blood or body fluids, and when performing venipuncture and other vascular access procedures. Change gloves after contact with each patient; do not wash or disinfect gloves for reuse. Wear masks and protective eyewear or face shields during procedures that are likely to generate droplets of blood or other body fluids to prevent exposure of mucous membranes of the mouth, nose, and eyes. Wear gowns or aprons during procedures that are likely to generate splashes of blood or other body fluids.

TABLE 4–1 **Universal Precautions to Prevent Transmission of HIV—cont'd**

2. Wash hands and other skin surfaces immediately and thoroughly following contamination with blood, body fluids containing blood, or other body fluids to which universal precautions apply. Wash hands immediately after gloves are removed.
3. Take care to prevent injuries when using needles, scalpels, and other sharp instruments or devices, when handling sharp instruments after procedures, when cleaning used instruments, and when disposing of used needles. Do not recap needles by hand; do not remove used needles from disposable syringes by hand; and do not bend, break, or otherwise manipulate used needles by hand. Place used disposable syringes and needles, scalpel blades, and other sharp items in puncture-resistant disposal containers, which should be located as close to the use area as is practical.
4. Although saliva has not been implicated in HIV transmission, the need for emergency mouth-to-mouth resuscitation should be minimized by making mouthpieces, resuscitation bags, or other ventilation devices available for use in areas in which the need for resuscitation is predictable.
5. Health care workers with exudative lesions or weeping dermatitis should refrain from all direct patient care and from handling patient care equipment until the condition resolves.

Universal precautions are intended to supplement rather than replace recommendations for routine infection control, such as hand washing and use of gloves to prevent gross microbial contamination of hands. In addition, implementation of universal precautions does not eliminate the need for other category- or disease-specific isolation precautions, such as enteric precautions for infectious diarrhea or isolation for pulmonary tuberculosis. Universal precautions are not intended to change waste management programs undertaken in accordance with state and local regulations.

Body Fluids to Which Universal Precautions Apply

Universal precautions apply to blood and other body fluids containing visible blood. Blood is the single most important source of HIV, hepatitis B virus, and other blood-borne pathogens in the occupational setting. Universal precautions also apply to tissues, semen, vaginal secretions, and the following fluids: cerebrospinal, synovial, pleural, peritoneal, and amniotic.

Universal precautions do not apply to feces, nasal secretions, sputum, sweat, tears, urine, and vomitus unless they contain visible blood. Universal precautions also do not apply to human breast milk, although gloves may be worn by health care workers in situations in which exposure to breast milk might be frequent. In addition, universal precautions do not apply to saliva. Gloves need not be worn when feeding patients or wiping saliva from skin, although special precautions are recommended for dentistry, in which contamination of saliva with blood is predictable. The risk of transmission of HIV, as well as hepatitis B virus, from these fluids and materials is extremely low or nonexistent.

Continued

TABLE 4–1 **Universal Precautions to Prevent Transmission of HIV—cont'd**

Use of Gloves for Phlebotomy

Gloves should be effective in reducing the incidence of blood contamination of hands during phlebotomy (drawing of blood samples), but they cannot prevent penetrating injuries caused by needles or other sharp instruments. In universal precautions, all blood is assumed to be potentially infectious for blood-borne pathogens. Some institutions have relaxed recommendations for the use of gloves for phlebotomy by skilled health care workers in settings in which the prevalence of blood-borne pathogens is known to be very low (e.g., volunteer blood donation centers). Institutions that judge that routine use of gloves for all phlebotomies is not necessary should periodically reevaluate their policy. Gloves should always be available for those who wish to use them for phlebotomy. In addition, the following general guidelines apply:

1. Use gloves for performing phlebotomy if cuts, scratches, or other breaks in the skin are present.
2. Use gloves in situations in which contamination with blood may occur—for example, when performing phlebotomy on an uncooperative patient.
3. Use gloves for performing finger or heel sticks on infants and children.
4. Use gloves when training persons to do phlebotomies.

TABLE 4–2 **First Aid After Blood or Body Fluid Exposure (Do Not Delay!)**

1. Immediately clean the exposed site. For skin sites, wash with detergent and water or a 1:10 bleach solution. For eyes and other mucous membranes, use saline or water. Wash for 5 minutes.
2. Save the instrument in a sharps container for testing later.
3. Seek out a supervisor for instructions. A specific protocol will be in place for your institution.
4. Serum probably will be drawn from you and the patient from whom the fluid originated.
5. Consent from the patient is often necessary.
6. Make sure tetanus and hepatitis B vaccinations are up to date.
7. Follow your institution's guidelines regarding prophylaxis against HIV.

Patient-Related Problems:
The Common Calls

Abdominal Pain

One of the most common calls, abdominal pain, is also one of the most difficult to evaluate. Whole textbooks have been written on the approach to abdominal pain in surgical patients. This chapter is not meant to replace those books, but it will cover many of the common calls in the hospital. Although most causes of abdominal pain are benign, some will require immediate attention and treatment. The first major decision to be made is whether the patient needs an operation immediately (acute abdomen). Once that is decided satisfactorily, the remainder of the evaluation may be performed. Recent abdominal surgery is a specific cause of abdominal pain, and it is often difficult to differentiate between expected incisional pain and a new process that needs attention.

PHONE CALL

Questions

1. How severe is the pain?
2. Is the pain localized or generalized?
3. Are there any changes in vital signs, such as fever, hypotension, or tachycardia?
4. Is the patient taking pain medications or steroids?
   Both of these may mask or alter pain perception.
5. Has the patient undergone a surgical procedure? If so, how long ago?
   Incision pain is normal immediately following an abdominal procedure. Also be mindful that adhesion formation following an abdominal procedure may cause bowel obstruction, even many years later, which may present with bloating and pain.
6. Is a nasogastric (NG) tube in place? Is it functioning normally? Have there been changes in the trends of volume output and fluid characteristics?
7. Are there any other symptoms, such as vomiting, dysuria, diarrhea, or bloating?

Orders

If an NG tube is in place for luminal decompression and it is not functioning, it may be flushed with 20 to 30 mL of normal saline (NS).

Do this yourself if the patient has had a luminal perforation or an anastomosis in the proximal GI tract.

If the patient is freshly post-op and you suspect that the incisional pain is being poorly controlled, consider additional pain meds at this time.

Degree of Urgency

If there is a significant change in vital signs or symptoms, or if the pain is a new symptom, the patient must be evaluated immediately. Recurrent and minor pain may be evaluated in 1 to 2 hours.

ELEVATOR THOUGHTS

Localized abdominal pain
    This is best organized by the location of the pain (Fig. 5–1).
Generalized abdominal pain
    Many etiologies of abdominal pain have aspects of both localized and generalized pain (Fig. 5–2), often with progression from one to the other over time.

MAJOR THREAT TO LIFE

    Luminal perforation
    Bowel infarction
    Sepsis associated with ruptured intra-abdominal abscess or ascending cholangitis
    Ruptured aortic aneurysm with exsanguinating hemorrhage

BEDSIDE

Quick Look Test

Mild abdominal pain is associated with only minor discomfort. The more severe the pain, the more uncomfortable the patient will appear. If the patient has an acute abdomen, impending hypovolemic shock may be present and the patient may be lethargic or even moribund. Patients receiving narcotic medication or steroids may be deceptively comfortable despite serious pathology; pain and inflammatory responses (including fever) may be blunted. Patients with peritonitis (acute abdomen) will be still, because any movement of their abdominal wall will cause pain. Patients with renal or biliary colic will be agitated and will often have "caged cat" restlessness as they try to find a comfortable position.

Airway and Vital Signs

Tachycardia and hypovolemia are associated with shock. Fever is an indication of infection or inflammatory etiology, although

RIGHT UPPER QUADRANT PAIN
Gallbladder and biliary tract
Hepatitis
Hepatic abscess
Hepatomegaly due to
congestive heart failure
Peptic ulcer
Pancreatitis
Retrocecal appendicitis
Renal pain
Myocardial ischemia
Pericarditis
Pneumonia
Empyema

LEFT UPPER QUADRANT PAIN
Gastritis
Pancreatitis
Splenic enlargement, rupture,
infarction, aneurysm
Renal pain
Myocardial ischemia
Pneumonia
Empyema

RIGHT LOWER QUADRANT PAIN
Appendicitis
Intestinal obstruction
Regional enteritis
Diverticulitis
Cholecystitis
Perforated ulcer
Leaking aneurysm
Abdominal wall hematoma
Ectopic pregnancy
Ovarian cyst or torsion
Salpingitis
Endometriosis
Ureteral calculi
Renal pain
Seminal vesiculitis
Psoas abscess

LEFT LOWER QUADRANT PAIN
Diverticulitis
Intestinal obstruction
Appendicitis
Leaking aneurysm
Abdominal wall hematoma
Ectopic pregnancy
Ovarian cyst or torsion
Salpingitis
Endometriosis
Ureteral calculi
Renal pain
Seminal vesiculitis
Psoas abscess

Figure 5–1 Common etiologies of localized abdominal pain by quadrant. (Modified from Schwartz SI, Shires GT, Spencer FC: Principles of surgery, 5th ed. New York, McGraw-Hill, 1989. With permission.)

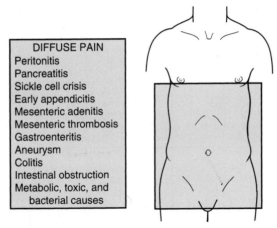

DIFFUSE PAIN
Peritonitis
Pancreatitis
Sickle cell crisis
Early appendicitis
Mesenteric adenitis
Mesenteric thrombosis
Gastroenteritis
Aneurysm
Colitis
Intestinal obstruction
Metabolic, toxic, and
    bacterial causes

Figure 5–2 Common etiologies of generalized abdominal pain. (Modified from Schwartz SI, Shires GT, Spencer FC: Principles of Surgery, 5th ed. New York, McGraw-Hill, 1989. With permission.)

it need not be present to make such a diagnosis. Tachypnea may be present due to a lower lobe pneumonia, or it may indicate progressive acidemia from necrosis of the bowel, which is more serious.

Initial Assessment

A preliminary assessment helps in making the final diagnosis and deciding if the patient needs surgery immediately.
1. Assess for an acute abdomen.
    A rapid examination of the ill-appearing patient is a prudent start. Questions may be asked of the patient while the examination is being performed. The presence of an acute abdomen is a surgical emergency, and exploratory laparotomy is indicated for diagnosis and potential repair of the problem. It is not an easy diagnosis, but some specific clues are helpful. The presence or absence of these symptoms individually does not make the diagnosis, but in combination, and taken in context with the history, a decision may be made. It is not unusual to have to make a rapid decision without having many pieces of the puzzle.

Abdominal distention
    May be present with acute obstruction or progressive ascites.

Quiet abdomen
    The lack of bowel sounds indicates a functional ileus or peritonitis. As a diagnostic symptom it is not very sensitive,

because bowel sounds are rarely completely absent; it may merely take several minutes to note them. High-pitched, rushing, or "tinkling" bowel sounds indicate possible obstruction.

Peritonitis

Severe pain to palpation or rigid abdominal musculature (involuntary guarding) is evidence of peritoneal irritation. This may be focal as in appendicitis, or it may be generalized as with rupture of the viscus. It may be apparent from gentle shaking of the bed or the patient, or by percussion or palpation of the abdomen. Rebound tenderness may be present but is a less specific finding.

Hypotension

A precipitous decrease in blood pressure associated with abdominal pain is a surgical emergency. You do not need to know the exact diagnosis before an exploratory laparotomy in a gravely ill patient.

2. Treat hypotension with aggressive fluid resuscitation, as necessary.

Do a complete fluid assessment (see Chapter 12). Orthostatic blood pressure and pulse measurements will aid in diagnosing intravascular volume deficits. If surgical treatment is required, the patient should receive aggressive fluid resuscitation as described in Chapter 17 while preparations for transfer to the operating room (OR) are being made.

3. If the patient does not have an acute abdomen, then the remainder of the history and physical examination may be performed.

4. Treat severe pain with narcotics if necessary. If a patient is in extreme distress, there is little value in delaying management of pain. True peritonitis will not be masked by judicious doses of narcotic medication, and the patient will be more comfortable during the evaluation.

Selective History and Chart Review

Gather a complete history of the pain.

Important features include the following:

1. Time of onset
   Many pain syndromes change over time. A classic example is the progression of appendicitis from periumbilical pain to right lower quadrant (RLQ) pain. The duration of the pain may suggest the location of the symptoms. Was the onset sudden or gradual? Did the pain awaken the patient?

2. Location
   Review Figures 5–1 and 5–2. Note whether pain is epigastric, umbilical, prepubic, right or left, and upper or lower; changes in location are important. Pain may also be difficult to localize

specifically; this is common in very old or very young patients. Most children will point at their belly buttons when asked to locate the pain.

3. Radiation

Pain can radiate to the back, groin, chest, and so on (Fig. 5–3). Radiation of pain occurs when the pain fibers from the affected organ are supplied by nerve roots that also have a cutaneous sensory distribution. Pain in the diaphragm from a left lower lobe pneumonia or perisplenic abscess is radiated to the left shoulder because of mutual innervation by the C-3, C-4, and C-5 nerve roots.

4. Quality of the pain

Pain can be stabbing, aching, cramping, burning, and so on.

5. Fluctuations in the pain

Pain can be constant, colicky, intermittent (at what intervals?), increasing, and so on. Solid organs tend to have constant ("solid") pain. Hollow organs will have pain only with paristalsis and therefore result in colicky pain.

6. Factors that lessen the pain

These can include position, meals, defecation, and time.

7. Factors that make the pain worse

8. Associated symptoms

Symptoms can include fever, nausea, vomiting, dizziness, dysuria, jaundice, and cough.

9. Character of the vomitus, if the patient is vomiting

Clear fluid indicates obstruction proximal to the sphincter of Oddi; bilious vomitus indicates a more distal obstruction. Feculent material indicates a distal colonic obstruction. Does the vomiting relate temporally to the pain?

10. Changes in the frequency or character of the stool

Changes can include diarrhea, constipation, or change in color or caliber.

11. Character of the stool, if the patient has diarrhea

Bloody stools or those containing mucus indicate an invasive enteritis or inflammatory bowel disease. Clear liquid may indicate a viral etiology. Diarrhea is sometimes associated with a high-grade obstruction, because fluid materials are the only types that may pass. Does the diarrhea relate temporally to the pain?

12. Time of the patient's last meal

Is the patient anorexic?

13. Whether the patient is passing gas

Passage of gas is largely due to swallowed air and indicates complete bowel continuity. A lack of flatus may indicate ileus or obstruction.

14. Prior abdominal procedures or infections

How long ago were procedures performed? Were any organs resected? Adhesions formed following an abdominal procedure or infection are a major cause of mechanical bowel obstruction.

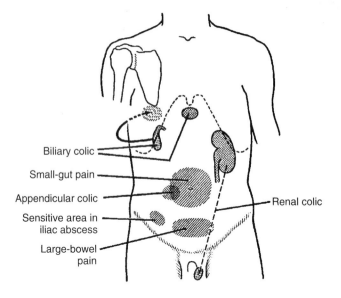

Biliary colic

Small-gut pain

Appendicular colic

Sensitive area in
iliac abscess

Large-bowel
pain

Renal colic

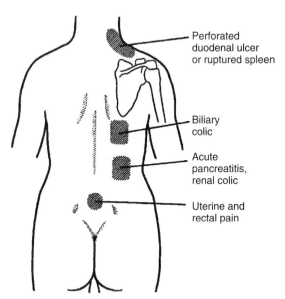

Perforated
duodenal ulcer
or ruptured spleen

Biliary
colic

Acute
pancreatitis,
renal colic

Uterine and
rectal pain

Figure 5–3 Common cutaneous sites of referred pain by etiology.
(From Cope Z: Cope's Early Diagnosis of the Acute Abdomen, Revised
by William Silen, 16th ed. Oxford, Oxford University Press, 1983, pp. 11,
141. With permission.)

15. Family history of abdominal pain syndromes
   These can include familial Mediterranean fever and sickle cell anemia.
16. What medications is the patient taking?
   Some medications can cause abdominal pain (antibiotics, NSAIDs, GI motility agents), and some may mask the symptoms of pain (steroids, pain medications).
17. Does the patient have a past medical history of abdominal pain (see Figs. 5–1 and 5–2)?
   The most common recurrent abdominal pain syndromes include
   a. Peptic ulcer disease
      Does the patient use histamine H_2 blockers or other antacids routinely?
   b. Alcoholic pancreatitis
      Any prior admission for ascites or abdominal pain?
   c. Gastritis
      This is common after steroid or NSAID administration.
   d. Nephrolithiasis
   e. Cholelithiasis or cholecystitis
   f. Inflammatory bowel disease
18. Is there a history of peripheral or cardiovascular disease?
   Atherosclerotic plaque formation may be present in the mesenteric vessels as well, resulting in mesenteric ischemia.

Selective Physical Examination

VS:	Repeat now.
MS:	Lethargy (hypotension and narcotic pain medication).
HEENT:	Icteric sclerae (hepatitis, cholangitis, and cholelithiasis).
	Flat neck veins (hypotension).
CVS:	New murmur or S_3 (myocardial infarction).
Resp:	Decreased breath sounds, dullness to percussion, rales (pneumonia or pleural effusion).
GU:	Dysuria (urinary tract infection [UTI]).
Skin:	Edema, jaundice, spider angiomata, caput medusae (liver failure).
Wound:	Discharge or erythema (wound infection).
Tubes:	NG tube in place? Functioning well?
Abd:	The aspects of a focused abdominal examination are as follows:

1. Observe: Look at the comfort of the patient. Look for distention. Occasionally the large colon may be seen in outline in cases of distal obstruction. Ascites may be evident by bulging flanks. Peristalsis or outlines of bowel loops may be visible. Look at the position of the patient. An agitated, moving patient probably has biliary or

renal colic. The still, quiet patient may have peritonitis. Look at the skin. Look for retroperitoneal bleeding and blood that extravasates along tissue planes, which may present as bruising along the back, flanks, or abdomen.

Grey Turner's sign: Ecchymosis noted in the groin or flanks.

Cullen's sign: Ecchymosis noted in the periumbilical region.

2. Position: The patient should be supine with the knees bent slightly to relax the abdominal musculature. Some examiners prefer to approach an abdominal examination from the same side of the bed each time.

3. Locate: Ask the patient to point to the location of the greatest pain. This is not always possible if the pain is generalized. If a point of maximal pain is identified, do not start the palpation at that spot or the patient will not trust you enough to relax for the remainder of the examination.

4. Auscultate: Listen for bowel sounds in all four quadrants. Note high-pitched or rushing sounds, which may indicate obstruction.

5. Percuss: This may elicit tenderness in peritonitis; if so, resort to light palpation. Determine the liver size and the tympanic quality of the abdomen. Distal obstruction may produce large gas pockets if the ileocecal valve is competent. Is there localizable percussion tenderness? (RLQ suggests appendicitis, prepubic suggests UTI.) Percuss for fluid waves and shifting dullness (ascites).

6. Palpate: Palpate gently at first, with gradual increase in pressure. Start at the least tender spot. Note tender areas and areas of referred pain. Note masses and regions of pulsation (as an artery). An acute abdomen may be rigid with "board-like stiffness," or tenderness may be more localized.

7. Rebound: Rebound tenderness is an insensitive finding associated with peritonitis.

Direct rebound is tenderness over a region when palpation pressure is quickly released.

Indirect rebound is pain referred elsewhere with the same movement. Appendicitis may have direct rebound over McBurney's point and may have indirect rebound to McBurney's point when pressure is released from elsewhere in the abdomen (Rovsing sign). Rebound itself does not make the diagnosis of peritonitis. An apprehensive patient usually has some element of rebound.

8. Guarding: Peritonitis is marked by guarding. *Voluntary guarding* is more insensitive and relates to the voluntary contraction of abdominal musculature to limit the pain anticipated by the patient (such as during an abdominal examination). Like rebound tenderness, this is present in many apprehensive patients in the absence of peritonitis. *Involuntary guarding* results in a rigid abdomen and is an ominous sign of acute peritonitis that requires immediate exploratory laparotomy. Guarding may be present only as unequal muscle tone in one region of the abdomen compared with another.

9. Hernias: Examine the abdomen and the groin for evidence of hernias.

10. Rectal examination: Rectal examination is absolutely necessary in the evaluation of abdominal pain. Evaluate for prostatic pain (prostatitis) and palpable, tender masses (appendicitis, tumor, or abscess). Guaiac-positive stool may be present with peptic ulcer disease, Meckel's diverticulum, inflammatory bowel disease, or intussusception.

11. Pelvic examination: Pelvic examination is absolutely necessary in the evaluation of lower abdominal pain in a woman. Discharge indicates vaginitis or cervicitis. Cervical motion tenderness is present in cervicitis and pelvic inflammatory disease (PID). Adnexal masses may be palpable and tender.

12. Special examination: *Murphy's sign:* Have the patient inhale while firm pressure is held under the costal margin on the right. A positive sign is pain and abrupt cessation of respirations with palpation of a tender gallbladder.
Psoas sign: With the patient prone or on the side, extend the leg at the hip. A positive sign is painful extension, as with psoas abscess or retrocecal appendicitis.
Obturator sign: With the patient supine, bend one knee creating 90-degree angles at the hip and knee, and rotate the foot outward (internal rotation at the hip). A positive sign is abdominal pain with this maneuver, as with retrocecal appendicitis.
Rovsing sign: Pain in the RLQ elicited by palpating the LLQ.

13. Additional tests:
Laboratory examination

a. Complete blood count (CBC) with differential
   An elevated white blood cell (WBC) count supports an infectious or inflammatory etiology.
b. Urinalysis (UA)
   WBCs with or without red blood cells (RBCs) are associated with UTI; occasionally, a retrocecal appendicitis that lies in contact with the ureter may cause minor pyuria. RBCs indicate nephrolithiasis.
c. Serum amylase or lipase
   Elevated levels suggest pancreatitis.
d. Liver function tests (LFTs)
   Useful in evaluating patients with suspected hepatitis and biliary tract disease.
e. Beta-human chorionic gonadotropin (β-hCG)
   Ectopic pregnancy is a cause of abdominal pain in women of child-bearing age. It is also necessary to consider whether a woman is pregnant before administration of anesthesia. In the first trimester, anesthetic agents are teratogenic, in the last trimester, they can stimulate preterm labor.
f. Stool studies
   If the patient has diarrhea, especially with evidence of microbial invasion (bloody stools, leukocytosis, and fever), send stools for fecal leukocytes, culture and sensitivities of all pathogens, and analysis for ova and parasites (O&P). Send stool for *Clostridium difficile* toxin titer if the patient has had recent antibiotic treatment.
g. Other tests as symptoms dictate

Three-way abdominal films
This includes a posteroanterior (PA) chest x-ray, and kidney, ureter, bladder (KUB) films done in the supine and upright positions. The important features to note are as follows:

a. Extra-luminal air under the diaphragm ("free air")
   This is most likely seen under the right diaphragm on an upright CXR, as this is the higher side. This indicates a rupture in a viscus such as perforated ulcer or diverticulum. Extra-luminal air is normally noted on x-ray after an abdominal procedure and may be seen for up to 7 days postoperatively. Air may also be noted in the biliary tree. A lateral abdominal x-ray may also demonstrate intraperitoneal air.
b. Dilation of loops of bowel
   This may be in the small or large intestine. The dilation occurs proximal to an obstruction. The obstruction need not be complete to cause dilation.
c. Air/fluid level
   This may occur throughout the intestinal tract and denotes stasis or ileus. It may be functional or secondary to obstruction.

d. Gas pattern
Is the gas equally distributed all the way to the rectum?
Rapid transit of luminal contents, such as in diarrhea, will
leave little gas in the bowel.
e. Inflammation of the bowel wall
This is most easily seen where two loops of bowel are side
by side.
f. Air in the bowel wall
Also called pneumatosis intestinalis, it is a characteristic of
necrotizing enterocolitis, but may also be a benign finding.
g. Stones
Nephrolithiasis and occasionally cholelithiasis may be
diagnosed on plain films.
h. Loss of the psoas shadow
This may indicate a retroperitoneal process.
i. Thumb printing
This is evidence of edema or thickening of the bowel wall.

Ultrasonography
This is used to evaluate specific complaints where indicated,
such as in cases of suspected pancreatitis, cholecystitis,
nephrolithiasis, appendicitis, or ovarian pathology. Liver
and spleen may also be readily visualized in cases of trauma.

Computed tomographic (CT) scan with contrast
This is useful to evaluate mass lesions in the abdomen
and to assess the patency and continuity of the intestines.
A noncontrast abdominal CT may be used to diagnose
appendicitis.

Angiography
Where indicated, selective vessel angiography can aid in the
evaluation of aneurysms, arterial obstructions, or ruptures.

MANAGEMENT

Definitive management of the patient is dictated by the suspected
diagnosis.

Gastritis or Peptic Ulcer Disease (Non-Perforated)

Mucosal injuries in the stomach and duodenum have a spectrum of
severity ranging from gastritis to acute or chronic peptic ulcer disease. The hallmark is GI bleeding.

Clues to Diagnosis:

History: Common in men in their 30s and 40s. History of
stress, NSAID use, steroid use, or tobacco or alcohol abuse. Dyspepsia is a common symptom.

Pain:	Sudden onset. Constant. Burning or stabbing. Relieved with food.
Location:	Epigastrium, occasionally radiating to the back.
Exam:	Epigastric tenderness. Stool may be guaiac positive.
Studies:	Evaluation for *Helicobacter pylori*. Upper endoscopy in the stable patient is diagnostic greater than 90% of the time.
Acuity:	Routine to urgent.
Treatment:	Bland diet.
	Medications (Table 5–1).
	Treat *H. pylori* if present. Many regimens are used. An inexpensive and effective one is:
	Clarithromycin 500 mg PO BID × 14 days, *and*
	Amoxicillin 1 gm PO BID ×14 days, *and*
	Prevacid 30 mg PO BID × 14 days
	Evaluation for coagulopathy and hyperacidity states.
	Do not administer antacids before endoscopy, as this will obscure the examination.
	Surgical therapy is reserved for treatment of chronic or severe symptoms or of bleeding that continues for 6 to 8 units over 48 hours.
Notes:	If hematemesis is the prominent symptom, an urgent upper endoscopy is required to rule out esophageal varices.

Perforated Peptic Ulcer

Perforated peptic ulcer disease occurs more frequently in the duodenum than in the stomach.

Clues to Diagnosis:

History:	Common in men in their 30s and 40s. History of peptic ulcer disease. Use of NSAIDs, steroids, or sympathomimetic drugs. Tobacco or alcohol abuse. Stress.
Pain:	Sudden onset. Severe burning or stabbing.
Location:	Localized to epigastrium but generalizes over time. Often radiates to the back or shoulder. Occasionally in RLQ.
Exam:	Peritonitis is common with severe epigastric tenderness caused by the chemical burn of gastric acids on the peritoneum. Stool may be guaiac positive. Impending shock and hypovolemia are the norm. Intestinal fluids may travel down to the RLQ, and symptoms may mimic acute appendicitis. Abdominal distention.
Studies:	Elevated WBCs. Free air under diaphragm on chest x-ray in 75% of cases.

TABLE 5–1 Common Medications Used to Treat Gastritis

	Secretion Blockade	
Medication[1]	Receptor Blockade	Dose[2]
Cimetidine (Tagamet)	H_2	300 mg IV every 6–8 hr, or 400 mg PO every 6 hr, may be given 800 mg PO twice per day
Ranitidine (Zantac)	H_2	50 mg IV every 8 hr or 150 mg PO twice per day may be given 300 mg PO qHS
Famotidine (Pepcid)	H_2	20–40 mg PO or IV every day, IV form divided twice per day
Nizatidine (Axid)	H_2	300 mg PO every day (or may be divided twice per day)
Omeprazole (Prilosec)	H^+K^+-ATPase	20 mg PO every day
Lansoprazole (Zoton)	H^+K^+-ATPase	15 mg PO every day
Pantoprazole (Protonix)	H^+K^+-ATPase	40 mg PO every day
Esomeprazole (Nexium)	H^+K^+-ATPase	20 mg PO every day
Rabeprazole (Pariet)	H^+K^+-ATPase	20 mg PO every day

Acid Neutralization[3]		
Magnesium Containing	Aluminum Containing	Combination Agents
Milk of magnesia	ALternaGEL	Alka-Seltzer
Mag-Ox 400	Alumina	Maalox
Uro-Mag	Alu-Cap or Alu-Tab	Mylanta
	Amphojel	Bicitra

Protective Coating	
Medication	Dose
Sulcralfate (Carafate)	1 g PO 4 times per day
Bismuth subsalicylate (Pepto-Bismol[4])	2 tbsp or tablets PO every 0.5–1 hr as needed. Do not exceed 8 doses/24 hr

[1]Higher doses of secretion blockade medications may be required to treat hypersecretion states such as Zollinger–Ellison syndrome. Check gastric pH frequently to monitor therapy; aim for pH >5.

[2]All H_2-receptor antagonist doses must be reduced in patients with renal failure.

[3]These may be administered in doses of 1–2 tbsp PO every 2–4 hr with "holds" for side effects, such as for diarrhea with magnesium-containing antacids and for constipation with aluminum-containing antacids.

[4]In patients with guaiac-positive stools, avoid the use of Pepto-Bismol, as the bismuth will turn the stool black and may be confused with melena. Note also that Pepto-Bismol contains salicylates.

IV, intravenously; PO, by mouth.

Bicarbonate deficit >4 mEq/L.

Differential diagnosis:	Acute appendicitis with perforation
	Acute cholecystitis
	Acute pancreatitis
	Intestinal obstruction
	Perforated diverticulitis
Acuity:	**Emergency.**
Treatment:	Nothing by mouth (NPO)
	Fluid resuscitation as necessary
	Emergency exploratory laparotomy with repair

Biliary Colic/Chronic Cholecystitis

The spectrum of gallbladder disease includes biliary colic, chronic cholecystitis, acute cholecystitis, and ascending cholangitis. Biliary colic describes intermittent pain in the RUQ after ingestion of fatty foods. This starts as discomfort, then crescendos into severe pain, which resolves in a short time (2 to 4 hours). It is caused by intermittent obstruction of the duct with a stone. It is treated with fluids and pain relief measures. Only if the pain is unremitting do these patients require admission. Chronic cholecystitis is the result of multiple inflammatory attacks on the gallbladder resulting in scar tissue and impaired function.

Acute Cholecystitis

Acute cholecystitis is a current inflammatory attack on the gallbladder. It is associated with complete occlusion of the duct by stones in 90% of the cases.

Clues to Diagnosis:

History:	Common in women in their 30s to 60s. Often a known history of biliary tract disease or symptoms of biliary colic. Pain tends to increase 1 to 2 hours after fat intake. About 75% of patients have had gallbladder symptoms in the past. The common mnemonic aid used to identify patients at risk is the "5 Fs:" fair, female, fat, forty, and fertile. Pain often wakes patient.
Pain:	Dull to colicky, may be constant. Onset may be sudden.
Location:	RUQ with radiation to the right subscapular region. Often the pain begins in the midline, then resolves and recurs in 6 to 8 hours in the RUQ. May generalize with gallbladder rupture or severe infection.
Other signs and symptoms:	Nausea, vomiting, fever, and jaundice if significant obstruction exists.
Exam:	Hypoactive bowel tones. Often signs of peritonitis, but some patients present with colicky pain. Right rectus muscle spasm may be present. RUQ tenderness with a positive *Murphy's sign* (see page 26).

Studies:	Elevated WBCs, bilirubin, and LFTs. Stones are uncommonly seen on plain films (<15%). Ultrasonography is the imaging study of choice and may reveal thickening of the gallbladder wall, pericholecystic fluid, stones in the gallbladder or the bile ducts, and dilation of the gallbladder or the biliary tree. Nonurgent gallbladder function tests include technetium Tc-99m radionuclide scanning. Liver is visualized within 5 to 10 minutes, followed by visualization of the gallbladder and the bile ducts. Failure or delay of gallbladder filling is abnormal. Ninety five percent of patients with nonvisualization of the gallbladder who are symptomatic have acute cholecystitis. A nonfilling gallbladder noted in a patient whose symptoms have resolved indicates chronic cholecystitis.
Differential diagnosis:	Acute appendicitis. Coronary artery disease. Fitz–Hugh–Curtis disease. Hepatitis. Obstructive jaundice due to cancer. Pancreatitis. Peptic ulcer disease. Pyelonephritis. Renal colic. Pneumonia.
Acuity:	Urgent.
Treatment:	NPO. Fluid resuscitation as necessary. Appropriate antibiotic therapy. Pain relief. If ducts are dilated, transhepatic cholangiography with placement of an external drainage tube may be palliative. Likewise, endoscopic retrograde cholangiopancreatography (ERCP) with sphincterotomy may allow passage of an obstructing stone. Emergency surgical management is reserved for rupture or gangrene of the gallbladder, indicated by impending sepsis.
Notes:	Many patients with acute cholecystitis is "cooled off" with antibiotic treatment until the WBC count normalizes prior to attempting cholecystectomy.

Ascending Cholangitis

Results from bacterial infection of the bile in settings of stasis or biliary obstruction.

Clues to Diagnosis:

History:	Often history of surgery on the biliary tract or adjacent structures. History of biliary colic.
Pain:	Sharp, colicky.
Location:	Right upper quadrant (RUQ) with radiation to the back.
Other signs and symptoms:	Nausea, vomiting, jaundice, fever, and chills. *Charcot's triad* of fever with chills, RUQ pain, and jaundice is variably present and should not be relied on. The addition of hypotension and mental status changes makes up *Reynold's pentad* and is an indication of sepsis.
Exam:	Hypoactive bowel tones. Often signs of peritonitis. RUQ tenderness with a positive *Murphy's sign* (see page 26).
Studies:	Elevated WBCs and bilirubin. Blood cultures may demonstrate growth of the causative microbe. Ultrasonography may reveal dilation of the gall-bladder or the biliary tree with or without stones. ERCP may demonstrate dilated and ectatic bile ducts but may not visualize beyond the obstruction. Transhepatic cholangiography is also diagnostic, and a tube may be left in place for external drainage.
Acuity:	**Emergency.** Sepsis is likely.
Treatment:	NPO. Fluid resuscitation as necessary. Appropriate antibiotic therapy. Biliary tract drainage, either by ERCP or transhepatic cholangiography. Emergency surgical management is reserved for rupture or gangrene of the gallbladder, signified by evidence of sepsis. Emergent surgery may also be warranted if biliary tract drainage procedures are unsuccessful.

Pancreatitis

Pancreatitis may be acute, chronic, or relapsing.

Clues to Diagnosis:

History:	Patients in their 20s to 50s with prior pancreatitis or alcohol abuse or a history of cholelithiasis.
Pain:	Rapid onset; severe, deep, constant, and progressive. May be colicky.
Location:	Epigastric with radiation to the back and both costal margins.

Other signs and symptoms:	Nausea, vomiting, and anorexia.
Exam:	Hypoactive to absent bowel tones. Epigastric tenderness. Hemorrhagic pancreatitis may be associated with retroperitoneal bleeding and blood that extravasates along tissue planes (*Grey Turner's sign* or *Cullen's sign,* see page 25).
Studies:	Elevated WBCs and serum amylase are diagnostic. P-amylase is specific to the pancreas, and isoenzymes are useful in differentiating from salivary amylase. Serum lipase is also a highly specific test, thought to be more sensitive in cases of long-standing alcoholic pancreatitis. Plain films may reveal calcification of the pancreas, pleural effusion, or a "sentinel loop" of bowel. CT or ultrasonographic scanning may be useful in assessing complications such as pseudocyst, and assessing perfusion of the pancreas. Order a "pancreatic protocol CT."
Differential diagnosis:	Acute appendicitis. Acute cholecystitis. Acute renal failure. Choledocholithiasis. Peptic ulcer disease. Mesenteric ischemia or thrombosis. Myocardial infarction. Small-bowel obstruction.
Acuity:	Urgent. **Emergent** if shock is apparent.
Treatment:	NPO. NG suction. Fluid resuscitation. Pain management. **Meperidine (Demerol) 50 to 150 mg intramuscularly (IM) every 3 to 4 hours, as necessary,** is thought to be more appropriate than morphine sulfate, because it causes less spasm of the sphincter of Oddi. Support respiration. Surgery is rarely required except for complications such as phlegmon, hemorrhagic pancreatitis, or pseudocyst.
Notes:	Patients with fever should be assessed with a pancreatic protocol CT scan to rule out pancreatic abscess. The severity of acute pancreatitis may be predicted by *Ranson's criteria,* which are summarized in Table 5–2. The larger the number of positive signs, the more severe the case. Patients demonstrating more than 4 positive

TABLE 5–2 **Ranson's Criteria for Predicting the Severity of Acute Pancreatitis**

Initial	Over the First 48 Hr
Age >55 yr	Hct drop >10%
WBC >16,000/mm^3	BUN rise >5 mg/dL
Blood glucose >200 mg/dL	Serum calcium <8 mg/dL
Serum LDH >350 IU/L	Bicarbonate deficit >4 mEq/L
Serum SGOT >250 sigma	PaO$_2$ <60 mm Hg
Frankel U/dL	Fluid gain >6 L
1-2 criteria met:	Mortality rare
3-4 criteria met:	Mortality 15%, half will require ICU care
5-6 criteria met:	Mortality 50%
7-8 criteria met:	Mortality >> 50%

WBC, white blood cell (count); LDH, lactate dehydrogenase; SGOT, serum glutamic-oxaloacetic transaminase; Hct, hematocrit; BUN, blood urea nitrogen; PaO$_2$, arterial partial pressure of oxygen.

signs are at greater risk of developing hemorrhagic pancreatitis.

Hepatitis

Hepatitis may be acute, chronic, or relapsing. Etiologies include viral infection and alcohol or other toxin ingestion.

Clues to Diagnosis:

History:	Exposure to known infectious agent or toxin.
Pain:	Gradual onset of severe, achy pain.
Location:	RUQ with radiation to the back and right costal margin.
Other signs and symptoms:	Nausea, vomiting, anorexia, jaundice, and fever.
Exam:	Normal to hypoactive bowel tones. Epigastric and RUQ tenderness. Note that the entire liver will be tender, including the lateral aspect. Palpate the low lateral intercostal spaces; this will be useful in differentiating hepatitis from acute cholecystitis.
Studies:	Elevated WBCs and LFTs are suggestive in viral etiologies. Serologies are available to diagnose the specific causative agent.
Acuity:	Routine to urgent.
Treatment:	Fluid resuscitation and pain management. Enteric or blood precautions as necessary. Acyclovir may have a role in chronic hepatitis B (HBV) infection. Surgery is rarely required.

Notes: Five distinct viruses cause hepatitis: Hepatitis A (HAV, formerly infectious hepatitis), Hepatitis B (HBV, formerly serum hepatitis), Hepatitis C (HCV, formerly a subset of non-A, non-B hepatitis), Hepatitis D (HDV, also known as delta-associated hepatitis, which requires concomitant HBV infection for replication), and Hepatitis E (HEV, viral cause of non-A, non-B hepatitis). HAV and HEV are transmitted in a fecal or oral manner, and the remainder of the Hepatitis viri are transmitted parenterally.

Hepatic reserve is estimated by the *Child–Pugh classification* (Table 5–3), which estimates risk based on biochemical and physical examination findings.

Acute Appendicitis

Clues to Diagnosis:

History: Characteristic pattern of pain progression.

Pain: Initially a generalized ache, which progresses within 6 to 8 hours to localized severe ache.

Location: Epigastric, then periumbilical, then RLQ (McBurney's point). As the appendix is variable in its location, the origin of the localized pain may vary.

Other signs and symptoms: Anorexia is the most frequent associated symptom. Nausea and vomiting are more variable. Fever may be present, but up to one-third of patients will be afebrile.

Exam: RLQ point tenderness, tenderness to percussion. Peritonitis is common. Other findings may include RLQ hyperesthesia, indirect (referred) rebound, or *psoas, Rovsing* or *obturator signs* (see page 26).

TABLE 5–3 **Child–Pugh Classification of Hepatic Reserve**

	Class A (Minimal Risk)	Class B (Moderate Risk)	Class C (Advanced Risk)
Bilirubin (mg/dL)	<2	2–3	>3
Albumin (g/dL)	>3.5	3–3.5	<3
Ascites	None	Easy to control	Difficult to control
Encephalopathy	None	Minimal	Advanced
Nutritional status	Excellent	Good	Poor
Mortality in shunting procedures	<2%	10%	50%

Studies:	Elevated WBCs, but one-third of patients may have a normal WBC count. Infrequently WBCs in the UA. Ultrasonography is a valuable tool to diagnose appendicitis and may find a thickened, noncompressible appendix, luminal stones, or rupture. Plain films are not usually helpful but may occasionally show a fecalith in the appendix.
Differential diagnosis:	See Table 5–4.
Acuity:	Urgent. **Emergent** if signs of sepsis or obstruction.
Treatment:	NPO. Exploratory laparotomy. If the appendix is found to be normal, it is removed anyway, to avoid future confusion. The presence of a McBurney's incision scar (commonly used in open appendectomy) will suggest to future examiners that the appendix has been removed. Removing the appendix also eliminates future risk of appendicitis.
Notes:	Especially difficult to diagnose in the very young (<3 years old) and in the elderly. The orientation of the appendix relative to the cecum may drastically alter the presenting symptoms.

Meckel's Diverticulitis

This results from persistence of a portion of the vitelline duct. It is found on the antimesenteric border of the distal ileum, usually two feet proximal to the cecum. Pain may be caused by inflammation (diverticulitis) or by obstruction and may be difficult to differentiate from acute appendicitis. A technetium-99m pertechnetate scan, which identifies gastric mucosa, may aid in diagnosis if the patient presents with lower GI bleeding. Patients who are symptomatic with pain or bleeding will require exploration and resection.

TABLE 5–4 **Common Diagnoses That May Mimic Appendicitis**

Intestinal	Renal
Crohn disease	Nephrolithiasis
Ulcerative colitis	Pyelonephritis
Gastroenteritis	Perinephric abscess
Mesenteric lymphangitis	Hydronephrosis
Inflamed Meckel's diverticulum	
Diverticulitis	Gynecologic
Psoas abscess	
Cecal tumor	Salpingitis
Intestinal obstruction	Ovarian torsion
Acute cholecystitis	Ovarian cyst (ruptured)
Perforated duodenal ulcer	Ectopic pregnancy

Acute Diverticulitis

Inflammation of congenital or acquired diverticuli in the large intestine. The spectrum includes mild inflammation, severe inflammation, and perforation (abscess, extra-luminal air, colovesicular fistula).

Clues to Diagnosis:

History:	Documented diverticulosis, a prior bouts of diverticulitis.
Pain:	Severe ache, crampy pain.
Location:	Left lower quadrant (LLQ) > RLQ.
Other signs and symptoms:	Fever and chills. Diarrhea with blood or mucous.
Exam:	LLQ tenderness. A mass may be palpable and peritonitis may be apparent if a diverticulum has ruptured resulting in an abscess.
Studies:	Elevated WBCs. CT scan may show abscess or mass. Contrast enema will fill the diverticuli and may show areas of perforation.
Acuity:	Urgent.
Treatment:	Fluid resuscitation and pain management. Appropriate antibiotic therapy. Mild inflammation may be treated as an outpatient, but if the patient is infirm or the inflammation is severe, hospitalization may be required. Emergency surgical management is reserved for complete obstruction or perforation with impending sepsis.
Notes:	Surgical options may include exploratory laparotomy with colonic diversion, resection with primary anastomosis, or transcutaneous drainage of the abscess.

Acute Obstruction of the Small Intestine

Lack of recognition and correction of this problem will lead to bowel infarction. The major etiologies include postoperative adhesions, hernias, tumors, intussusception, strictures, and volvulus.

Clues to Diagnosis:

History:	Prior abdominal surgery, GI neoplasm, history of hernia.
Pain:	Sudden, crampy, or colicky. The patient may be pain-free between bouts.
Location:	Periumbilical or generalized.
Other signs and symptoms:	Vomiting. The character of the vomitus will give clues as to the location of the obstruction. Clear vomitus indicates obstruction proximal to the bile duct. Bilious vomitus indicates obstruction

	distal to the sphincter of Oddi. Brown or feculent vomitus indicates a distal colonic obstruction and is a late finding.
Exam:	Hyperactive bowel tones with rushes. Distention. Generalized tenderness.
Studies:	Elevated WBCs. Three-way abdominal series is diagnostic and may show dilated loops of bowel or air/fluid levels. The colon distal to the obstruction may be empty of gas or stool.
Differential diagnosis:	Acute appendicitis. Acute cholecystitis. Acute pancreatitis. Ascites. Large-bowel obstruction. Mesenteric ischemia or thrombosis. Paralytic ileus. Peptic ulcer disease.
Acuity:	Urgent.
Treatment:	NPO. NG decompression. Fluid resuscitation. This is important, as patients tend to secrete fluid into obstructed bowel loops. Emergent surgical management is reserved for complications of bowel obstruction such as perforation, or complete closed-loop obstruction.

Acute Obstruction of the Large Intestine

Most common causes include carcinoma, diverticulitis, fecal impaction, and volvulus.

Clues to Diagnosis:

History:	Age older than 40 years of age. History of prior abdominal surgery.
Pain:	Gradual onset, crampy, and intermittent. Cramps less frequent than in small-bowel obstruction.
Location:	Generalized.
Other signs and symptoms:	Constipation, nausea, and vomiting. Vomitus may be brown or feculent. Alternating diarrhea and constipation may indicate a partial obstruction.
Exam:	Distended and tympanitic. Generalized tenderness. Stool may be guaiac positive in cases of carcinoma. A mass may be palpable. "Rushing" bowel tones differentiate obstruction from the quiet abdomen of paralytic ileus.
Studies:	Elevated WBCs. Three-way abdominal series is diagnostic and may show dilated loops of bowel or air/fluid levels. The proximal small bowel may be normal if the ileocecal valve is competent.

A cecum acutely measuring 10 to 12 cm in diameter is an indication of impending perforation. Contrast enema may aid in diagnosis.

Differential diagnosis:	Metastatic cancer.
	Ogilvie syndrome.
	Paralytic ileus.
	Endometriosis.
Acuity:	Urgent.
Treatment:	NPO.
	NG decompression.
	Fluid resuscitation.
	Sigmoidoscopy may be palliative to relieve pressure. If a lesion is found, diagnosis is possible. A rectal tube may be left in place to facilitate decompression.
	Intravenous antibiotics are indicated in settings of fever, leukocytosis, or evidence of perforation.
	Emergent surgical management is reserved for complications of bowel obstruction such as perforation.

Volvulus

This is a form of large-bowel obstruction caused by a twisting of the cecum or the sigmoid colon. The sigmoid is more commonly affected (80% to 85%). Cecum is more commonly affected in younger patients.

Clues to Diagnosis:

History:	Greater than 65 years of age. History of chronic laxative use and chronic constipation.
Pain:	Rapid onset, crampy, and intermittent.
Location:	Sigmoid volvulus: generalized to LLQ. Cecal volvulus: generalized to RLQ.
Other signs and symptoms:	Nausea and vomiting. Vomitus may be brown or feculent.
Exam:	Distended and tympanitic. Generalized tenderness.
Studies:	Three-way abdominal films. In sigmoid volvulus, the sigmoid colon looks doubled in a characteristic "bent inner tube" or "omega" sign. The convexity of the loop lies away from the site of obstruction. In cecal volvulus, the gas-filled cecum may be noted in the left upper quadrant (LUQ) and may appear as a "coffee bean" sign with the apex pointing toward the RLQ.
	Contrast enema will show the point of obstruction and may occasionally aid in the reduction of the obstruction.
Acuity:	**Emergency.** Rapid reduction will decrease the risk of infarction.

Treatment: NPO.
               Fluid resuscitation.
               Sigmoidoscopy. This will be diagnostic and cura-
               tive in sigmoid volvulus. Cecal volvulus may
               require contrast enema or surgical reduction.

Mesenteric Ischemia

This may be an acute or chronic disorder. The acute form is usually
due to arterial embolization and is associated with a high mortality
rate despite surgical resection.

Clues to Diagnosis:

This is often a difficult diagnosis to make.

History:	Known arteriosclerotic disease. Taking medications known to decrease intestinal blood flow (Table 5–5).
Pain:	Crampy, postprandial, especially after large meals.
Location:	Epigastric or generalized.
Exam:	Generalized tenderness, but the pain is usually well out of proportion to the physical findings.
Other signs and symptoms:	Nausea and vomiting. Weight loss or change in bowel habits. Look for evidence of cardiovascular or peripheral vascular disease. If infarction is present, then melena and peritonitis will be evident.
Studies:	Elevated WBCs. Angiography may locate the arterial lesion, but degree of occlusion may not correlate with degree of symptoms.
Acuity:	Urgent. **Emergent** if sepsis or peritonitis are evident.
Treatment:	NPO.

TABLE 5–5 **Medications Known to Decrease Intestinal Blood Flow**

Angiotensin
Digoxin
Dopamine (high dose)
Epinephrine
Halothane
Indomethacin
Metaraminol
Methoxamine
Norepinephrine
Ouabain
Phenylephrine
Prostaglandins E_1, E_2, and F_2 (α or β)
Vasopressin

Emergency surgical management is reserved for infarction.

Arterial reconstruction is curative in cases of chronic mesenteric ischemia.

Bowel Infarction

This may be due to intussusception, volvulus, herniation, mesenteric ischemia, thrombosis, or ischemic colitis.

Clues to Diagnosis:

History:	Preexisting condition such as inflammatory bowel disease or prior abdominal surgery.
Pain:	Gradual onset, crampy, and sharp.
Location:	Generalized.
Exam:	Distention, generalized abdominal tenderness.
Studies:	Elevated WBCs. Progressive acidemia and shock. Plain films may show stasis or obstruction.
Acuity:	**Emergency.**
Treatment:	NPO.
	Fluid resuscitation.
	Exploratory laparotomy with bowel resection.

Abdominal Abscess

Clues to Diagnosis:

History:	History of diverticulitis, inflammatory bowel disease, or other ruptured viscus. Recent abdominal procedure, especially biliary, pancreatic, or gastric.
Pain:	Gradual onset, sharp, and constant.
Location:	Depends on the location of the abscess. Pain from subphrenic abscesses may radiate to the shoulders.
Exam:	Distention. Tenderness to palpation. Rupture of an abscess may result in peritonitis.
Other signs and symptoms:	Nausea, vomiting, anorexia, and fever.
Studies:	Elevated WBCs. CT scan or ultrasonogram may localize the mass.
Acuity:	Urgent. Ruptured abscess is an **emergency.**
Treatment:	NPO.
	Fluid resuscitation.
	Appropriate antibiotic therapy.
	Emergency transcutaneous drainage of intact abscesses.
	Emergency surgical management is reserved for ruptured abscesses.
Notes:	Abdominal abscesses may form even in the setting of broad-spectrum antibiotic therapy.

Renal Calculi

Clues to Diagnosis:

History:	Prior renal stones, hypercalcemia, or hypercalciuria.
Pain:	Sudden, severe, and colicky.
Location:	Location of the pain depends on the location of the stone. High ureteral stones are felt in the right or left flank. As they move down the ureter, pain may radiate into the groin, the perineum, or the testicle.
Other signs and symptoms:	Dysuria, hematuria, and dehydration.
Exam:	Abdomen may be benign.
Studies:	RBCs in the UA. Eighty percent of stones are visible on plain films of the abdomen. CT scan with IV contrast or intravenous pyelography will determine the degree of obstruction and size of the stone.
Acuity:	Urgent.
Treatment:	Fluid resuscitation.
	Pain management.
	Strain urine to ensure passage of the stone.
	Most stones pass on their own, but stones of greater than 1 cm or stones that do not move with time may need surgical removal, transurethral basket extraction, or lithotripsy.

Pyelonephritis

Clues to Diagnosis:

History:	Recent UTI.
Pain:	Gradual, severe, and constant with colicky increases.
Location:	Right or left flank into back, abdomen, groin, perineum, or testicle.
Other signs and symptoms:	Dysuria, frequency, hematuria, fever, chills.
Exam:	Abdomen may be benign. Tenderness over the affected flank.
Studies:	Elevated WBCs. WBCs and RBCs in the UA. WBC casts may be seen.
Acuity:	Urgent.
Treatment:	Fluid resuscitation.
	Pain management.
	Culture urine.
	Appropriate empirical antibiotic therapy.
	Focus antibiotic therapy as culture results dictate.

Ruptured Abdominal Aortic Aneurysm

Clues to Diagnosis:

History:	Known abdominal aneurysm, hypertension, or arteriosclerotic disease.
Pain:	Sudden, severe, and tearing.
Location:	Epigastric or periumbilical with sharp radiation to the back or groin.
Exam:	Hypoactive bowel sounds. Peritonitis. Pulsatile abdominal mass. Decreased femoral and lower extremity pulses. Progressive shock.
Studies:	CT scan, angiogram, or ultrasonogram will confirm the diagnosis in a stable patient. An unstable patient should be evaluated on the OR table.
Acuity:	**Emergency.**
Treatment:	NPO.
	Fluid and pressor resuscitation.
	Emergency exploratory laparotomy with repair of the rupture.
Notes:	These patients are critically ill and require immediate surgery. Send a crossmatch immediately for 5 to 10 units of whole blood. Be prepared to transfuse with type O, Rh negative uncrossmatched blood until crossmatched blood is available. Advise the blood bank that a "high volume" case is in progress.

Acute Salpingitis

(Pelvic Inflammatory Disease)

Clues to Diagnosis:

History:	Occurs before menopause, usually just after a menstrual period. History of chlamydial or gonorrheal infection.
Pain:	Sharp or achy.
Location:	RLQ or LLQ with radiation to the back and umbilicus.
Other signs and symptoms:	Nausea, vomiting, fever, and vaginal discharge.
Exam:	Hypoactive bowel tones. RLQ or LLQ tenderness. Cervical motion tenderness. Possibly adnexal mass.
Studies:	Elevated WBCs. Ultrasonography may be useful in differentiating ovarian pathology or ectopic pregnancy.

Differential diagnosis:	Acute appendicitis.
	Ovarian torsion.
	Tubal pregnancy.
Acuity:	Urgent.
Treatment:	Fluid resuscitation.
	Appropriate antibiotic therapy.
	Emergency surgical management is reserved for tubo-ovarian abscesses.
Notes:	This is often treated by a gynecologist.

Ovarian Cyst

Usually present with pain if in association with torsion or rupture.

Clues to Diagnosis:

History:	Prior cysts.
Pain:	Of sudden onset and constant.
Location:	RLQ or LLQ.
Exam:	Palpable mass on pelvic examination.
Studies:	Ultrasound is diagnostic and is useful in ruling out acute appendicitis.
Acuity:	Urgent.
Treatment:	Fluid resuscitation and pain management.
	Emergency surgical management is reserved for acute hemorrhage or torsion.
Notes:	This is often treated by a gynecologist.

Ectopic Pregnancy

Almost 95% of ectopic pregnancies are tubal.

Clues to Diagnosis:

History:	Suspected pregnancy.
Pain:	Sudden onset, sharp, and persistent.
Location:	RLQ or LLQ.
Other signs and symptoms:	Occasionally nausea and vomiting. Signs of early pregnancy: softening and cyanosis of the cervix, and amenorrhea.
Exam:	Mass on abdominal or pelvic examination and point tenderness.
Studies:	Positive β-hCG. Ultrasonogram is diagnostic. Progressive anemia is possible.
Differential diagnosis:	Acute appendicitis.
	Ovarian cyst.
	Salpingitis.
Acuity:	**Emergency.**
Treatment:	NPO.
	Exploratory laparotomy or laparoscopy with removal of the conceptus.
Notes:	This is often treated by a gynecologist.

Special Surgical Considerations

Postoperative considerations

1. Table 5–6 lists common postoperative conditions associated with abdominal pain and fever.
2. After antral resection of the stomach, and less commonly with other gastric resections, a "dumping" syndrome results in which partially digested highly osmotic foods are transported into the small intestine. This leads to hypermotility of the small intestine and rapid absorption of carbohydrates. The syndrome presents with early symptoms of abdominal pain after meals and diarrhea, and late symptoms of hypoglycemia due to hypersecretion of insulin in response to the carbohydrate bolus. It is treated by instituting a "postgastrectomy diet" consisting of frequent, small, low-carbohydrate meals.
3. Diarrhea is also common with onset of feeding after any bowel resection, as there is a measurable loss of absorptive surface. An extensive resection will result in a higher chance of feeding intolerance. Antibiotic-associated diarrhea and *C. difficile* pseudomembranous colitis are common postoperative complications. See Chapter 6.

TABLE 5–6 **Common Causes of Postoperative Abdominal Pain and Fever**

Condition	Common Cause	Diagnostic Study	Treatment
Abdominal abscess	Anastomotic leak	CT scan	Drainage, antibiotics
Peritonitis	Anastomotic leak, peritoneal soilage	PE, paracentesis, CT scan	Antibiotics, reoperation
Pancreatitis	Surgical trauma	CT scan, amylase	Fluid support, drainage of pseudocyst as necessary
Cholangitis	Surgical trauma	US, transhepatic cholangiogram	T-tube drainage, antibiotics, surgical repair
Perforated peptic ulcer	Stress ulceration	Contrast swallow, endoscopy	Surgical repair
Acute cholecystitis	Perioperative stasis	US, LFTs, scintiscan	Antibiotics, surgical resection
Wound infection	Dehiscence	PE	Debridement, antibiotics

CT, computed tomography; PE, physical examination; US, ultrasonography; LFT, liver function test.

4. Major abdominal procedures cause severe pain. This is generally treated with narcotic medication. Every patient differs in his or her response to narcotics, so a common cause of postoperative abdominal pain is inadequate narcotic administration. Consider giving a small bolus of morphine or fentanyl and reassess the patient.

Remember

Keep in mind the following "nonabdominal" causes of abdominal pain:

1. Myocardial infarction
2. Pneumonia
3. Diabetes mellitus
4. Porphyria
5. UTI
6. Sickle cell disease

Female patients of child-bearing years should be considered pregnant until proven otherwise.

Bowel Function—
Constipation and Diarrhea

Phone calls regarding the bowel functions of your patients will be frequent; fortunately, many of these problems can be managed over the phone. Patients may have changes in bowel function while hospitalized because of dietary changes, less mobility, narcotic analgesics, other medications, and abdominal surgery with functional ileus. You should be familiar with the major causes of these changes and feel comfortable with the range of options for treating these problems. Many patients become distressed with bowel function changes and appreciate being made to feel more comfortable.

CONSTIPATION

PHONE CALL

Questions

1. **Has this patient had surgery? If so, what was the operation and when was it performed?**

    Patients undergoing abdominal surgery develop a functional ileus that lasts 4 to 5 days or more. These patients should *not* be given a laxative. They must wait for their gastrointestinal (GI) function to return. Ambulation appears to help GI function return postoperatively. Also, postoperative appendectomy patients should not receive rectal suppositories. Some surgeons believe that this may cause contractions in the colon and increase the risk of appendix stump leaks.

2. **Why does the patient want a laxative? When was the last bowel movement (BM)? What is the normal bowel routine for this patient?**

    Some people have up to three BMs per day, while others have a BM as infrequently as once a week. These ranges are normal. You should know a patient's normal routine before prescribing a laxative.

3. **Is the patient nauseated or has he or she been vomiting?**

    Be hesitant to prescribe a laxative to a patient who has signs of upper GI dysfunction. The patient could have another problem, such as intestinal obstruction or appendicitis. Constipation alone does not lead to upper GI symptoms unless the patient is impacted and has a significant ileus.

4. Does the patient have abdominal pain?

A patient with abdominal pain and who requests a laxative should be examined. An ileus, and hence constipation, results from many serious surgical problems of the abdomen. For example, a perforated viscus often presents with abdominal pain and ileus.

5. Has a rectal examination been performed on the patient?

Fecal impaction is diagnosed by rectal examination. Laxatives do not usually help patients who are impacted. Manual disimpaction may be necessary.

6. Does the patient routinely use laxatives?

Some patients may abuse laxatives; these patients develop GI dysfunction.

Orders

Once you have determined that it is safe and appropriate to prescribe a laxative or an enema, you must think about what type of agent to use (Table 6–1). Laxatives can be delivered by mouth or rectum; enemas are delivered by rectum.

Oral Laxatives

Laxatives that are usually considered stool softeners include surface-active agents (docusate sodium [Colace]) and bulk-forming agents (psyllium [Metamucil, Konsyl]). These agents tend to soften the stool for the foodstuffs eaten at about the same time that the agent is taken. For example, a patient with constipation who begins taking Metamucil is unlikely to benefit until the older hard stool has been cleared and the bulk-forming agent can soften the newly formed stool. In a similar fashion, surface-active laxatives such as Colace take a day or more to show significant stool-softening action.

The osmotic laxatives include magnesium citrate. This is a pleasant tasting, carbonated liquid. Most patients have a BM within several hours of taking this agent. You can repeat the dose if no results are obtained with the first dose. Commonly used in bowel preparation before surgery is the osmotic agent GoLYTELY. This agent contains polyethylene glycol, circumvents fluid absorption cleanses the bowel. It is not used routinely good bowel-preparation agent.

Rectal Laxatives

Glycerin is an osmotic laxative given of action is usually 30 to 60 minutes. [Dulcolax]) is a stimulant of defecatio is popular in hospitals. If the first bisa tive, the dose can be repeated.

TABLE 6–1 **Common Laxatives and Enemas for Use in Surgical Patients**

Type of Agent	Name of Agent	Dose	Cautions
Bulk-forming laxative	Psyllium seed Metamucil Konsyl	1 tsp in liquid PO each day up to 3 times per day	Some drugs may be bound by the cellulose
Surface-active laxative	Docusate (Colace)	100 mg PO 3 times per day	
Lubricant laxative	Mineral oil	10–15 mL PO twice daily	Decreases fat-soluble vitamin absorption
Osmotic laxatives	Magnesium citrate	100 mL of a 15 g/300 mL solution PO	Do not use in patients with renal dysfunction
	Glycerin	1 preformed suppository PR	
Stimulant laxatives	Dulcolax	5–15 mg PO or 10 mg PR	
Hypertonic enema	Fleet enema	60–120 mL PR from a disposable container	Do not use in patients with nausea, vomiting, or abdominal pain
Mineral oil enema	Fleet mineral oil enema	60–120 mL PR from a disposable container	Good for fecal impaction

PO, by mouth; PR, rectally.

Enemas

Enemas deliver agents directly to the rectum. This is useful to help the patient evacuate hard stool. Options include the hypertonic enemas (Fleet enemas), oil-retention enemas, and soapsuds enemas.

What to Use and When—Some Suggestions

Usually, it is best to put most hospitalized patients on an oral stool softener, especially if any narcotic analgesic is to be used. Most patients prefer Colace or a bulk-forming agent such as Metamucil or Frequently, a stool softener will eliminate the need for other

patients who are constipated prefer a stimulatory supposi- Dulcolax. This stimulatory suppository is safe and may til results are achieved. If the stimulatory suppository fails, an osmotic agent such as magnesium citrate may be effective. However, some patients develop some abdominal cramping with osmotic agents.

Finally, enemas can be used if attempts with an osmotic agent are unsuccessful. A fleet enema or a mineral oil enema usually gives profound evacuation. Mineral oil enemas are especially good for softening impacted feces.

Notes

A common cause of constipation is medication. Psychotropic drugs and diuretics can cause severe constipation, which may also be exacerbated if the patient is institutionalized.

DIARRHEA

PHONE CALL

Questions

1. **Has the patient had surgery? If so, what was the operation and when was it performed?**
2. **Does the patient have abdominal pain or a fever? Is there blood in the stool?**

    A patient may have infectious diarrhea. Signs that suggest an infectious etiology are abdominal pain, fever, and bloody diarrheal stools. Never give an antidiarrheal agent to a patient you suspect may have an infectious GI process.
3. **Does the patient have a history of diarrhea? Are there any known or suspected medical problems?**

    Perhaps the patient has a history of lactose intolerance, intestinal malabsorption, short-bowel syndrome, Crohn disease, ulcerative colitis, or ischemic colitis. These are common causes of diarrhea.
4. **Did the patient eat foodstuffs recently that did not agree with him or her?**

    The patient may have developed food poisoning or may have food intolerances. Are there any friends or family members with similar symptoms?
5. **Does the patient have any flu symptoms?**

    A major cause of diarrhea is viral gastroenteritis.
6. **Is the patient on tube feedings?**

    A major cause of diarrhea in patients taking tube feedings is administration of feedings at a rate or an osmolarity greater than what the small intestine can tolerate.
7. **Is the patient taking broad-spectrum antibiotics?**

    Always suspect *Clostridium difficile* if severe diarrhea begins in a patient taking broad-spectrum antibiotics. Remember that ordinary antibiotic-induced diarrhea is more common than that caused by *C. difficile*.

Orders

Regardless of the cause of diarrhea, make sure that the patient is well hydrated. Ask the nursing staff if the patient has been able to take adequate fluids orally. A good oral fluid for repletion is an isotonic glucose-containing electrolyte solution. Prolonged, severe diarrhea in a patient unable to take oral fluids leads to dehydration. If a patient is unable to take oral fluids and has significant diarrhea, the patient should be rehydrated intravenously. Monitor urine output and electrolytes.

MANAGEMENT

Diarrhea may or may not be associated with abdominal pain. It is not uncommon for the initial resumption of bowel function following an abdominal procedure to be diarrheal stools. This is usually without other symptoms and is self-limited. There are other syndromes of diarrhea, which must be differentiated to appropriately treat the symptom.

Clues to Diagnosis:

Pain:	Gradual or sudden onset, mild to severe intermittent cramps.
Location:	Generalized but occasionally will be localized.
Other signs and symptoms:	Vomiting, fever, and chills may also be present. Diarrhea mixed with blood or mucus suggests a bacterial or parasitic etiology.
Exam:	Diffuse tenderness. Stool may be guaiac positive.
Studies:	Elevated WBCs. Stool cultures should be sent for O&P, rotozyme, *C. difficile* toxin titer, and fecal leukocyte studies, as appropriate.
Acuity:	Routine to urgent.
Treatment:	Enteric precautions as indicated. Antibiotics as indicated. See treatments under specific diarrhea etiologies below.

Antibiotic-Induced Diarrhea

A greater understanding of this problem has made this common entity easier to anticipate, diagnose, and treat. This can happen with any antibiotic and is not associated with colitis (tissue invasion).

Signs and symptoms:	May be symptomless or may present with crampy abdominal pain. Evidence of tissue invasion (fever, bloody stool, or leukocytosis) is rarely present.
Stool characteristics:	Watery, rarely bloody, or containing fecal leukocytes. Usually *C. difficile* toxin titer negative.

Treatment:	Discontinue the identified antibiotic.
	Fluid support.
	Avoid antidiarrheal and narcotic medications.

Antibiotic-Induced Colitis

This occurs in about 1 per 1000 antibiotic-treated patients and is associated with evidence of invasive disease (fecal leukocytes, fever, and leukocytosis). The most likely antibiotics include ampicillin, clindamycin, and cephalosporins. *C. difficile* toxin-positive colitis represents about 25% of cases of antibiotic-associated colitis. Diagnosis is confirmed by the presence of *C. difficile* toxin in the stool. Sigmoidoscopy may show characteristic pseudomembranes.

Signs and symptoms:	Crampy abdominal pain, fever, and leukocytosis occurring within days after the beginning of antibiotic therapy. Evidence of peritonitis may indicate megacolon or perforation, often associated with marked leukocytosis in excess of 20,000.
Stool characteristics:	Watery, occasionally bloody, fecal leukocytes, and possibly *C. difficile* toxin-positive.
Treatment:	Mild colitis:
	Discontinue the identified antibiotic.
	Fluid and electrolyte support.
	Avoid antidiarrheal and narcotic medications.
	Moderate to severe colitis, and *C. difficile* toxin-positive cases:
	Vancomycin (Vancocin) 125 to 500 mg by mouth 4 times per day for 7 to 14 days or metronidazole (Flagyl) 500 mg by mouth or intravenously 3 times per day for 10 days.
	Discontinue the identified antibiotic.
	Fluid and electrolyte support.
	Avoid antidiarrheal and narcotic medications.
	Bowel rest for severe cases.
Notes:	Relapse rate is high, up to 20%, and requires additional treatment. IV vancomycin is ineffective.

Noninvasive Gastroenteritis

Usually viral in etiology. The associated risk is of dehydration and electrolyte abnormalities, greatest in pediatric or elderly patients.

Signs and symptoms:	Crampy abdominal pain, fever, and leukocytosis.
Stool characteristics:	Watery, rarely with blood or fecal leukocytes, and may be rotozyme positive if rotavirus is the causative agent.
Treatment:	Fluid and electrolyte support.
	Antidiarrheal medications **only** if no intestinal anastomoses are present (Table 6–2).

TABLE 6–2 **Antidiarrheal Therapies**

Generic	Brand Name	Dose
Diphenoxylate HCl (2.5 mg) with atropine sulfate (0.025 mg)	Lomotil	2 tablets PO 4 times per day (may take up to 48 hr to work)
Loperamide HCl	Imodium	4 mg PO initial dose followed by 2 mg PO with each unformed stool (not to exceed 16 mg/day)
Difenoxin HCl (1 mg) with atropine sulfate (0.025 mg)	Motofen	2 tablets PO initial dose followed by 1 tablet PO 3 to 4 times per day as needed, or 1 tablet with each unformed stool (not to exceed 8 tablets/day)
Phenobarbital (16.2 mg), with atropine sulfate (0.02 mg), hyoscyamine sulfate (0.1 mg), scopolamine hydrobromide (6.5 mcg)	Donnatal	1–2 tablets PO every 6–8 hr as needed
Belladonna (16.2) with opium powder (30–60 mg)	B&O supprette	1 suppository PR every day or twice daily as needed (not to exceed 4 doses/day)
Bismuth subsalicylate	Pepto-Bismol	2 tbsp or tablets PO every 0.5–1 hr as needed (not to exceed 8 doses/day) (may take up to 24 hr to work)
Morphine (2 mg/5 mL)	Paregoric*	5–10 mL PO 4 times/day as needed with anise oil (0.02 ml), benzoic acid (20 mg), camphor (0.2 mL), and alcohol (45%)
Kaolin (975 mg/5 mL) and pectin (22 mg)	Kaopectate	60–120 mL PO after each loose stool

Notes: Diphenoxylate HCl and difenoxin HCl are related to meperidine HCl; they are considered Schedule V medications and are habit forming. Opium powder is a Schedule II medication and is habit forming. Do not exceed recommended dosage.

PO, by mouth; PR, rectally.

*No brand name.

NPO if abdominal pain is severe. Clear liquids when tolerated, with slow advancement to a bland diet.

Avoid milk and milk by-products because lactase is not as readily available in settings of acute gastroenteritis, which increases intraluminal concentrations of milk sugars, contributing to an osmotic diarrhea.

Enteric precautions as necessary.

Often treated as an outpatient, but if the patient is infirm or dehydrated or if the inflammation is severe, hospitalization may be required.

Invasive Gastroenteritis

May be bacterial or parasitic. Often there is evidence of invasive disease. Bloody diarrhea is found with acute infections caused by *Shigella*, enterotoxic *Escherichia coli*, *Campylobacter*, *Salmonella*, *Yersinia*, and *Entamoeba*.

Signs and symptoms:	Crampy abdominal pain, fever, and leukocytosis.
Stool characteristics:	Watery, with blood and mucus. Fecal leukocytes, specific culture, or O&P positivity.
Treatment:	Fluid and electrolyte support.
	Appropriate antibiotic therapy.
	NPO if abdominal pain is severe.
	Clear liquids when tolerated, with slow advancement to a bland diet.
	Avoid milk and milk by-products.
	Fluid resuscitation as needed.
	Enteric precautions as needed.

Inflammatory Bowel Disease

Ulcerative colitis and Crohn disease are characterized by recurrent bouts of symptoms. They may reactivate perioperatively and complicate pre- or postoperative care.

Signs and symptoms:	Crampy abdominal pain, fever, and leukocytosis.
Stool characteristics:	Watery, occasionally bloody, fecal leukocytes. Negative stool cultures and O&P.
Treatment:	Bowel rest as indicated.
	Corticosteroids. Enemas may be sufficient for localized disease. Oral or intravenous doses may be required for more severe symptoms.
	Mesalamine (Asacol, Pentasa) 400 to 800 mg by mouth three times daily is useful for mild-to-moderate symptoms.

Feeding-Associated Diarrhea

This is especially associated with tube feedings. Volumes and concentrations of feedings should be increased slowly, or the bowel will not tolerate the osmotic load.

Signs and symptoms:	May be symptomless or may be associated with crampy abdominal pain.
Stool characteristics:	Watery to milky, Clinitest positive.
Treatment:	Slow or stop current feeding regimen. Maintain hydration with intravenous fluids if necessary.

Other Causes of Diarrhea

1. Laxative use
2. Other malabsorption, e.g., sprue or Whipple disease
3. Pancreatic insufficiency
4. Lactase deficiency (lactose intolerance)
5. Irritable bowel syndrome
6. Diabetic enteropathy
7. Visceral scleroderma

The most common antidiarrheal agents used in the hospital are Kaopectate, Imodium, and Lomotil. These medications are safe and well tolerated by patients. Kaopectate is an absorbent, which decreases stool content. It exerts local action and is not absorbed. Onset is within 30 minutes and duration is 4 to 6 hours. Imodium has a slower onset of action but is well tolerated and effective. The manufacturer does not recommend continuing the maximum dosage of 8 mg/day for more than 2 days. Lomotil is a highly effective drug that can be titrated to control moderate to serious diarrhea. Although the suggested dose is up to 5 mg every 4 to 6 hours, a patient with chronic diarrhea can usually tolerate higher doses. Safe doses for many patients can be titrated to 10 mg every 6 hours.

Remember that diarrhea in a pediatric patient is a frequent cause of dehydration. Many diarrheal illnesses in pediatric patients are caused by very contagious viruses. Although the diarrhea is usually self-limited, the fluid and electrolyte status of these patients must be monitored carefully and replaced appropriately.

Intermittent diarrhea may also be caused by Zollinger–Ellison syndrome and postgastrectomy dumping syndrome.

Chest Pain

Chest pain is one of the most concerning calls you will receive. Chest pain may represent a nonserious problem such as heartburn or a life-threatening problem such as acute myocardial infarction (MI). To best handle chest pain calls, follow a logical progression in the evaluation and management of the patient. Always assume that chest pain represents a serious medical problem until proven otherwise.

PHONE CALL

Questions

1. **What is the pain like and how severe is it (on a scale of 1 to 10)?**

   The greatest concern is that the patient has a life-threatening problem such as myocardial ischemia. The spectrum of diseases spans from angina pectoris to acute MI, and often presents with diverse pain manifestations and severities. However, many types of noncardiac pain syndromes exist, which can be distinguished by history physical examination. For example, burning chest pain between meals often represents esophageal reflux or peptic ulcer disease, whereas substernal pain after exertion is more suggestive of myocardial ischemia.

   Patients with any significant chest pain, chest pressure, or chest pain radiating to the jaw, neck, shoulder, or arm should have an electrocardiogram (ECG). Always think about a cardiac source of pain, and rule this out before proceeding in the differential diagnosis.

2. **Are there any changes in vital signs?**

   Hemodynamic instability or respiratory compromise associated with chest pain represents a life-threatening emergency. Begin resuscitation efforts immediately.

3. **Is there any shortness of breath (SOB)?**

   Shortness of breath (SOB) is commonly associated with myocardial ischemia. However, SOB may also be the initial symptom of pulmonary problems such as pneumothorax or pulmonary embolus. Ask if the SOB developed before or after the chest pain.

4. **Does the patient have a history of coronary artery disease (CAD), angina, MI, dyspepsia, reflux, or peptic ulcer disease?**

   The best way to ascertain the cause of chest pain is to obtain a good history. Frequently, patients presenting with chest pain have a history of similar pain episodes already known to be of a cardiac or gastrointestinal (GI) cause. If a postoperative patient has had an MI in the last 6 months, he or she is more likely to have another MI than a patient who has not had a prior infarction.

5. **Did the patient have surgery? If so, what operation was performed and when was it performed?**

   Surgery and anesthesia stress the heart. Thus, it is understandable that postoperative patients may develop cardiac complications of surgery. Postoperative MIs occur in 0.4% of all patients who have undergone surgery. For some patient groups, the risk is much higher. Patients who have significant atherosclerosis of the lower extremities, carotid vessels, or aorta have a risk of postoperative MI in the range of 5% to 10%. Always consider postoperative myocardial ischemia as a cause of chest pain. In general, the longer the duration of the operation and the greater the blood loss, the greater the risk of postoperative MI in those patients with CAD. The use of perioperative β-blockade is recommended in selected patients to decrease the risk of cardiac event (see Chapter 24).

Orders

Unless the pain is clearly related to a musculoskeletal or GI cause, myocardial ischemia should be suspected until disproved.

1. Obtain an ECG immediately.
2. Obtain a portable chest x-ray immediately. Especially if the patient has a chest tube or a history of chest trauma or has had chest surgery.
3. Place the patient on a pulse oximeter.
4. Give **sublingual nitroglycerin 0.4 mg every 5 minutes** until pain resolves. Hold medication for a systolic blood pressure (SBP) of less than 90 mm Hg.
5. If the pain is severe or associated with vital sign changes, ask the RN to stay with the patient and monitor the vital signs until you arrive.
6. Ask the RN to have the patient's chart at the bedside.

Inform RN

Will arrive at the bedside in … minutes.

You must assume that every chest pain call may represent a medical emergency. Assess the patient immediately, and remember that the best evidence for the cause of the pain will come from the patient's history.

ELEVATOR THOUGHTS

What Causes Chest Pain?

There are many possible causes of chest pain. Some of the more common causes are as follows:

Cardiac	Angina
	Infarction
	Aortic dissection
	Pericarditis
Pulmonary	Pleuritis
	Pneumonia
	Pneumothorax
	Pulmonary embolus
	Pulmonary contusion
	Severe asthma attack
GI	Esophageal reflux
	Esophagitis
	Peptic ulcer disease
	Diaphragmatic hernia
Musculoskeletal	Costochondritis
	Rib fracture
	Muscle spasm
	Chest tube-associated pain

MAJOR THREAT TO LIFE

- Acute MI
- Pulmonary embolus
- Aortic dissection
- Tension pneumothorax

It is often difficult to distinguish these serious problems from one another quickly at the bedside. A severe MI leading to cardiogenic shock often is associated with respiratory failure. Pulmonary embolus or pneumothorax may lead to circulatory arrest if not treated appropriately. Frequently, the initial presentation is the best evidence. MI and aortic dissection often begin with pain. Pulmonary embolus and pneumothorax often begin with SOB and hypoxia.

BEDSIDE

Quick Look Test

Does the patient look well (comfortable), sick (uncomfortable or distressed), or critical (about to die)?

The overall appearance of the patient provides important evidence to the severity of the problem. A conversant, relatively comfortable patient is more likely to have a nonthreatening cause for chest pain (e.g., costochondritis or reflux). A pale, anxious patient is more likely to have a serious problem (e.g., myocardial ischemia or pulmonary embolism). Evaluating the patient's appearance and taking a quick history will help to best identify and manage the problem.

Airway and Vital Signs

What is the blood pressure (BP)?

Most patients with chest pain will have normal BP. Hypotension suggests cardiogenic shock, pulmonary embolus, cardiac tamponade, or tension pneumothorax. The hypotension must be treated. Hypertension may be associated with an anxious patient with chest pain. Severe hypertension (systolic BP >180 mm Hg, diastolic BP >110 mm Hg) should also be treated, because it may worsen myocardial ischemia or it may help to expand an aortic aneurysm.

What is the heart rate (HR)?

Bradycardia may be associated with acute MI, in particular an inferior MI. It may also represent cardiogenic shock or a blockade due to drugs (e.g., beta blockers or calcium channel blockers). Treat only if the patient is hypotensive or the HR is less than 40 beats/minute (see Chapter 9).

Tachycardia may be a response to anxiety and pain. However, tachycardia may also represent a tachyarrhythmia. The key tachyarrhythmias to look for include supraventricular tachycardia, wide-complex tachycardia, atrial fibrillation, atrial flutter, and ventricular tachycardia. Many of these arrhythmias require immediate and emergent treatment (see Chapter 9).

What is the breathing pattern?

Tachypnea associated with hypoxia may signify acute MI, pulmonary edema, pulmonary embolus, or pneumothorax. Patients usually are in distress. Shallow breathing associated with splinting is more suggestive of a musculoskeletal cause (e.g., costochondritis, rib fracture, or pain from a recent surgical incision) or of a pleural cause (e.g., pneumothorax or pleuritis).

What does the ECG show?
1. **Normal ECG**

   A normal ECG does not rule out myocardial ischemia. Further work-up may be indicated if the chest pain by history is suggestive of a cardiac cause. Compare the new ECG to any previous ECG studies; look for new findings.
2. **An ECG with ST segment changes and T wave changes**

   ST segment changes with peaked upright or inverted T waves suggest acute MI. ST depression may indicate a non-Q wave MI.

3. **An ECG with Q waves**
> New Q waves may suggest MI or prolonged myocardial ischemia.

If an acute MI is suggested by the evaluation, consult with a cardiologist immediately. Begin treatment with oxygen, aspirin, nitrates, beta blockade, and analgesics. Thrombolytic therapy or coronary angiography with angioplasty is usually managed by the cardiology team. The patient will need continuous ECG monitoring, usually in a cardiac care unit (CCU).

What does the CXR show?
1. **Normal CXR**
> The CXR may be normal in settings of acute MI (without congestive heart failure [CHF]), aortic dissection, pericarditis, and pulmonary embolism.
2. **Pneumonia**
> A pulmonary infiltrate suggests the presence of pneumonia.
3. **Pneumothorax**
> Pneumothorax may be simple, with collapse of a lung on one side, or may present as tension pneumothorax with mediastinal shift away from the affected side, SOB and hypotension. Immediate treatment with thoracostomy is necessary to treat symptomatic pneumothoraces (see Chapter 30).
4. **Pulmonary edema**
> Pulmonary edema may be present in patients with a history of congestive heart failure, or may represent the sequellae of an acute MI.

Is the patient hypoxic?
This may have pulmonary or cardiac etiologies but is associated with a more severe process and requires immediate treatment.

If the Patient Is Hypotensive

Immediate steps must be taken:
1. Confirm that the pressure is real and differs from the patient's normal pressure.
2. Ensure that the patient is receiving oxygen.
3. Ensure that the patient has a functioning IV; obtain IV access if none is available.
4. Ensure that the patient is on a cardiac monitor, if dysrhythmias are noted, begin ACLS protocols (see Appendix A).
5. Refer to Chapter 17 for a full discussion on the evaluation and treatment of hypotension and shock.
6. A fluid bolus is appropriate in most cases.

Selective History and Chart Review

Ask the patient if he or she has known heart disease. Ask angina, MI, reflux problems, and similar episodes of pain in the past. Skim the history and physical examination in the chart, paying special attention to the past medical history, medicines, and current problems.

If this is an episode of a recurring chest pain for the patient, ask if this pain is similar and how the pain has been managed in the past.

Ask if the pain radiates to the back, jaw, or arm. Are there associated symptoms of nausea, vomiting, or dizziness?

Selective Physical Examination

The objective of the physical examination is to find a cause of the chest pain or any sequellae of the chest pain. Focus on the vital signs, the nature of the pulse, the heart sounds, and the breath sounds.

VS:	Measure HR, BP, and respiratory rate. Take the pulse and assess if it is regular or irregular, strong or weak. Evaluate for pulsus paradoxus (associated with cardiac tamponade).
CVS:	Evaluate if there is a murmur or rub. Assess the heart sounds carefully.
Resp:	Listen for the quality of the breath sounds. Evaluate the symmetry of the breath sounds of right and left lungs. Nonsymmetric breath sounds may indicate pneumothorax or postsurgical change. Listen for regions of nonaeration, hyperaeration, wheezes, rhonchi, and crackles.
Neck:	Look for jugular venous distention (JVD). Measure any JVD to assess right-sided heart filling pressures. If there is elevated JVD, consider heart failure, fluid overload, cardiac tamponade, and constrictive pericarditis. Confirm that the trachea is midline. Deviation of the trachea may represent tension pneumothorax.
GI:	Bowel sounds in the chest are indicative of diaphragmatic hernia. Assess for abdominal tenderness, softness of abdomen, liver edge position, and masses. Some forms of abdominal pain (e.g., epigastric pain) may be described by the patient as chest pain.
Extremities:	Evaluate pulses for presence, strength, and evidence of dysrhythmias. Evaluate perfusion with capillary refill.

MANAGEMENT

Initial Management

Initial management includes providing oxygen, relieving ischemic pain, and preventing and treating life-threatening complications of the major serious causes of chest pain.

1. Place the patient on oxygen. Run oxygen at 4 L/minute. If the patient retains CO_2, run oxygen at 2 L/minute. SaO_2 saturations should be in excess of 93%.

2. Provide **sublingual nitroglycerin 0.4 mg every 5 minutes** until pain resolves. Take care to monitor BP while treating with nitroglycerin.

3. Order a portable chest x-ray (CXR) immediately if there are abnormal or unequal breath sounds, if the patient has a chest tube or is at high risk for a pneumothorax, or if aortic pathology (aneurysm) is suspected.

4. Provide analgesia, especially during an active MI. Patients with an active MI will not obtain pain relief with nitroglycerin alone. **Intravenous (IV) morphine sulfate 2 to 4 mg** is an appropriate starting dosage. You may repeat every 2 to 3 minutes and titrate until pain is relieved.

5. Treat rhythm disturbances that are associated with hemodynamic instability or are at high risk for deteriorating into life-threatening arrhythmia (e.g., ventricular tachycardia, see Chapter 9).

6. If acute MI is suspected, administer aspirin (325 mg PO/PR).

Definitive Management

This stage of management involves definitive treatment or triage after stabilizing the patient.

Myocardial Ischemia

RESOLVING ANGINA

If the chest pain has been relieved with sublingual nitroglycerin and the patient has a history of angina, an adjustment of the patient's cardiac medications may be the only definitive treatment to be rendered. Discuss the case with your chief resident or attending physician. Nonemergent consultation with the patient's cardiologist or internist may be appropriate.

NEW-ONSET OR UNSTABLE ANGINA

A patient with no prior cardiac history who develops chest pain of cardiac origin must be evaluated by cardiology (CCU/intensive care unit [ICU] team). In addition, a patient who develops angina at rest should be evaluated by a cardiologist whether or not the pain can be resolved with sublingual nitroglycerin. These consultations should be performed promptly.

Order serial ECGs, troponin, and cardiac isoenzyme tests every 8 hours for a total of 3 times for any patient that you suspect may have had a small infarction not readily detectable on your initial evaluation. Any patient who does not have relief of ischemic cardiac pain with sublingual nitroglycerin or morphine should be transferred to the ICU or the CCU for continuous cardiac monitoring. These patients may need an IV nitroglycerin drip, aspirin administration, and beta-blockade therapy.

ACUTE MYOCARDIAL INFARCTION

Patients who are having a suspected MI need emergent evaluation by the cardiology (CCU or ICU) team. The treatment of these patients is becoming standardized. Treatment options include noninvasive therapy such as IV nitroglycerin, beta blockers, aspirin, anticoagulation, and thrombolytic therapy. Invasive treatment options include coronary angiography and angioplasty. Treatment decisions are best made by the attending surgeon and the attending cardiologist. Clear recommendations include administration of aspirin within 24 hours, and subsequent discharge of the patient on aspirin. Also recommended are early administration of beta-blockers and the use of ACE inhibitors in settings of myocardial dysfunction.

ACUTE PERICARDITIS ASSOCIATED WITH MI

Patients with large infarctions often develop acute pericarditis. Symptoms include substernal chest pain with pain radiating to the back. Pain is often relieved with sitting up. A pericardial friction rub may be heard. Echocardiography may be useful to diagnose the condition. Unless there is hemodynamic compromise (which is unusual), an echocardiogram may be performed nonemergently to arrive at the definitive diagnosis. Aspirin is useful to relieve pain. Do not use glucocorticoids or other nonsteroidal anti-inflammatory drugs (NSAIDs) because they retard myocardial scar formation and may increase the incidence of ventricular rupture after a large MI. For pericarditis that is *not* associated with MI, the treatment of choice is **indomethacin 50 mg PO three times per day.**

Aortic Dissection

An acute, proximal aortic dissection is an emergency requiring rapid stabilization and antihypertensive therapy. Most of these patients are hypertensive.

1. Transfer the patient to the CCU/ICU.
2. Start therapy by placing the patient on a **sodium nitroprusside** drip.

    Start at **0.5 to 1. mcg/kg/minute** and titrate the dose to achieve an SBP of about 100 mm Hg or the minimum BP to maintain organ perfusion. The maximum dose of nitroprusside is about 10 mcg/kg/minute. Above this dosage, cyanide toxicity can develop, and it is a good idea to check thiocyanate levels if you are going to use higher doses.
3. In addition to nitroprusside, start the patient on a beta-blocker.

    The use of nitroprusside alone is inadequate to avoid intimal shearing. Add a beta-blocker even if the hypertension is resolved with nitroprusside. Esmolol is a good cardioselective beta-adrenergic antagonist to use. It has a short half-life (9 minutes). Dosing ranges from 50 to 200 mcg/kg/minute.
4. If nitroprusside or esmolol is not available, use a single agent, labetalol, to lower BP and intimal shearing.

    Dosing of **labetalol** is **20 mg IV every 10 minutes to a total of 300 mg.**

5. Arrange an emergent thoracic computed tomographic (CT) scan or a transesophageal echocardiogram.

A transthoracic echocardiogram provides less information than a CT scan or transesophageal echocardiogram; however, it is better than no diagnostic study if the others are not available.

Acute aortic dissections may be classified as involving the ascending aorta with or without the descending aorta (Stanford A) or limited to the descending aorta (Stanford B).

Type A dissections almost always require surgical repair, whereas many type B dissections may be managed expediently (Fig. 7–1).

6. Type and crossmatch the patient for 6 to 8 units of packed red blood cells.

Obtain a platelet count, a prothrombin time, a partial thromboplastin time, electrolytes, and a renal panel.

7. Obtain an emergent cardiac surgical consultation.

Whether the dissection is Stanford type A or B, a cardiac surgical consultation is warranted. Be prepared to arrange aortography if the surgical consultant believes it is needed.

8. Obtain a 12-lead ECG to rule out acute MI.

Pneumothorax

A pneumothorax can be life threatening when tension or pressure is exerted against the heart, the great vessels, and the lung tissue. In a pneumothorax, air is usually trapped in the pleural space. If there is a parenchymal lung tear or leak, air continues to collect in the pleural space and the pneumothorax worsens. If you suspect a pneumothorax and the patient is stable and well oxygenated, obtain a

Stanford
type A

Stanford
type B

Figure 7–1 Stanford classification of aortic dissection. Type A includes the ascending aorta and the aortic arch. Type B includes the descending aorta only.

CXR. Have the patient sit upright for the CXR so that any air in the pleural space can rise to the apex of the thoracic cavity.

A significant pneumothorax in the presence of a parenchymal air leak requires chest tube drainage. If a patient demonstrates agitation, progressive hypoxia, hypotension, or electromechanical dissociation, and you suspect a tension pneumothorax, emergency needle aspiration should be performed before chest tube placement. Insert a 14-gauge catheter or needle into the second or third intercostal space, mid-clavicular line, to acutely decompress the tension pneumothorax. Once the tension component of the pneumothorax is released, a chest tube can be inserted into the fifth or sixth intercostal space (see Chapter 30).

Pulmonary Embolism

A patient who develops sudden-onset SOB, hypoxia, and chest pain may have a pulmonary embolism. The details of diagnosis and management are presented in Chapter 28. Surgical patients are at high risk for this problem. Pulmonary embolism is common in patients with pelvic trauma, lower abdominal surgery, lower extremity surgery, prolonged immobilization, and venous disease of the lower extremities.

Reflux Esophagitis or GERD

Symptoms of reflux include heartburn, chest pain, dysphagia, and sore throat. The following treatments can be useful:

1. Have the patient propped up in bed.

    Keeping at least a 30-degree head elevation is important.
2. Have the patient avoid alcohol, chocolate, fat, and caffeine.

    These foods frequently make reflux worse.
3. Consider using an antacid.

    Maalox and Mylanta are useful, and both contain aluminum and magnesium hydroxide. These agents may cause diarrhea. The dosage is **30 mL PO every 4 hours as needed.** Amphojel contains only aluminum hydroxide. The dosage is **5 mL PO every 4 hours as needed.** This agent may cause constipation. Tums tablets contain calcium carbonate. The dosage is **500 mg PO as needed.**
4. Patients with ongoing or recurrent reflux problems are best treated with histamine H_2-receptor antagonists or proton pump inhibitors (PPIs). See Table 5–1 for a list of these agents.
5. Metoclopramide improves gastric emptying and increases lower esophageal sphincter tone.

    It is most effective when used in combination with histamine H_2-receptor antagonists.
6. Severe recurring reflux symptoms are best evaluated by a gastroenterologist.

Pneumonia

Chest pain caused by pneumonia is usually focal and mild, but occasionally severe and pleuritic. NSAIDs or low-doses of narcotic medications are usually sufficient to treat the pain. Treatment of the pneumonia with appropriate antibiotics will usually eliminate the pain. For full discussion of treatment of pneumonia, please refer to Chapter 28.

Musculoskeletal Pain

Costochondritis and rib pain are best treated with NSAIDs. **Ibuprofen 400 to 600 mg PO every 6 to 8 hours** or **naproxen 250 mg PO twice daily** is usually helpful. For more severe musculoskeletal pain, ketorolac (Toradol) is useful. The dosage is a 30- to 60-mg intramuscular (IM) loading dose, followed by 15 to 30 mg IM every 6 hours. Due to the antiplatelet effects of NSAIDs, they should not be given to patients with active peptic ulcer disease or multiple traumatic injuries, or to patients who are anticoagulated. In addition, NSAID use should be avoided in patients with congestive heart failure or renal insufficiency. Toradol should not be used for more than three days.

Drug Reactions

Reactions to medications may be wide ranging, from complaints of bad aftertaste to more serious problems with allergic reactions and anaphylaxis. Most calls will encompass three major groups of symptoms: rashes, anaphylaxis, and other complaints of patient intolerance of medication. All drugs have side effects, and many calls may be eliminated by explaining to the patient what to expect before administering the drug. This is especially important when the side effects are severe or require additional management to control.

Many drug combinations may augment side effects, be frankly dangerous, or change the biologic action of one or the other medication. If you have any questions about drug interactions, contact your pharmacist.

RASHES AND ANAPHYLAXIS

Rash is a common manifestation of drug reaction. The first step to management is to rule out anaphylaxis, because urticarial rash is a primary symptom.

PHONE CALL

Questions

1. **How long has the rash been present?**
2. **Is the rash urticarial?**
   Rule out anaphylaxis, symptoms of which include an urticarial rash (hives), wheezing, shortness of breath (SOB), and decreased blood pressure.
3. **Is the patient taking any new medications?**
   This includes any recent intravenous (IV) contrast dye.
4. **Does the patient have any known allergies or intolerances?**
5. **Has the patient undergone a surgical procedure, and if so, how long ago?**
6. **Are there any other symptoms?**
   Rashes are also associated with upper respiratory infection symptoms or other irritant exposures.

7. **Are there any changes in vital signs such as hypotension or fever?**

Orders

If the patient has signs of anaphylaxis:
1. Start an IV with normal saline (NS) if not already in place.
2. Have at the bedside the following medications:
   Epinephrine (1:1000) for SC administration and epinephrine (1:10,000) for IV administration. (Label these carefully by their route of administration, so no mistake is made. Either may be necessary depending on the severity of the reaction.)
   Diphenhydramine (Benadryl) 50 mg for IV administration.
   Hydrocortisone (Solu-Cortef) 250 mg for IV administration.
3. Support SOB with oxygen if necessary as described in Chapter 28.

Degree of Urgency

If the patient is anaphylactic, the patient must be evaluated immediately. Most other rashes may be seen in 1 to 2 hours.

ELEVATOR THOUGHTS

Drug eruptions follow patterns specific to their medication class.

Urticaria

Lesion: The lesion is well circumscribed, raised, irregularly bordered, firm, blanching, transient, mobile, and often erythematous with central pallor.
   Etiologies include the following:
1. Histamine-releasing drugs
   a. IV contrast
   b. Narcotics
   c. Antibiotics
      i. beta lactams (penicillins and cephalosporins)
      ii. sulfonamides
      iii. tetracycline
      iv. isoniazid
      v. polymyxin
   d. Anesthetic agents (curare)
   e. Vasoactive agents (atropine, amphetamine, and hydralazine)
   f. Miscellaneous (thiamine, dextran, deferoxamine)
2. Nonhistamine releasers (aspirin and other nonsteroidal anti-inflammatory drugs [NSAIDs])
3. Nondrug (hereditary angioedema, food allergies, and idiopathic reactions)

Maculopapular (Morbilliform)

Lesion: The lesion may be raised or nonraised, erythematous, irregularly bordered, and firm.

Etiologies include the following:
1. Antibiotics
   a. Beta lactams (penicillins and cephalosporins)
   b. Sulfonamides
   c. Chloramphenicol
2. Antihistamines
3. Antidepressants (amitriptyline)
4. Diuretics (thiazides)
5. Oral hypoglycemics
6. Sedatives (barbiturates)
7. Anti-inflammatory agents (gold and phenylbutazone)
8. Nondrug (bacterial or viral infection, Reiter syndrome, inflammatory bowel disease, sarcoidosis, and serum sickness)

Vesicular

Lesion: The lesion is well circumscribed, elevated, and blister-like and may be filled with clear fluid (vesicle) or purulent material (pustule).

Etiologies include the following:
1. Antibiotics (sulfonamides and dapsone)
2. Anti-inflammatory agents (penicillamine)
3. Sedatives (barbiturates)
4. Halogens (iodides and bromides)
5. Chemotherapeutic (cetuximab)
6. Nondrug (bacterial or viral infection, toxic epidermal necrolysis, and inflammatory bowel disease)

Purpuric

Lesion: The lesion is erythematous to purplish, large, macular or papular, and nonblanching.

Etiologies include the following:
1. Antibiotics (sulfonamides and chloramphenicol)
2. Diuretics (thiazides)
3. Anti-inflammatory agents (phenylbutazone, salicylates, and indomethacin)
4. Drug-induced thrombocytopenia, i.e., after heparin administration
5. Vasculitis (sepsis, bacterial or viral infection, and Henoch-Schönlein purpura).

Exfoliative Dermatitis

Lesion: The lesion is typified by flaky patches.

Etiologies include the following:
1. Antibiotics (streptomycin)

2. Anti-inflammatory agents (gold and phenylbutazone)
3. Antiepileptic agents (carbamazepine and phenytoin)

Fixed Drug Reactions

Lesion: The lesion is specific to a region of the body. Repeated administration of the same agent will cause return of the rash in the same region.
Etiologies include the following:
1. Antibiotics (sulfonamides and metronidazole)
2. Anti-inflammatory agents (phenylbutazone)
3. Analgesics (phenacetin)
4. Sedatives (barbiturates and chlordiazepoxide)
5. Laxatives (phenolphthalein)

MAJOR THREAT TO LIFE

Anaphylactic shock
This is associated with urticaria but not with other forms of skin rash.

BEDSIDE

Quick Look Test

A patient in anaphylaxis may be hypoxic (agitated) or in hypovolemic shock (lethargic and comatose).

Airway and Vital Signs

Hypotension is a sign of anaphylaxis. Fever is often associated with drug reactions.

Selective History and Chart Review

Review the patient's allergy and intolerance profile.
Review the patient's medications, both current and discontinued.
Has the patient recently undergone a procedure requiring IV contrast?

Selective Physical Examination

VS:	Repeat now; hypotension (anaphylaxis)
MS:	Agitation (hypoxia) or lethargy (shock)
HEENT:	Facial edema (urticaria)
CVS:	Tachycardia (anaphylaxis)
Resp:	Wheezing or SOB (anaphylaxis)
Skin:	Rash or itching
Neuro:	Decreased mental status (anaphylaxis)

MANAGEMENT

Initial Management

If the patient is in anaphylaxis
1. Have someone notify the chief resident immediately.
    Anaphylaxis is a medical emergency.
2. Support respirations. If wheezing is present:
    Supply oxygen to keep oxygen saturation of arterial blood (SaO_2) at 93%.
    Epinephrine 0.3 mg (0.3 mL of 1:1000 solution SC, or 3 mL of 1:10,000 solution IV); may repeat the dosage every 10 to 15 minutes as needed; if the skin is cool or clammy, give epinephrine IV to ensure adequate delivery.
    Albuterol (Ventolin or Proventil) nebulizer treatment, 2.5 mg in 3 mL NS; may repeat the treatment every 4 to 6 hours as needed, more frequently if adequate cardiovascular monitoring is available.
    Diphenhydramine (Benadryl and others) 50 mg IV push.
    Hydrocortisone (Solu-Cortef and others) 250 mg IV push, followed by hydrocortisone 100 mg IV every 6 hours.
3. Support blood pressure. If hypotension is present:
    Start a large-bore IV and begin aggressive replacement of crystalloid (NS); continue the fluid resuscitation until the patient is normotensive.
    Elevate the patient's legs, which is preferable to having the patient assume Trendelenburg's position.
    Reassess the fluid status frequently.
4. Arrange the transfer of the patient to the intensive care unit or the coronary care unit.
    Anaphylaxis is a potentially fatal, multiorgan disease and should be treated by an experienced team.

If the patient is NOT in anaphylaxis:
1. Treat associated symptoms.
    a. Pruritus
        Cool compresses
        Topical moisturizing creams; topical steroid preparations may add some relief if the rash is long-standing
        Diphenhydramine (Benadryl and others) 25 to 50 mg IV or PO every 6 hours, as needed or
        Hydroxyzine (Atarax and Vistaril) 25 to 50 mg PO every 6 hours, as needed
    b. Secondary lesions, resulting from scratching or if lesions are large bullae resulting in skin loss, require wound care lesions

Refer to Chapter 32 for principles of wound care; treat large erosions as thermal burns.

The best dressing on a firm blister is the existing skin; if the blister is not firm or is leaking, it must be debrided and dressed with a burn dressing such as bacitracin ointment and xerofom gauze.

Update the patient's tetanus booster as necessary.

Watch for evidence of infection; routine antibiotics are not necessary for treatment of nonerythematous erosions, but open skin is a common entry site for bacteria and fungi.

2. Note and document the character of the rash, including the following important features:
   Distribution on the body
   Skin color
   Primary lesion (macule, papule, or vesicle)
   Secondary changes (erosion, flaking, crust, and ulcer)
   Special features (annular, groupings, and pruritus)

Definitive Management

If the rash is urticarial, stop the offending medication and treat the associated symptoms.

If the rash is not urticarial, the medication may be safely continued until the morning if necessary for the care of the patient, and associated symptoms should be treated.

SPECIFIC IMPORTANT RASHES

Urticaria

This is discussed above. Its importance is reiterated because of its association with anaphylaxis, albeit a rare complication.

Herpes Zoster

Lesion: The lesion is composed of grouped vesicles on an erythematous base, with dermatomal distribution. This disease is especially problematic in immunosuppressed patients such as transplant recipients. To avoid disseminated disease, immediate treatment with IV acyclovir may be indicated.

Petechiae

Lesion: The lesion is composed of pinpoint purple to red macules and is associated with platelet malfunction. Along with searching for and treating the causative agent, patients may also need platelet transfusions.

Purpura

Lesion: This lesion is erythematous to purplish, large, and non-blanching and may be macular or papular (palpable purpura). Purpura may have a hematologic cause, and complete blood count, prothrombin time, and activated partial thromboplastin time should be obtained as indicated.

REMEMBER

1. History of a drug reaction does not need to be present to make the diagnosis. Drug allergies may present at any time.
2. Drug reactions may be delayed by 1 to 2 weeks after the administration of a drug. Be sure to review the discontinued medication list as well as the active list.
3. Drug reactions may present as almost any type of rash. The rash itself may be polymorphic. Always suspect a medication reaction if rash is present.

OTHER DRUG REACTIONS

Nonrash reactions range from the harmless (bad aftertaste and dry mouth) to the serious (hepatitis, thrombocytopenia, and leukopenia). These symptoms may not be immediately associated with the medication, and they should be considered independently until a clear link is established. Each medication has a variety of side effects and idiosyncratic reactions associated with it, and these may be found in a pharmacology text or by discussion with a pharmacist. These are valuable resources; do not hesitate to use them. It is important to know and anticipate the potential complications of the medications and then the therapies used.

Remember that drugs often interact with each other and polypharmacy is a major cause of drug reactions.

Some symptoms present in the absence of a drug that the patient normally takes (tachycardia during beta blockade withdrawal, recurrence of heartburn if a PPI is withheld). Be sure to review medications taken at home to see if one was omitted from the admission or post operative orders.

Dysrhythmias

Abnormalities of heart rate (HR) and rhythm include both harmless processes and potentially life-threatening processes. Rate and rhythm disturbances include bradycardias, tachycardias, and irregular rhythms. Bradycardias are rhythms resulting in a ventricular rate of lesser than 60 beats/minute. Tachycardias are defined as rhythms with an HR of greater than 100 beats/minute. As the on-call physician, you must identify the type of rate and rhythm disturbance and the likely cause. This will require that you be familiar with basic electrocardiographic (ECG) techniques and tracings (see Appendix C). The first section of this chapter will cover bradycardias. Tachycardias and irregular rhythms are covered in the second section of this chapter.

BRADYCARDIAS

PHONE CALL

Questions

1. **What is the HR?**
2. **What is the blood pressure?**
    Hypotension with bradycardia is a medical emergency. A normotensive BP in the presence of a bradycardia may require no acute treatment.
3. **Is the patient taking any medications for HR or BP control?**
    Ask the nurse if the patient is taking digoxin, calcium channel blockers, or beta-blockers. These drugs, if taken in overdose, may result in bradycardia.
4. **Does the patient have a history of bradycardia?**
    The patient may have a long-standing, stable bradycardia. If this is the case, ask if the current HR is slower than the past recorded HRs.
5. **Does the patient have a pacemaker?**
    Bradycardia in patients with pacemakers may indicate pacemaker dysfunction. A pacemaker-dependent heart may require

external pacing or emergent pacemaker replacement. Postoperative cardiac surgery patients may have epicardial pacing leads in place.

Orders

1. If the patient is hypotensive (systolic blood pressure [SBP] lesser than 90 mm Hg), ask the RN to place the patient in Trendelenburg's position.
2. If no intravenous (IV) line is present, have the RN place an IV immediately. Instruct the nurse to instill a bolus of 250 to 500 mL normal saline.
3. Ask the RN to obtain a 12-lead ECG immediately.
4. Have the RN bring the crash cart to the bedside and connect the patient to a continuous ECG monitor.
5. If the HR is lesser than 40 beats/minute or is lesser than 50 beats/minute and associated with hypotension (SBP lesser than 90 mm Hg), have the RN obtain 1 mg of atropine sulfate and bring it to the bedside.
6. Supply oxygen, 4 liters by nasal cannula.

Inform RN

Will arrive at the bedside in ... minutes.
Hypotension needs immediate attention.

ELEVATOR THOUGHTS

What causes slow HR?
1. Sinus bradycardia
   - Sick sinus syndrome
   - Vasovagal episode
   - Acute myocardial infarction (MI) (inferior wall)
   - Pacemaker malfunction
   - Conduction system disease
   - Electrolyte abnormalities
   - Hypothyroidism
2. Drug induced (digoxin, calcium channel blockers, beta-blockers, and antiarrhythmic agents). Note that drugs may induce either sinus bradycardia, first, second, or third degree heart blocks.
3. High level of cardiac fitness (athletic heart)
4. Atrial fibrillation (AF) with slow ventricular rate
5. First-degree heart block
6. Second-degree heart block
   - Mobitz type I (Wenckebach) block
   - Mobitz type II block
7. Third-degree AV block
8. Elevated intracranial pressure (ICP).
   Sinus Bradycardia: Sinus bradycardia (Fig. 9–1) occurs when the sinus rate slows to lesser than 60 beats/minute but

Figure 9–1 Sinus bradycardia.

the activation of atria and ventricles is normal (as documented on 12-lead ECG).

First-Degree Atrioventricular (AV) Block: First-degree AV block (Fig. 9–2) is associated with conduction delay through the AV node and a prolonged PR interval on ECG tracings (greater than 200 msec).

Second-Degree AV Block: Second-degree AV block occurs when atrial impulses are not conducted to the ventricle during times in which the AV node is not refractory.

Mobitz Type I (Wenckebach) Block: Mobitz type I block (Fig. 9–3) is associated with a progressive elongation of AV conduction before blocking an impulse. ECG tracings show gradual prolongation of the PR interval coming before a nonconducted P wave. Common causes include myocardial ischemia, conduction system abnormalities, drug toxicity, and electrolyte disturbances.

Figure 9–2 First-degree atrioventricular block.

Figure 9–3 Second-degree atrioventricular block; Mobitz type I (Wenckebach).

Mobitz Type II Block: Mobitz type II block (Fig. 9–4) is associated with conduction block without conduction delays. No prolongation of PR intervals is noted. Common causes include those of first-degree heart block and acute inferior MI.

Third-Degree Heart Block (Complete Heart Block): Third-degree heart block (Fig. 9–5) results when there is no transmission of atrial impulses to the ventricles. The atrial rate is frequently greater than the ventricular rate. ECG analysis shows no relationship between atrial and ventricular activity. Causes include major MI, conduction system disease, sarcoidosis, amyloidosis, Chagas' disease, aortic valvular disease, trauma, and infection (endocarditis and myocarditis). Also medications such as beta-blockers, calcium-channel blockers, digoxin, amiodarone and sotalol.

MAJOR THREAT TO LIFE

- Progression to life-threatening arrhythmia
- Hypotension
- MI

Bradycardia may cause hypotension secondary to low cardiac output. Poor perfusion of the myocardium secondary to hypotension may result in myocardial ischemia and infarction. Myocardial ischemia may predispose the patient to life-threatening arrhythmias.

Figure 9–4 Second-degree atrioventricular block; Mobitz type II.

Figure 9–5 Third-degree atrioventricular block; complete heart block.

BEDSIDE

Quick Look Test

Does the patient look well (comfortable), sick (uncomfortable or distressed), or critical (about to die)?

Patients who are bradycardic and hypotensive appear pale and sick. These patients should be monitored with continuous ECG tracings. If the patient is not in an intensive care unit (ICU), connect the patient to a bedside monitor and evaluate rhythm strips. Be prepared to treat symptomatic bradycardia with drugs or pacing techniques.

Airway and Vital Signs

What is the HR?

This absolute rate gives clues to the etiology. Review the ECG.

What is the BP?

The BP of the patient determines whether acute treatment is necessary. A patient who is bradycardic but normotensive requires no treatment. However, a patient who is both bradycardic and hypotensive needs urgent care. Bradycardia and hypotension may precede cardiac arrest.

Selective History and Chart Review

Focus your history and chart evaluation on looking for probable causes for bradycardia. Look for a history of bradycardia, heart block, or ischemic heart disease. Evaluate cardiac medications carefully. Careful attention to the following areas is helpful:

1. Drugs
   - Digoxin
   - Calcium channel blockers
   - Beta-blockers
   - Antiarrhythmic agents such as amiodarone and satalol
2. Heart disease
   - Silent ischemia
   - Acute MI
   - History of angina or MI
   - History of sick sinus syndrome
   - Risk factor analysis: diabetes and peripheral vascular disease

Selective Physical Examination

Examination may provide information leading to a likely etiology for the bradycardia.

VS:	HR, BP, temperature (hypothermia may indicate hypothyroidism)
HEENT:	Fundi changes associated with hypertension or diabetes

Papilledema may suggest increased ICP. Carotid bruits

CVS: New S_3, S_4, or heart murmur (suggestive of acute MI)
Resp: Rales, evidence of CHF
Abd: Evidence of aortic, renal, or femoral bruits (suggestive of atherosclerotic disease with possible concurrent coronary disease)
Extrem: Absent pulses or ischemic changes (diabetes and peripheral vascular disease with concurrent coronary disease)
Neuro: Dizziness, agitation, confusion, and other evidence of decreased cerebral perfusion

MANAGEMENT

If the Patient is Hypotensive

Immediate steps must be taken:
1. Confirm that the pressure is real and differs from the patient's normal pressure.
2. Ensure that the patient is receiving oxygen.
3. Ensure that the patient has a functioning IV; obtain IV access if none is available.
4. Ensure that the patient is on a cardiac monitor, if dysrhythmias are noted, begin ACLS protocols (see Appendix A).
5. Refer to Chapter 17 for a full discussion on the evaluation and treatment of hypotension and shock.

Sinus Bradycardia

Asymptomatic patients require no treatment. However, the HR should be followed closely. Adjustments in medications or workup may be required if the HR continues to slow or the patient becomes symptomatic. Patients who are symptomatic require **atropine 0.5 to 1 mg IV push** (dose may be repeated, as needed, up to 3 mg) or cardiac pacing. External transthoracic pacing or transvenous pacing provides temporary pacing. Cardiac surgery patients may have existing pacing wires. If pacing equipment is not available, a dopamine or epinephrine drip may provide relief of symptomatic bradycardia. Dosing is **5 to 15** mcg/kg/minute for dopamine or **2 to 15** mcg/minute for epinephrine. Transfer the patient to the ICU/CCU. Hold or adjust doses of medications known to slow the heart rate.

Atrial Fibrillation with Slow Ventricular Response

Asymptomatic patients do not require treatment. Hypotension or hypoperfusion associated with this condition requires ICU or coronary care unit transfer and pacemaker placement. Often, patients with atrial fibrillation are anti-coagulated to prevent blood clot formation in the atrium.

AV Block

First-degree AV block requires no treatment if the patient is asymptomatic. In symptomatic patients, make sure that the serum electrolytes are within normal limits and that drugs known to cause AV conduction delays are withdrawn (digoxin, calcium channel blockers, and beta-blockers). Atropine or cardiac pacing is used to treat symptomatic AV block.

Symptomatic Mobitz I block can be managed with **atropine 0.5 to 1 mg IV.** Dose may be repeated as needed, up to 2 mg. Temporary pacing or pressor drips, as described above, may be required if atropine is ineffective. Mobitz II block is treated similarly as Mobitz I block; however, permanent pacemaker placement should be considered early in this condition. In both types of second-degree block, discontinue any medication that might have contributed to the block.

Third-degree AV block should be treated with **atropine 0.5 to 1 mg IV** (dose may be repeated), **dopamine (5 to 15** mcg/kg/minute), or **epinephrine (2 to 15** mcg/minute). If a rapidly reversible cause for the complete heart block is not found, pacemaker insertion is appropriate. Cardiac surgery patients may be directly paced via the epicardial leads, if still present.

Drug Overdose

Grossly elevated digoxin levels are associated with bradycardia and toxicity. A single dose of only 2 mg of digoxin is likely to be toxic. If a patient has bradycardia associated with an elevated digoxin level, the patient should be transferred to a monitored bed. Any unabsorbed digoxin may be removed with gastric lavage or activated charcoal administration. Serum digoxin levels should be monitored. Digoxin-immune Fab fragments should be given for life-threatening complications of digoxin toxicity, including ventricular tachycardia, ventricular fibrillation (VF), or heart block associated with hypotension.

TACHYCARDIAS AND IRREGULAR RHYTHMS

PHONE CALL

Questions

1. **What is the HR?**
   Very high HRs may be associated with poor perfusion and hypotension.
2. **Is the rhythm regular or irregular?**
3. **What is the BP?**
   Hypotension with tachycardia is a medical emergency. This could represent either a compensatory mechanism (e.g.,

hypovolemia) or a life-threatening arrhythmia (e.g., ventricular tachycardia [VT]).

4. Does the patient have chest pain or shortness of breath?

Myocardial ischemia or pulmonary embolism may be associated with tachycardia.

5. Does the patient have a fever?

Fever is a common cause of tachycardia in surgical patients.

6. Is the patient taking any medications for HR, BP, or rhythm control?

Ask the RN if the patient is taking digoxin, calcium channel blockers, beta-blockers, procainamide, or other antiarrhythmic drugs. Patients taking these drugs for rate or rhythm control may have subtherapeutic levels or a rebound tachycardia from sudden medication discontinuation.

7. Does the patient have a history of tachycardia or arrhythmia?

If the patient has a history of recurrent tachycardia or arrhythmia, see what prior treatments have been effective.

8. Does the patient have pacing wires or an automatic defibrillation device?

Pacing wires are placed at the time of cardiac surgery. They are useful when temporary pacing is necessary. Automatic defibrillator devices are implanted in patients with recurrent, life-threatening arrhythmias.

Orders

1. If no IV is present, have the RN place an IV immediately (preferably 16 gauge or greater).
2. If the patient is having chest pain and tachycardia, ask the RN to bring the crash cart into the room and attach the patient to the continuous ECG monitor.
3. Ask the RN to obtain a 12-lead ECG.
4. If otherwise appropriate and if the patient is hypotensive (SBP lesser than 90 mm Hg), ask the RN to place the patient in Trendelenburg's position.
5. Supply oxygen, 4 liters by nasal cannula.

Inform RN

Will arrive at the bedside in . . . minutes.

Tachycardia associated with hypotension or an irregular rhythm requires that you examine the patient immediately. Beware that chest pain associated with tachycardia may represent acute MI or pulmonary embolus. Your rapid intervention may be lifesaving for the patient.

ELEVATOR THOUGHTS

What causes rapid HRs or irregular rhythms?

Tachycardias with regular rhythms
  1. Sinus tachycardia
  2. Atrial tachycardia (supraventricular tachycardia [SVT])
      a. Paroxysmal atrial tachycardia (PAT)
      b. Ectopic atrial tachycardia
      c. Atrial flutter
      d. AV nodal reentrant tachycardia (AVNRT)
      e. Wolff–Parkinson–White syndrome (WPW)
  3. Ventricular tachycardia (VT)
Tachycardias with irregular rhythms
  1. Atrial fibrillation
  2. Atrial flutter with variable block
  3. Multifocal atrial tachycardia
  4. Sinus tachycardia with premature atrial contractions (PACs) or premature ventricular contractions (PVCs)
Irregular rhythms not compatible with life
  1. Ventricular fibrillation (VF) (prolonged)
  2. Asystole (prolonged)

MAJOR THREAT TO LIFE

- Arrhythmia progressing to cardiac arrest
- Hypotension
- MI
- Hypoxemia

The tachyarrhythmias may deteriorate to VF and asystole. Rapid diagnosis and treatment of tachyarrhythmias will improve outcome. In addition, it is important to quickly treat any reversible cause of tachycardia associated with hypotension. Hypotension results in coronary hypoperfusion, myocardial dysfunction, and MI.

BEDSIDE

Quick Look Test

Does the patient look well (comfortable), sick (uncomfortable or distressed), or critical (about to die)?

With the quick look test, assess tissue perfusion. Patients who are hypoperfused will be pale and lethargic, but patients with a normal BP will have normal color and mental status. Patients who are normotensive with a tachycardia or arrhythmia often look well. However, patients with rapid HRs or abnormal rhythms associated with hypotension usually look sick or critical.

When assessing a patient with tachydysrhythmia, the quick look test is done with a hand on the patient's pulse.

Airway and Vital Signs

What is the HR, and is it regular or irregular?

Assess the HR by taking the patient's pulse and reading the rhythm strip. Feel for the strength of the pulse and its regularity. Also estimate the HR from the strip recording.

What is the BP?

This is the most important issue to consider. If the patient is hypotensive, you must determine if it is related to hypovolemia (in which the tachycardia is a compensatory mechanism) or if hypotension is the result of the tachycardia.

Compensatory tachycardia is most common after bodily injuries and "third-spacing" of intravascular volume. Bleeding is also a common cause of compensatory tachycardia. Surgical patients may develop hypovolemia and a compensatory tachycardia after major surgery, blunt and sharp trauma, burns, and postoperative bleeding. Tachycardia as a compensatory response to hypovolemia will usually show sinus tachycardia on the rhythm strip. Treat with a crystalloid challenge (**500 mL normal saline** or **lactated Ringer solution,** repeat as appropriate) or transfusion.

Tachycardia may cause hypotension. If there is not enough time for diastolic filling of the ventricle, the cardiac output falls. This may lead to hypotension. The most common tachyarrhythmias that are associated with hypotension include the following:
1. AF with rapid ventricular response (Fig. 9–6)
2. SVT (Fig. 9–7)
3. VT (Fig. 9–8)

Accurately diagnose these tachyarrhythmias on rhythm strip or ECG. The treatment for these arrhythmias is outlined below.

What is the temperature?

Patients with fever often have a tachycardia. As the body temperature rises, the HR rises. Be aware that persistent fever greatly increases insensible fluid losses. Tachycardia in the presence of infection or sepsis may be a response of both elevated body temperature and hypovolemia.

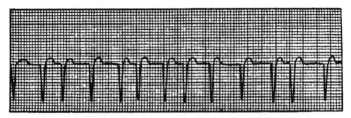

Figure 9–6 Atrial fibrillation with rapid ventricular response. (From Marshall SA, Ruedy J: On Call: Principles and Protocols, 2nd ed. Philadelphia, WB Saunders, 1993, p. 116.)

Figure 9–7 Supraventricular tachycardia.
(From Marshall SA, Ruedy J: On Call: Principles and Protocols, 2nd ed. Philadelphia, WB Saunders, 1993, p. 117.)

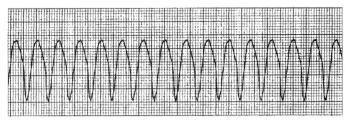

Figure 9–8 Ventricular tachycardia.

MANAGEMENT

If the Patient Is Hypotensive

Immediate steps must be taken:
1. Confirm that the pressure is real and differs from the patient's normal pressure.
2. Ensure that the patient is receiving oxygen.
3. Ensure that the patient has a functioning IV; obtain IV access if none is available.
4. Ensure that the patient is on a cardiac monitor, if dysrhythmias are noted, begin ACLS protocols (see Appendix A).
5. Refer to Chapter 17 for a full discussion on the evaluation and treatment of hypotension and shock.

Tachycardia is a HR of greater than 100 beats/minute. There are two sites of origin of tachycardias: supraventricular (SVT), and ventricular (VT). These two sites yield very different types of tachycardias, with different treatments and outcomes.

TACHYCARDIAS WITH REGULAR RHYTHMS

SINUS TACHYCARDIA

Sinus tachycardia (Fig. 9–9) occurs when the normal sinus mechanism increases its rate of firing under the influence of the autonomic nervous system. Many of the causes of tachycardia are directly or indirectly linked to the autonomic nervous system. Sinus tachycardia may be caused by any of the following:

1. Hypovolemia
2. Hypoxemia
3. Increased sympathetic tone
4. Decreased parasympathetic tone
5. Catecholamine release
6. Drugs that mimic endogenous catecholamines (e.g., cocaine and amphetamines)
7. Myocardial ischemia
8. Pain
9. Pulmonary embolism
10. Sepsis or shock
11. Anxiety

The best way to treat sinus tachycardia is to treat the cause. Hypovolemia should be treated with intravenous hydration. Hypoxemia should be treated with oxygen. Use 100% oxygen unless the patient has chronic obstructive pulmonary disease (COPD) and retains CO_2. In these cases, use 30% oxygen. A cause of the hypoxemia should be investigated. Pain should be treated with appropriate analgesics. Myocardial ischemia associated with tachycardia may be treated with oxygen, analgesics, and beta-adrenergic antagonists (see Chapter 7). Sepsis is treated with fluid resuscitation, intravenous antibiotics, and pressor agents as needed.

Figure 9–9 Sinus tachycardia.

Atrial Tachycardia

Paroxysmal Atrial Tachycardia (PAT)

PAT frequently occurs in patients with pulmonary disease, coronary artery disease, digoxin toxicity, and acute alcohol overdose. It also may occur due to reentry pathways. Treatment is targeted at the underlying process.

- If the cause is digoxin toxicity

    Stopping digoxin and maintaining normal potassium levels is often all that is needed. If PAT continues, consider loading and treating with lidocaine. Propranolol may also be useful.

- If the cause is not digoxin toxicity

    Calcium channel blockers, beta-adrenergic antagonists, or digoxin is helpful in slowing the ventricular response rate.

Atrial Flutter

The ECG (Fig. 9–10) shows a classic sawtooth pattern with an atrial rate of 275 to 350 beats/minute.

STABLE HEMODYNAMICS

If the patient is stable (SBP greater than 90 mm Hg), consider IV verapamil. **A dose of 2.5 to 5 mg can be given slowly over 2 minutes. The dose may be repeated in 5 to 10 minutes** if there is little or no clinical response. Be aware that verapamil (a calcium channel blocker) is a negative inotropic agent and may worsen congestive heart failure (CHF) or hypotension.

Digoxin may also be useful in treating atrial flutter. First, rule out that the atrial arrythmia is not due to digoxin toxicity. Once you decide to treat with digoxin, start by loading with **0.25 to 0.5 mg digoxin IV. Then, give 0.25 mg every 6 hours until a total of 1 mg digoxin is given. A maintenance dose of 0.125 to 0.25 mg PO or IV every day is usually required** to maintain therapeutic levels. You will need to lower the digoxin dose for patients with abnormal renal function. Check daily digoxin levels for all patients until a steady state is achieved. Digoxin works by slowing AV nodal conduction and ventricular response.

Figure 9–10 Atrial flutter.

Additional medications that may be useful include:
Metoprolol 1 to 2 mg/minute IV up to a dose of 5 mg if necessary.
If successful, convert to an oral dose of **25 to 50 mg PO BID.**
Esmolol 0.5 mg/kg IV over one minute
If successful, follow with an infusion of **0.05 to 0.2 mg/kg/minute.**
Diltiazem 0.25 mg/kg IV (usual dose 15 to 25 mg) over 2 minutes.
If successful, convert to a short- or long-acting preparation.

UNSTABLE HEMODYNAMICS
Patients with unstable atrial flutter (SBP lesser than 90 mm Hg) require cardioversion (Table 9–1).

AV Nodal Reentrant Tachycardia (AVNRT)

AVNRT occurs when there is reentry of two different pathways, one of which is faster than the other. The pathways link the right atrium

TABLE 9–1 **Protocol for Elective Cardioversion**

1. Ensure that all antiarrhythmic drugs are at their therapeutic levels.
2. Obtain informed consent.
3. Ensure that a functional IV is present.
4. Connect patient to continuous ECG monitor. Have a crash cart in the patient's room.
5. Check final ECG to ensure that the atrial arrhythmia is still present.
6. Place oxygen (nasal cannula) on the patient.
7. Ensure that intubation equipment and a ventilation bag are at the bedside. If possible, have an anesthesiologist at the bedside to monitor the airway.
8. Patient should be sedated with IV medications. Consider **midazolam 1–2 mg IV every 2 minutes, maximum 5 mg.** Monitor BP and oxygen saturation.
9. Place anterior electrode several centimeters to the right of the sternum at the 3rd or 4th interspace. For ventricular arrhythmias, the second electrode should be placed at the cardiac apex or more posteriorly. For atrial arrhythmias, place the second electrode just inferior to the left scapula.
10. Energy requirements:
    Atrial fibrillation usually requires at least 100 J; 200–360 J may be required.
    Atrial flutter often responds to 25–50 J.
    Reentry SVTs respond to 25–100 J.
    Ventricular tachycardia associated with hemodynamic compromise should be cardioverted with 200 J, followed by 360 J if initial shock is unsuccessful.
    Ventricular fibrillation should be treated with a rapid 200-J shock, followed by 360-J shocks.

ECG, electrocardiographic; IV, intravenous; BP, blood pressure; SVT, supraventricular tachycardia.

to the AV node. A narrow complex tachycardia results. The ECG (Fig. 9–11) shows an HR of 150 to 250 beats/minute, with the P wave either not visible or inverted in the T wave. The PR interval may be either normal or prolonged.

There are several therapeutic options for the treatment of this type of tachycardia. Vagal maneuvers may help break the tachycardia.

VALSALVA'S MANEUVER

Ask the patient to take a deep breath and hold it. Have the patient bear down as if having a bowel movement. Holding the breath while bearing down for 10 seconds increases vagal tone and may slow the tachycardia.

CAROTID MASSAGE

This is an effective technique to increase vagal tone. Proceed as follows:

1. Turn the patient's head to the side.
2. Locate the carotid sinus.
    The carotid sinus is located between the thyroid cartilage and the sternomastoid muscle (Fig. 9–12).
3. Apply moderate pressure with several fingers to the neck directly over the carotid pulse.
4. Massage for about 10 seconds.

Warning: This maneuver must be done carefully. Always perform carotid massage with ECG monitoring. Have atropine available if a bradycardia results from the massage. Never perform this maneuver on a patient with hypotension. The vagal stimulation may lower the HR and further depress the BP. Also, avoid carotid massage in a patient with carotid bruits. It is possible to dislodge a carotid plaque and have it embolize to the brain. Finally, never perform bilateral, simultaneous carotid massage. This may lead to cessation of carotid blood flow to the brain.

Drug therapy options for the treatment of AVNRT include **adenosine 6 to 12 mg IV**, or **verapamil 5 mg IV** given over 2 minutes (may repeat dose once in 5 minutes), or **diltiazem 0.25 mg/kg IV** given

Figure 9–11 Rapid regular rhythms; supraventricular tachycardia, atrioventricular nodal reentry, or Wolff–Parkinson–White tachycardia. (From Marshall SA, Ruedy J: On Call: Principles and Protocols, 2nd ed. Philadelphia, WB Saunders, 1993, p. 120.)

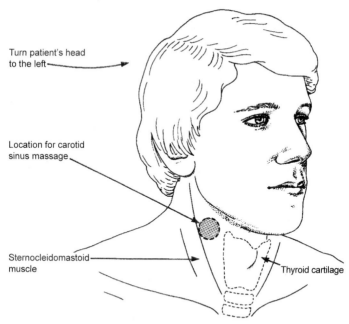

Figure 9–12 Carotid sinus massage.
(From Marshall SA, Ruedy J: On Call: Principles and Protocols, 2nd ed. Philadelphia, WB Saunders, 1993, p. 126.)

over 2 minutes, or **digoxin 0.25 to 0.5 mg IV,** followed by **0.125 mg to 0.25 mg IV every 4 to 6 hours** until a loading dose of 1 gm is given (if the rhythm is not due to digoxin toxicity). Remember that before any of these drug regimens are attempted, the patient must have oxygen in place and appropriate monitoring (ECG and oxygen saturation monitors). Have a crash cart nearby. Notify your resident.

Wolff–Parkinson–White Syndrome

WPW syndrome is caused by preexcitation involving a bypass tract or accessory pathway between the atria and the ventricles. ECG findings include a short PR interval (0.12 second), a QRS complex (greater than 0.11 second), and a delta wave (Fig. 9–13).

Treatment of WPW syndrome is similar to the drug treatment for AVNRT. However, much care must be used when giving adenosine, calcium channel blockers, or digoxin to these patients. Atrial fibrillation (AF) or a rapid ventricular response may be triggered, requiring direct current (DC) cardioversion. Additional options include **amiodarone 150 mg IV** bolus over 10 minutes, or **procainamide 20 mg/minute IV** until the dysrhythmias cease or hypotension is

Delta wave

Figure 9–13 Wolff–Parkinson–White syndrome. This condition is characterized by a regular rhythm, a PR interval of less than 0.12 second, a QRS complex of greater than 0.11 second, and a delta wave (i.e., slurred beginning of the QRS complex).
(From Marshall SA, Ruedy J: On Call: Principles and Protocols, 2nd ed. Philadelphia, WB Saunders, 1993, p. 121.)

present or the QRS widens by greater than 50. **The total dose of procainamide should not exceed 17 mg/kg.**

Ventricular Tachycardia

VT (see Fig. 9–8) is defined as three or more consecutive premature ventricular beats. The ventricular rate is usually 160 to 250 beats/minute. The rhythm is usually regular. Classic ECG appearance includes ventricular complexes with a wide QRS complex (greater than 120 msec) and T waves with an opposite polarity to the QRS complexes. Pulseless VT is the most common life-threatening arrhythmia. MI, electrolyte abnormalities, reentry pathways, cardiomyopathy, myocardial infarction, or inflammation predispose the patient to VT.

A patient with VT may be asymptomatic and normotensive. Symptomatic patients have shortness of breath, presyncope, palpitations, and angina. A patient with symptomatic VT must be treated immediately and definitively. If untreated, VT commonly degenerates into VF.

Sustained VT associated with compromise requires immediate DC cardioversion (see Appendix A). Compromise includes hypotension, angina, altered level of consciousness, or shortness of breath. Pharmacologic cardioversion may be attempted in patients with clinically stable VT. Drug choices include the following:

Amiodarone 150 mg IV bolus over 10 minutes, or

Lidocaine 1 mg/kg IV followed by repeat doses of 0.5 mg/kg every 8 minutes, or

Procainamide 20 mg/minute IV until the dysrhythmias ceases or hypotension is present or the QRS widens by more than 50. **The total dose of procainamide should not exceed 17 mg/kg.** Continue with a drip of the effective agent.

TACHYCARDIAS WITH IRREGULAR RHYTHMS

ATRIAL FIBRILLATION

AF is the most common sustained arrhythmia (Fig. 9–14; see Fig. 9–6). It is also the most common sustained arrhythmia seen in postoperative patients. AF occurs when multiple waves of activation occur simultaneously in different parts of the atria. The ECG shows ill-defined P waves, with irregular spacing between R waves. The ventricular response is irregular and varies from 80 to 160 beats/minute. AF is associated with variable periods of diastolic filling, and thus, each ventricular beat is often not associated with a palpable pulse.

Factors predisposing to the development of AF include atrial stretch (fluid overload and cardiomyopathy), rheumatic heart disease, hypertension, trauma, and cardiac surgery. Complications arising as a result of AF include embolic events such as strokes and peripheral thromboembolisms.

If AF is associated with a rapid ventricular response in conjunction with hypotension, myocardial ischemia, MI, or rapidly worsening CHF, DC cardioversion should be performed (see Appendix A). Patients with stable AF not associated with cardiac decompensation may be loaded with **digoxin (0.25 to 0.5 mg IV, followed by 0.25 mg IV every 6 hours for total of 1 mg)** or treated with calcium channel blocking drugs. The calcium channel blocking drugs (e.g., **verapamil 5 mg IV**) slow the ventricular rate quickly and may alleviate hypotension due to rapid ventricular rates. However, long-term control of AF or the treatment of AF in patients with heart failure is best done with digoxin.

Additional medications that may be useful include:

Metoprolol 1 to 2 mg/minute IV up to a dose of 5 mg if necessary. If successful, convert to an oral dose of **25 to 50 mg PO BID.**
Esmolol 0.5 mg/kg IV over one minute.
If successful, follow with an infusion of **0.05 to 0.2 mg/kg/minute.**
Diltiazem 0.25 mg/kg IV (usual dose 15 to 25 mg) over 2 minutes. If successful, convert to a short- or long-acting preparation.

Figure 9–14 Atrial fibrillation with slow ventricular response.

Multifocal Atrial Tachycardia

Multifocal atrial tachycardia (Fig. 9–15) is characterized by variable P wave morphology and irregular PP intervals. The rate is usually between 100 and 150 beats/minute. Patients usually have an underlying pulmonary illness, such as COPD. Treatment for this arrhythmia is best done by treating the underlying cause. Check that the patient does not have the following problems: hypoxia, hypercapnia, hypokalemia, CHF, theophylline toxicity, or acute alcohol toxicity. If the underlying problem has been corrected and the patient is still tachycardic, consider:

> **verapamil 5 to 10 mg IV or 80 mg PO, or**
> **diltiazem 30 to 90 mg PO QID**

Sinus Tachycardia with Premature Atrial Contractions or Premature Ventricular Contractions

Patients with PACs and sinus tachycardia (Fig. 9–16) may not require treatment. However, PACs may degenerate into multifocal

Figure 9–15 Rapid irregular rhythms; multifocal atrial tachycardia. (From Marshall SA, Ruedy J: On Call: Principles and Protocols, 2nd ed. Philadelphia, WB Saunders, 1993, p. 118.)

Figure 9–16 Rapid irregular rhythms; sinus tachycardia with premature atrial contractions. (From Marshall SA, Ruedy J: On Call: Principles and Protocols, 2nd ed. Philadelphia, WB Saunders, 1993, p 118.)

atrial tachycardia or AF. Therapy should be directed toward correction of any underlying abnormality (electrolytes and drugs). If desired, a patient with sinus tachycardia and PACs may be treated electively as Multifocal Atrial Tachycardia earlier, with a calcium channel blocker such as verapamil or diltiazem.

PVCs are premature beats originating in the ventricles (Fig. 9–17). Single PVCs are frequently seen in patients without structural heart disease. However, the presence of complex forms such as couplets and triplets may indicate myocardial ischemia, infection, inflammation, or drug use.

Isolated PVCs require no therapy. If a patient is symptomatic, therapy should be directed at correcting the underlying cause. Common causes of PVCs include the following:

1. MI
2. Myocardial ischemia
3. Hypokalemia
4. Hypoxia
5. Acidosis
6. Alkalosis
7. Cardiomyopathy
8. Drug toxicity (antiarrhythmics)
9. Hyperthyroidism
10. Mitral valve disease

If a patient has runs of PVCs (couplets, triplets, or greater than 5 PVCs/minute), consider transferring the patient to a cardiac monitored bed. Hold or reduce any medications known to affect the heart rate and look for reversible causes of the rhythm. IV lidocaine is effective in suppressing PVCs, but it is associated with toxic effects and is reserved for use in severe cases or in patients with documented VT.

Figure 9–17 Rapid irregular rhythms; sinus tachycardia with premature ventricular contractions.
(From Marshall SA, Ruedy J: On Call: Principles and Protocols, 2nd ed. Philadelphia, WB Saunders, 1993, p. 119.)

IRREGULAR RHYTHMS NOT COMPATIBLE WITH LIFE

VENTRICULAR FIBRILLATION

VF occurs when uncoordinated electrical activity within the ventricle occurs, producing ineffective mechanical contraction. Patients with VF generally have no significant blood pressure and die rapidly unless resuscitated aggressively. Baseline ECG (Fig. 9–18) shows rapid oscillations (250 to 400 beats/minute), without evidence of distinct P waves, QRS complexes, or T waves.

Implement immediate cardiopulmonary resuscitation (CPR) with bag ventilation or intubation and immediate unsynchronized DC cardioversion (see Appendix A). If DC cardioversion alone is unsuccessful, IV epinephrine, lidocaine, and bretylium are used one at a time with cardioversion in an attempt to restore a stable cardiac rhythm.

Asystole

Asystole (Fig. 9–19) carries a very poor prognosis for resuscitation. Start resuscitation attempts by beginning CPR and intubation. Then,

Figure 9–18 Ventricular fibrillation.

Figure 9–19 Asystole.

confirm an ECG reading of asystole in more than one lead. Sometimes, fine VF can appear as asystole. VF has a much better prognosis for resuscitation than asystole. Thus, if VF is suspected or cannot be ruled out, consider attempted unsynchronized cardioversion as per the VF protocol (see Appendix A). If the rhythm strip shows a true asystole, give **1 mg epinephrine IV push.** Follow with **atropine 1 mg IV push.** Consider **high-dose epinephrine (10 mg) IV push** if there is no response to lower dose epinephrine or atropine after 5 to 10 minutes. Consider transcutaneous pacing if early resuscitation of the asystole was initiated.

SPECIAL SURGICAL CONSIDERATIONS

Postoperative tachycardia is common. In the normotensive patient, always evaluate the intravascular volume status, level of pain or anxiety, and oxygen saturation.

Falls

When a patient falls it is a serious event. Whether the patient falls from bed or falls elsewhere in the hospital, be mindful of the following two questions after the fall: Is the patient injured? And, what was the cause of the fall?

PHONE CALL

Questions

1. **Was the fall witnessed?**
   Anyone who witnessed the fall should be contacted, and his or her story should be documented.
2. **Is there an emergent injury?**
   Head injuries and fractures are particularly worrisome.
3. **Is there a change in the patient's mental status?**
   A computed tomographic (CT) scan of the head immediately is indicated if a significant head injury or change in mental status is apparent.
4. **Was there an obvious identifiable cause?**
   The cause of a fall is often multifactorial.
5. **Has the patient undergone a surgical procedure, and if so, how long ago?**
   Protection from falls is an important part of postoperative management in neurosurgical and orthopedic patients.
6. **Are there any other symptoms?**
7. **Are there any changes in vital signs?**

Orders

1. Ensure the safety of the patient, and respond to any injuries present.
2. Instruct the bedside caregiver to call if there are any further changes in vital signs or mental status.

Inform RN

Will be at the bedside in . . . minutes.

If there is a significant change in vital signs or symptoms, especially if the patient has an obvious injury such as a fracture or if there is a significant change in mental status, the patient must be evaluated immediately. Also, if the baseline condition of the patient was serious before the fall, it is important to evaluate the situation quickly.

ELEVATOR THOUGHTS

What are the causes of falls?
1. Mental status changes

    Organic causes include Alzheimer disease, multi-infarct dementia, delirium, confusion, and other organic brain syndromes. Acute changes such as stroke, transient ischemic attack, and epileptic seizure may also cause falls. Patients may also have vasovagal reactions in response to anxiety, severe coughing, or sustained Valsalva's maneuver.

2. Medications

    Medications include sedatives, opiate pain relievers, muscle relaxants, antihypertensive medications, and sleeping aids. Be mindful of any newly started medications.

3. Cardiac events

    Cardiac events include myocardial infarction, dysrhythmias, and hypotension. Be mindful that postoperative patients are often fluid depleted and are predisposed to orthostatic hypotension.

4. Infections

    Infections include sepsis associated with hypotension, delirium associated with fever, or primary central nervous system infections such as meningitis.

5. Respiratory

    Respiratory causes include hypoxia due to pulmonary edema or embolism.

6. Metabolic derangements

    Metabolic derangements include azotemia, hypoglycemia, liver failure, and electrolyte abnormalities.

7. Environment

    Patients are often unfamiliar with their surroundings, and in addition, they are surrounded by inconvenient obstacles such as intravenous (IV) poles, tubes, wires, catheters, and bed rails. It is amazing that falls do not happen more often. A little preventive organization in the patient's room is helpful, for example, putting the telephone or call button within the patient's reach. Bed rails are a safety measure for alert or comatose patients.

MAJOR THREAT TO LIFE

Causes of Falls

- Myocardial infarction
- Stroke
- Hypoxia

Result of Falls

Head Injury

Any patient who has had a fall, especially an unwitnessed fall, must have a full neurologic evaluation. Compare your findings with other documented neurologic examinations in the chart to identify significant changes. Significant changes must be evaluated by CT scan to rule out intracranial bleeding.

Fractures

These are especially prevalent in the elderly. Hip fractures carry a high morbidity.

BEDSIDE

Quick Look Test

Most patients are well after an uncomplicated fall, although specific complaints are often present. Patients can often tell you exactly what happened.

Airway and Vital Signs

Repeat taking vital signs when at the bedside. Is there a change in the trends?

Is the patient alert and oriented?
Are there symptoms of mental status change?

What is the heart rate, and is there a change in the rhythm?
Perform an electrocardiogram (ECG) as necessary.

What is the blood pressure?
Orthostatic BP and pulse trends may be helpful when assessing fluid status.

How is the patient's breathing, and does the patient appear agitated (a sign of hypoxia)?
Do a spot pulse oximetry reading or chest x-ray as indicated.

Initial Management

1. Look for the cause of the fall.

   Gather as much information as possible. Ask the patient what happened, talk with witnesses, and observe the fall site. Be especially mindful of any symptoms the patient noted before the fall, such as dizziness, palpitations, or pain. These may be clues to the cause.

2. Do a complete neurologic examination on patients, especially those who had unwitnessed falls and those with evidence of head injury.

   If a significant mental status change or a new neurologic sign is present, a head CT scan is indicated immediately.

3. Treat other apparent injuries.

   A patient with mental status changes may not be able to identify other injuries. Have a high level of suspicion, and do a thorough examination. Obtain x-rays to evaluate painful or swollen areas as indicated.

4. Ensure that the patient is as safe as possible from further falls.

   An identifiable cause may be treated or prevented in the future. If the problem is more unpredictable, such as a delirium, keeping the patient safe may include sedatives or soft restraints, depending on the situation.

Selective History and Chart Review

Is there a condition predisposing to disorientation, lightheadedness, or postural instability?

1. Look for previous falls.

   What prior workup has been done? Is there an unidentified trend? Does the patient have a history of nighttime disorientation ("sundowning")?

2. Are there any new medications?

   Adverse reactions can include BP derangements and mental status changes.

3. Does the patient have a history of heart disease or arrhythmia?

4. Look for laboratory abnormalities.

   Is the patient diabetic? A glucose determination immediately by finger stick is useful. Also review any insulin therapy. Are there other treatable metabolic abnormalities?

5. Does the patient have a seizure disorder?

   Are antiepileptic medication levels within therapeutic range?

6. Does the patient have nocturia?

   Urinary tract infection, overhydration, diuretic therapy, or prostate enlargement may predispose a patient to urinate at night. Often the route to the bathroom is a maze of tubes and wires. Is a urinal available at the bedside?

Has the patient's surgical procedure contributed to the fall?

1. Assess the patient's fluid status.

Is the patient well hydrated? What fluid has the patient already received? If the patient is taking nothing by mouth and has been started on total parenteral nutrition, often glucose abnormalities are present. Check the finger stick.

2. Is the patient taking pain medications?

If disorientation or sedation is too great with the current regimen, consider other combinations of medicines or delivery schemes.

3. Look for other surgery-related changes.

Thyroid or autonomic storm can exacerbate arrhythmias. Pain can slow reflexes and change ambulation patterns.

Is the patient anticoagulated?

This adds to the danger of any fall. If significant bleeding is present, reversal of the anticoagulation must be considered. It is imperative to reverse anticoagulation if the bleeding is intracranial.

Selective Physical Examination

VS:	Repeat now with orthostatic measurements as necessary.
MS:	Any changes may be significant as a cause or as a result of a fall.
HEENT:	Look for bruises or lacerations to the head indicating significant injury. Tongue or cheek lacerations may be present and may result from seizure activity.
CVS:	Current rate and rhythm should be compared with recent trends.
Resp:	Labored breathing, evidence of hypoxia.
Skin:	Bruising or painful regions associated with the fall.
Extrem:	Evidence of fracture.
Neuro:	A complete neurologic examination is absolutely necessary. Any changes require further evaluation and treatment.
Wound:	Ensure that suture lines are intact and there is no new bleeding.
Tubes:	Are all necessary tubes still in place and secure?
Additional tests:	ECG is indicated to assess rhythm or cardiac symptoms. Finger stick glucose or electrolytes as indicated.
	Radiographs as indicated to assess injury
	Consider checking levels of anticonvulsant or antiarrhythmic medications as necessary.

MANAGEMENT

1. Identify a cause for the fall and treat this as necessary.

Sometimes the cause is obvious, but often it is multifactorial. Stop unnecessary medications.

2. Identify all sequelae from the fall and treat these as necessary.

   Patients who are alert and oriented may be embarrassed and only mildly hurt after a fall. They may still require a mild anti-inflammatory and local ice therapy. Other injuries must be evaluated as indicated.

3. Take steps to avoid the next fall.

   Correct identifiable causes, and treat reversible conditions as indicated. If the cause is not apparent or is irreversible, make the patient's environment as safe as possible.

4. Document the fall completely including time, place, circumstances, obvious injuries, complete neurologic examination, and appropriate changes in care and follow-up.

   Falls in an institution are a medicolegal issue. As much as possible, patients are kept in a safe environment, but occasionally accidents happen. Be complete in your documentation!

Special Surgical Considerations

Preoperative Considerations

The cause of the fall or any resultant injuries may affect a scheduled procedure. Check with the chief or attending physician if there is any question about needing to reschedule the case.

Postoperative Considerations

1. Postoperative patients are often disoriented because of the combination of intravascular depletion, pain, and pain medication treatment, in addition to whatever underlying causes may already be present. Very sick or febrile patients are also more likely to fall.

2. After intracranial procedures, neurosurgical patients are often neurologically impaired and their mental status changes very quickly. The advantage is that neurologic examinations are performed frequently on these patients, and trends are often readily identifiable. Do not give antiepileptic medications to a postoperative neurosurgical patient unless specifically told to do so by the chief resident or attending physician. Intractable seizures are an indication for a repeat head CT immediately, first, and antiepileptic medication, second. Have a low threshold for considering a head CT scan in these patients.

3. Orthopedic patients who have fractures or repairs of their lower extremities will often have weight-bearing instructions written. Make sure that these were followed. If the patient has walked inappropriately on a cast or dressing, examine the wound and consider x-rays to assess the repair.

4. It is important for most postoperative patients to ambulate. Make sure that the patient is still safe to perform this activity, then encourage it with assistance as necessary.

Fever

All patients with fever warrant clinical investigation. Although most febrile patients in the postoperative period are not infected, the evaluation is directed toward the discovery of infection, as this is the most threatening cause.

PHONE CALL

Questions

1. **How high is the temperature?**
   A core temperature of greater than 38.5°C is considered significant.
2. **What was the route of measurement?**
   Temperatures taken orally are about 0.5°C higher than those taken in the axilla or the ear and are about 0.5°C below those taken rectally. Rectal temperature is considered core.
3. **Has the patient been febrile before?**
4. **Has the patient undergone a surgical procedure, and if so, how long ago?**
5. **Are there any other symptoms?**
6. **Are there any changes in vital signs?**
   Be concerned about early sepsis.

Orders

1. If there are changes in vital signs, support hemodynamics and oxygenation.
2. Other orders depend on other symptoms.

Inform RN

Will be at the bedside in . . . minutes.

The patient should be evaluated usually within the hour if the patient is stable. If there is a significant change in vital signs or symptoms, then the patient must be evaluated immediately.

ELEVATOR THOUGHTS

The timing of the fever relative to the postoperative day will indicate the most likely cause (Table 11–1). Noninfectious causes must be considered with infectious causes in the postoperative patient.

MAJOR THREAT TO LIFE

- Sepsis
- Other life-threatening infection
- Pneumonia
- Meningitis
- Pulmonary embolus

TABLE 11–1 **The Timing of Common Causes of Postoperative Fever**

	POD 1	POD 2–3	POD 3 and Up
Infectious			
Respiratory	Atelectasis[†]	Pneumonia	Pulmonary embolus
Wound	*Streptococcus* sp.	*Clostridium* sp.	*Staphylococcus* sp., mixed aerobic and anaerobic species
GU	—	UTI	UTI, pyelonephritis
IVs, drains	—	Staph./Strep.	Staph./Strep.
Surgical bed	—	—	Abscess
Noninfectious*			
Malignant hyperthermia			
Thyroid storm			
Multiple trauma			
Hematoma			
Devitalized tissue			
Contaminated IV fluids			
Blood product transfusion			
Deep venous thrombosis			
Malignancy			
DT			
Drug fever			

POD, postoperative day; GU, genitourinary system; IV, intravenous; UTI, urinary tract infection; Staph./Strep., *Staphylococcus/Streptococcus;* DT, delirium tremens.

*Noninfectious etiologies may occur at any time.

†Strictly speaking, atelectasis is not an infectious cause of fever, but it is included in this list to emphasize the timing.

BEDSIDE

Quick Look Test

Most patients will be comfortable. If early sepsis is present, then the patient may appear agitated or delirious.

Airway and Vital Signs

Is the patient in shock?
>Note the heart rate (HR) and the blood pressure (BP).
>What is the patient's fluid status?
>Note the perfusion and the respiratory rate (RR).

Selective History and Chart Review

- What brought the patient to the hospital? Is fever an expected part of the disease process such as with ruptured appendices or cholecystitis? Does the patient have specific complaints?
  This often leads to the source of the infection.
- Surgical procedure or recent anesthetic, if any
- Postoperative complications
- Medications including antibiotics, immunosuppressants, chemo-therapeutics, and antipyretics
  Especially note any recent change in antibiotic therapy.
- Temperature curve pattern
  Patients with abscess complications often have repetitive, high, spiking fevers.
- Recent cultures and blood work
  The primary care team may have a plan outlined if a patient has continued fevers.
- Any underlying condition that may have fever as a component, such as colitis, collagen vascular disease, and malignancy
- Recent blood product administration
- What lines, tubes, or foreign bodies are present, and how long have they been in?
  This includes any prosthetic joints or devices.
- Is the patient diabetic (uncontrolled)?
  This condition increases the susceptibility to bacterial and yeast infection.
- Is the patient otherwise immunosuppressed, for example, an acquired immunodeficiency syndrome (AIDS) patient or transplant recipient?
- Does the patient have an existing seizure disorder?
  Seizure activity (witnessed or unwitnessed) can raise temperature, but rarely above 38.5°C.

Selective Physical Examination

VS:	Repeat now.
MS:	Delirium or agitation; think of early sepsis or hypoxia.
HEENT:	Headache. Is a nasogastric tube in place? Check for evidence of sinusitis, otitis, pharyngitis, or parotitis.
	Look for dental abscesses. Look for meningeal signs including nuchal rigidity or photophobia.
CVS:	Tachycardia, possible flow murmur, and skin perfusion.
Resp:	Tachypnea, aeration, rales, rhonchi, and wheezes.
Abd:	Evidence of distention and peritonitis.
GU:	Bladder discomfort, dysuria, and flank pain. Is a urinary catheter in place?
Extrem:	IV sites, redness or swelling, and calf tenderness.
Wound:	Redness, induration, tenderness, drainage, or purulence.
Tubes:	Redness, induration, tenderness, drainage, or purulence.
Special examinations:	Check IV fluids for evidence of contamination.
	Special examinations for meningitis; as follows: *Brudzinski's sign:* Positive if a patient flexes at the hip or knee in response to flexion at the neck. *Kernig's sign:* Positive if pain response is elicited with passive straightening of the knee from a position of 90 degree flexion at the hip. See Figure 15–2.

MANAGEMENT

Initial Management (If the Patient Is Unstable)

1. Order oxygen and pulse oximetry.
   Fever shifts the oxygen saturation curve such that a given arterial partial pressure of oxygen (PaO_2) results in a lower hemoglobin saturation.
2. Order cardiovascular monitoring.
3. Support hemodynamics with fluids and inotropes as necessary.
4. Provide adequate intravenous (IV) access.
5. Prevent shivering.
   Fever is already a high metabolic state. Further muscle contractions may result in increased myocardial oxygen demand and increased HR and RR and may produce metabolic acido-

sis. Cooling blankets are not as useful in this setting as judicious use of paralytic agents.

Definitive Management

For the first episode of fever without an obvious source (preoperative or postoperative), an ardent search for the site of infection is undertaken and the following preliminary measures are begun.

Patients will often have symptoms to direct your search. If a patient complaint leads to investigation of one area (i.e., UA in a patient with dysuria), it is unnecessary to subject that patient to "pan-culturing." In an unstable or uncommunicative patient, you may have no choice but to "cast your net widely."

1. Obtain a complete blood count with differential analysis.
2. Take blood cultures; two distant sites.
3. Obtain a UA, microscopic analysis, and culture.
4. Obtain a wound or a drain site culture.
   IV sites may be "milked" by gently stroking from proximally to distally, to attempt to express purulence.
5. Obtain a sputum analysis and culture as indicated.
   If the patient is intubated, obtain a Gram stain of the endotracheal tube aspirate. This site will be chronically colonized, so culture only if there are significant white blood cells (WBCs) present. A suction lavage may be useful to obtain a deeper pulmonary sample.
6. Obtain a chest x-ray.
7. Consider a finger stick glucose measurement.
   Often early septic patients will exhibit glucose instability.
8. Consider a lumbar puncture as symptoms dictate.
   This is especially important to consider in the obtunded patient. Also consider computed tomographic (CT) scan of the head to rule out central nervous system (CNS) abscess if fevers are prolonged and unremitting in an unconscious patient.
9. Perform a vaginal examination with cervical cultures as indicated.
10. Obtain a throat culture.
11. Change IV and central line sites.
    Some hospital protocols advocate changing central lines over a wire, maintaining the original site. This is useful when IV access is problematic. The safest approach is the removal of central access catheters and replacement at a clean site after the resolution of the fevers. This is especially important if there is purulence evident at the IV site. When a central line is removed, send the tip for culture by sterilely clipping the distal inch or so off and placing it in a sterile container (e.g., a urine specimen cup). Suspect any IV line that is still in place after a documented positive blood culture.
12. Remove the urinary catheter as indicated.
    Expect that patients with urinary catheters in place for more than 3 days will be colonized with bacteria. Use the

presence of WBCs and leukocyte esterase in the UA to interpret the significance of a positive culture.
13. Perform a pulmonary toilet as indicated.

Especially in the intubated or the obtunded patient, improving mobilization and expulsion of secretions will decrease the risk of pulmonary infection. This includes the use of mucolytics such as acetylcysteine, bronchodilators, and chest physical therapy (CPT) as indicated. In awake patients, hourly use of incentive spirometry will decrease atelectasis. Make sure postoperative patients have adequate pain control to ensure comfort during CPT or incentive spirometry.
14. Use antipyretics as a comfort measure only. Their use may obscure the temperature curve and may mask other symptoms.
15. Antibiotic therapy as outlined below.

Patients Who Require Empirical Broad-Spectrum Antibiotic Therapy

1. Febrile patients without a source who are becoming more ill, which especially applies to early septic, hypotensive, or hypermetabolic patients, require empirical broad-spectrum antibiotic therapy. Start with broad-spectrum antibiotic coverage, and narrow the therapy if the microorganism, specificities, and site of infection become known.
2. Patients with suspected serious infections such as meningitis or pneumonia with associated hypoxia also require broad-spectrum antibiotic therapy. Narrow the therapy as the microorganism, sensitivities, and site become known.
3. Immunocompromised patients such as transplant recipients, patients with AIDS, or patients treated with high-dose steroids or chemotherapy also require broad-spectrum antibiotic therapy. Remember that patients with low absolute neutrophil counts may have fever without a documentable source. This does not preclude them from empirical treatment. It is prudent to assume infection in these patients.

Patients Who Require Directed Antibiotic Treatment

Those patients with an identifiable source and who are currently stable require directed antibiotic treatment. A choice of antibiotic coverage can be made based on a knowledge of common pathogens and based on Gram stain information when available. See Table 11–2 for typical sites, pathogens, and antibiotic regimens for common infections. As each hospital has a different spectrum of bacteria that are common to wards and intensive care units, it is wise to check with the clinical microbiology division to find out the local nosocomial flora and any sensitivity idiosyncrasies.

TABLE 11–2 **Empirical Treatment for Common Infections**

Site	Common Pathogens	Empirical Treatment
Lungs		
Community acquired	*Streptococcus pneumoniae*	Penicillin, ampicillin, co-trimoxazole, or 2nd-generation cephalosporin
	Hemophilus influenzae	
	Mycoplasma pneumoniae	Erythromycin
	Legionella pneumophila	
Hospital acquired	*Escherichia coli*	Synthetic penicillin, carbapenem, or 3rd-generation cephalosporin **plus** aminoglycoside (or aztreonam)
	Klebsiella pneumoniae	
	Proteus sp.	
	Pseudomonas aeruginosa	
	Enterobacteriaceae	
	Staphylococcus aureus	Add clindamycin, synthetic penicillin, or 1st-generation cephalosporin
	Bacteroides	
Urine	Enterobacteriaceae (including *E. coli*)	Aminoglycosides (or aztreonam) with or without ampicillin; co-trimoxazole, fluoroquinolone
	Enterococci	Penicillin **plus** aminoglycoside
Wound	*Streptococcus* sp.	1st-generation cephalosporin, synthetic penicillin, or clindamycin
	Staphylococcus sp.	
	Clostridium sp.	

Patients Who Require No Antibiotic Therapy Immediately

1. Nonsick patients in whom no source is readily identifiable and those for whom a fever workup is in progress require no antibiotic therapy immediately. These may include patients with a cause of fever other than infection such as malignancy, but it must be emphasized that infection must still be ruled out.
2. Patients with temperature spikes of less than 38.5°C require no antibiotic therapy immediately.
3. Patients with suspected atelectasis require no antibiotic therapy immediately.

Patients with Fever Already Taking Antibiotics

1. If a source has been identified, consider the natural history of the disease. Patients with abscesses and severe infections such

as pyelonephritis and meningitis often have spikes of fevers for several days after initiation of appropriate therapy.
2. Make sure that the current antibiotic therapy is appropriate for the pathogens identified (type of antibiotic, dose, and dosing interval).
3. Nonbacterial sources of infection (especially yeast) must be considered in the very ill or immunosuppressed patient, the patient on prolonged antibiotic therapy, and the patient treated with total parenteral nutrition.

Patients with Fever in Whom Surgical Intervention Should be Considered

1. Any acute abdomen patient with fever should be considered for surgical intervention.
2. Patients who have undergone abdominal surgery in whom there is a question of bowel viability or anastomotic leak should be considered for surgical intervention.
3. Those with documented abscesses should be considered for surgical intervention.
   These abscesses may often be drained by transcutaneous catheter placement under ultrasonographic or CT guidance by interventional radiology.
4. Those patients with infected foreign bodies such as septic prosthetic joints should be considered for prosthesis removal.

Special Surgical Considerations

Preoperative Considerations

1. A remote infection increases the risk of subsequent wound infection postoperatively; so, fever in the elective preoperative patient will most likely preclude the planned procedure pending evaluation of the symptoms.
2. A change in condition associated with fever, such as development of an acute abdomen, can require emergent surgery.
3. Consider the following factors, which predispose for infection in the preoperative patient:
   Immunosuppressants
   Protein malnutrition
   Inadequate hydration
   Uncontrolled diabetes
   Prolonged hospitalization
   Alcoholism
   Remote infection

Postoperative Considerations

1. Cardiopulmonary bypass is a frequent cause of fever in the postoperative cardiac patient.
2. Large spiking fevers 5 to 7 days after a surgical procedure may indicate abscess formation.

3. Devitalized tissue such as massive crush injuries and necrotic bowel can be a source of fever and may require repeat surgery for resection.
4. In transplant recipients, fever can be a sign of rejection.
5. Fever is a side effect of some medications (e.g., OKT-3, amphotericin).

Malignant Hyperthermia

- It generally occurs intraoperatively but may occur up to 25 hours after delivery of anesthesia.
- The incidence is 1:16,000 anesthetics and is higher in children (1:12,000).
- The most likely causes are volatile agents such as halothane, enflurane, or isoflurane, or the paralytic agent succinylcholine.
- Mortality is 10% even in appropriately treated patients.
- Symptoms include the following:

    Increased temperature, as high as 43°C at times. This may be a late finding. Do not wait for it to initiate therapy.

    Increased RR, HR, and BP

    Agitation

    Hypoxia

    Skin mottling

- Damage is to the CNS, and it occurs rapidly because of cerebral edema and hypermetabolism. When the diagnosis is suspected, the following treatment is emergent:

    Provide fluid support.

    Discontinue anesthetic agents.

    Hyperventilate with 100% O_2.

    Administer dantrolene (Dantrium) 1 mg/kg IV immediately and **every 5 minutes up to 10 mg/kg** until symptoms abate.

    Treat metabolic acidosis.

    Watch for evidence of muscle breakdown products. Maintain urine output with adequate hydration and furosemide. Check urine for myoglobin.

    Check serial creatine phosphokinase (CPK) levels.

    Watch for and treat disseminated intravascular coagulation.

    Watch for and treat arrhythmias.

    Control pyrexia.

Fluids, Electrolytes, and Acid–Base Status

Surgical disease and treatment is often associated with aberrations in fluids, electrolytes, and acid–base status. Rapid fluid status assessment is a constant exercise in the management of surgical patients, as well as the application of therapies best suited to treat respective abnormalities. The common denominator in all fluid management is the avoidance of shock or inadequate end-organ perfusion. Poor end-organ perfusion may lead to hypoxia and irreversible damage. This chapter discusses normal fluid distributions and describes the more frequent causes of changes in volume distribution, biochemical abnormalities, and their treatments. The chapter is organized to address aberrations in intravascular volume. The intravascular space is the smallest fluid compartment but is the most dynamic (i.e., changeable) and is of critical importance to the maintenance of end-organ perfusion.

NORMAL FLUID DISTRIBUTION

The body is composed mostly of water (Fig. 12–1). Total body water represents up to 60% of the weight of an adult male. This percentage is higher in infants and lower in adult women, elderly, and the obese. Total body water can be thought of as residing in two separate compartments; *intracellular* and *extracellular*. The extracellular compartment is further divided into *interstitial fluid*, which bathes the cells and tissues, and *intravascular fluid* which is in the blood and lymphatic vessels of the body. Fluid can be thought to be freely flowing between the compartments, constrained mostly by the ionic strength or osmotic pressure of the respective compartment. Intravascular fluid makes up only about 8% to 10% of the total body water and is essentially the only site at which fluid replacement can take place.

In addition to the compartments listed above, there is a potential space that is loosely termed the *third space*. The third space is a pathologic expansion of the interstitial space via capillary leak in response to injury and illness. The size of the third space is proportional to the severity of the illness or injury. It is the shift of fluid

TBW = Total body water (60% of body weight)
IC = Intracellular space (67% of TBW)
EC = Extracellular space (33% of TBW)
Interstitial space (22% of TBW)
Intravascular space (8–10% of TBW)

Figure 12–1 Normal body distribution of water.

between the intravascular space and the third space that is most important in the evaluation and care of surgical patients. The shift between intracellular and extracellular fluid spaces also becomes important in the management of some electrolyte imbalances.

Normal daily fluid requirements are about 1500 mL/m². This volume replaces the sensible (measurable) losses of urine, feces, and drain outputs, and the insensible (unmeasurable) losses from respiration, skin, and open wounds. Fluid resuscitation often refers to the replacement of fluid deficits in addition to these normal daily requirements. Remember that various metabolic states such as fever, tachypnea, diarrhea, burns, and large open wounds greatly increase insensible losses and will increase the daily requirement. Renal failure may decrease the sensible losses and may require a reduction of the daily maintenance fluid requirements.

PREOPERATIVE FLUID DEFICITS

Many surgical diseases cause shifts of volume out of the intravascular space. Examples include sepsis, bowel obstruction, mechanical bowel preparation, and blood loss due to trauma. These deficits need to be addressed prior to operative management if possible. Most anesthetic agents will decrease blood pressure. This effect is augmented in hypovolemic patients.

POSTOPERATIVE FLUID CHANGES

After surgery, especially major surgery, there are physical and neuroendocrine causes for changes in intravascular volume. The most common abnormality is a depletion of intravascular volume leading to inadequate perfusion of end-organs. This may be a total body depletion due to underhydration, or there may be functional depletion by fluid shifts away from the intravascular space. Various surgical factors influencing intravascular volume are listed in Table 12–1. The longer the surgical procedure, the greater the fluid losses. The anesthesiologist will do much of the fluid replacement intraoperatively, but there is often need for continued fluid replacement postoperatively. In addition to intraoperative losses, there are often postoperative losses through open wounds, naso-gastric (NG) or drainage tubes, or postoperative bleeding. These ongoing losses represent depletion of electrolytes as well as fluid.

RAPID FLUID STATUS ASSESSMENT

The assessment of fluid status should become a reflex maneuver. Practice it daily on rounds on both ill and non-ill appearing patients. Soon it will become a comfortable skill. The assessment is based on observation, examination of the patient and the chart, and vital signs and laboratory data. The following are the three basic states of total body fluid status: *normal*, *fluid overloaded*, and *fluid depleted*. The state of intravascular volume is described as *normovolemic*, *hypervolemic*, and *hypovolemic*. The intravascular volume is important in determining perfusion of organs, and a depletion of this space has readily apparent signs. The three most apparent signs are changes in the perfusion of the skin, the kidneys, and the brain. Confirm the following:

1. **The skin is warm and moist.**

    One response to hypovolemia is to decrease perfusion of the peripheral vascular beds. Skin that is cool, pale, and dry is poorly perfused. A capillary refill time of >1.5 seconds is highly suggestive of hypovolemia.

2. **The urine output (UO) is adequate.**

    Generally this is considered to be greater than 20 mL/hour. Less urine volume than that is considered oliguria and may be due to hypovolemia.

TABLE 12–1 **Perioperative Factors Resulting in Decreased Intravascular Volume**

Inadequate preoperative resuscitation
Insensible loss through an open surgical field
Blood loss
Suction loss (from nasogastric tube and from the surgical field)
Insufficient intraoperative fluid replacement
Postoperative antidiuretic hormone secretion
Medications (including diuretics)
Postoperative fluid shifts ("third spacing")
Urinary losses

3. The patient is mentating well or at least at the baseline level.

Hypovolemia is a cause of delirium and confusion.

These signs individually may have many causes but when considered together represent a rapid, effective scan of the adequate functional intravascular volume. Remember that the fluid need not be missing from the body; it may be displaced from the intravascular space into the interstitial space. That is, a patient does not need to be total body volume depleted to be hypovolemic.

COMMON FLUID IMBALANCES: THE FLUID-OVERLOADED PATIENT

ELEVATOR THOUGHTS

What causes fluid overload?
1. Sequestration of fluids
   - Systemic infection
   - Pancreatitis
   - Severe injuries, polytrauma, or burns
   - Ileus
2. Overzealous hydration
3. Renal failure
4. Hepatic failure

MAJOR THREAT TO LIFE

- Pulmonary edema (increased intravascular volume)
- Myocardial infarction (MI) (increased intravascular volume)

BEDSIDE

Quick Look Test

Patients with minor fluid shifts may be asymptomatic, but patients who are severely fluid overloaded may present with pulmonary edema causing tachypnea and hypoxia. Patients with hypoxia will be quite agitated and distressed.

Airway and Vital Signs

The first step in evaluating fluid status is to check the vital signs. Tachypnea may be present in settings of pulmonary edema. If you suspect pulmonary edema, check the oxygenation of the patient with pulse oximetry.

Tachycardia may also be present in fluid overload as the heart attempts to unload the fluid accumulation in the lungs.

Selective History and Chart Review

- Check the input and output measurements (I/Os) for the last day or so. Do not forget the output from drains and tubes. These measurements are notoriously inaccurate but may supply clues. Another clue is the daily weight.
- Has the patient had aggressive fluid resuscitation?
- Does the patient have a disease that would predispose to fluid sequestration?
- How are the renal function and the liver function?
- Is the patient taking medication or therapy that might alter fluid distribution?
- Is the patient improving?
  After a serious illness or major surgery a patient may sequester several liters of fluid by third spacing. This will return to the vascular space during the recovery phase and may cause transient fluid overload.
- Is the patient worsening, or is there a change in fluid status, indicating MI or systemic infection?

Selective Physical Examination

VS:	Tachycardia (pulmonary edema or atrial fibrillation)
MS:	Decreased mental status (hypoxia)
HEENT:	Moist mucous membranes
	Full neck veins

Evaluation of neck veins is often a reasonable assessment of central venous pressure (CVP). When the patient is evaluated while lying down, note the fullness of the external jugular vein. Then slowly raise the head of the bed until the neck veins lose their fullness and pulsations are noted. Note the distance between the point of pulsation and the approximate position of the right atrium on a vertical axis (measure to the sternal notch and add 5 cm; Fig. 12–2). The distance is a gross estimate of the CVP in centimeters of H_2O.

A measurement of 2 to 3 cm above the sternal notch is normal in adults. Patients with fluid overload may have jugular venous distention (JVD) at greater than 3 cm; lesser than 2 cm or consistently flat neck veins despite lying flat indicates fluid depletion.

Resp:	Rales and decreased aeration (fluid overload, congestive heart failure [CHF])
CVS:	S_3, irregular pulse
Abd:	Hepatomegaly (CHF)
Skin:	Dependent edema, especially over the sacrum in supine patients or in the calves of ambulatory patients; edematous skin may be taut.

Additional tests:

1. UA: Low specific gravity supports fluid overload if the kidneys are functioning normally.

Figure 12–2 Measurement of jugular venous pressure. A, The perpendicular distance from the sternal angle to the top of the column of blood; B, the distance from the center of the right atrium to the sternal angle, commonly accepted as measuring 5 cm, regardless of inclination. (From Marshall SA, Ruedy J: On Call: Principles and Protocols, 2nd ed. Philadelphia, WB Saunders, 1993, p. 12.)

2. Electrolytes: To assess for metabolic derangement and elevations in blood urea nitrogen (BUN) and creatinine.

3. Urine Na⁺:   Assessment of renal function (see Table 31–2).

MANAGEMENT

See Chapter 31 for a complete discussion of the fluid-overloaded patient.

Initial Management

1. Support oxygenation as necessary.
2. Order intravenous (IV) access if not already available.

Definitive Management

1. Correct the underlying cause if known.
2. Limit ongoing fluid replacement regimens.
3. If the patient is in respiratory distress, maintain oxygenation and monitor with pulse oximetry. Consider intubation if necessary. Notify your resident.
4. Consider diuretic therapy as outlined in Chapter 31.
5. Rarely, if diuretic therapy is ineffective, hemodialysis may be required.

COMMON FLUID IMBALANCES: THE FLUID-DEPLETED PATIENT

ELEVATOR THOUGHTS

What causes fluid depletion?
See Tables 12–1 and 12–2.

MAJOR THREAT TO LIFE

- Hemodynamic shock

TABLE 12–2 **Etiologies of Fluid Depletion**

GI losses	Vomiting
	Diarrhea
	Nasogastric suction
Urinary losses	Diuretics
	Diabetes mellitus
	Diabetes insipidus
	Osmotic agents (mannitol and hypertonic fluid)
	Postobstructive diuresis
	Adrenal insufficiency
	Mobilization of third-spaced fluid
	Recovery phase of acute tubular necrosis
Insensible losses	Open wounds (e.g., burns; large defects may lose up to 5 L/day)
	Respiratory tract (unhumidified oxygen; hyperventilation may lose up to 1.5 L/day)
	Increased sweating (may lose up to 3 L/day)
Third spacing	Systemic infection
	Pancreatitis
	Ileus
	Burns
	Postoperative
Blood losses	Perioperative
	GI bleeding
	Trauma
Iatrogenic	Insufficient maintenance fluids
	Insufficient replacement of losses
	Frequent blood sampling
Other	Poor PO intake

GI, gastrointestinal; PO, by mouth.

BEDSIDE

Quick Look Test

Patients with minor fluid shifts (<10%) may be asymptomatic. Greater losses are associated with stupor and drowsiness. Major fluid deficit can cause hypotension and shock (see Chapter 17).

Airway and Vital Signs

The first step in evaluating fluid status is to check the vital signs. Orthostatic vital signs are the most useful in determining a deficiency in intravascular volume. Orthostatics are heart rate (HR) and blood pressure (BP) taken while the patient is lying flat, while the patient is sitting, and while the patient is standing. Allow a minute or two to pass between each change in position so the patient may equilibrate. A rise in HR of 15 beats/minute or a drop in systolic blood pressure (SBP) of 15 mm Hg or any drop in diastolic blood pressure with a change in position is evidence of a significant intravascular deficit and may require fluid replacement. Also be mindful of any symptoms that the patient exhibits during changes in position. Dizziness on standing may also indicate loss of intravascular volume. In a young individual, BP is tightly controlled and may be maintained easily with only an increase in pulse rate despite dangerous hypovolemia. In these patients, tachycardia with a stable BP may be the last step before complete cardiovascular collapse. Also, beta blockade may mask increases in HR and result in profound drops in BP on changes in position.

Tachycardia itself is not sufficient to make the diagnosis of intravascular depletion, as it may also be present in fluid overload states.

Selective History and Chart Review

Check the I/Os for the last day or so. This measurement is notoriously inaccurate but may supply clues. Remember that UO is an indication of renal perfusion. Look carefully at the most recent changes in UO. Check the daily weights.

Has the patient had inadequate maintenance fluid replacement?

Does the patient have a disease that would predispose to fluid loss?

How is the renal function? (See Chapter 31.)

Is the patient taking medication or therapy that might alter fluid distribution?

Is the patient worsening, or is there a change in fluid status, indicating sepsis or another form of shock?

Selective Physical Examination

VS:	Tachycardia or postural BP changes (dehydration)
MS:	Decreased mental status (decreased perfusion)
HEENT:	Dry or sticky mucous membranes and flat neck veins (dehydration)
Skin:	Decrease in warmth or turgor and dry axilla (dehydration)
Tubes and drains:	Is the output from these tubes high? Is the output volume being added to replacement fluids?

Additional tests:

1. UA: High specific gravity supports fluid deficit if the kidneys are able to concentrate normally.
2. Electrolytes: To assess for metabolic derangement and elevations in BUN and creatinine (Cr). A BUN/Cr ratio of greater than 12 is an indication of dehydration.
3. CBC: Hemoconcentration
4. Urine Na^+: Assessment of renal function (see Table 31–2)

MANAGEMENT

Also see Chapter 17 for treatment of shock and hypovolemia.

Initial Management

1. Support perfusion and oxygenation as necessary.
2. Order orthostatics if not already done.
3. Order IV access if not already available.

Definitive Management

1. Correct the underlying cause if known (see Table 12–2 for a list of common etiologies).
2. Choose an appropriate fluid to replace the loss.

Gastric loss:	5% dextrose in one-half normal saline (NS) + 30 to 40 mEq/L KCl
Biliary loss:	Lactated Ringer's (LR)
Pancreatic loss:	LR + supplemental HCO_3
Small bowel loss:	LR
Diarrheal loss:	LR or one-half NS + 20 mEq/L KCl + 25 mEq/L HCO_3

3. Replace fluids with the goal of maintaining adequate end-organ perfusion.
4. Choose a rate of rehydration that the patient can tolerate and reevaluate frequently with examinations of respiratory rate (RR), lung fields for rales, skin for adequate perfusion, and I/Os for consistent UO.

REPLACEMENT OF FLUID DEFICITS

The major goal in replacement of fluids to the intravascular space is to maintain an adequate cardiac preload. This helps ensure end-organ perfusion and oxygenation to decrease the risk of ischemia or infarction. Remember that there are other aspects of delivery of oxygen to the end-organs, of which intravascular volume is one (see "Calculation of Oxygen Delivery" in Appendix G). Be sure to optimize the oxygen delivery to the patient, the cardiac output, and the vascular bed tone in addition to replacing the intravascular fluid.

When replacing fluids, there are a variety of products to choose from, and the correct choice is a matter of the pathophysiology of the fluid deficit, the goals of fluid replacement, and the preferences of the primary care team. In general, it is reasonable to rehydrate with a fluid whose characteristics closely match those of the fluid that is being lost. See Table 12–3 for a listing of common gastrointestinal (GI) fluids and their electrolyte compositions. If there is a question, consult the resident or attending physician.

The timing in which the fluid should be replaced is variable, depending on the severity of the deficit, the type of fluid lost, and the ability of the patient to tolerate large volumes of fluid replacement. Shock should be treated aggressively and rapidly until hemodynamics stabilize. Thereafter, further fluid deficits are generally replaced over 24 to 48 hours with the first 50% of the loss being replaced in the first 6 to 8 hours.

Monitoring the progress of the resuscitation is very important. The goal is to find the balance between adequate rehydration and overhydration. Rapid fluid replacement can be associated with peripheral and pulmonary edema and with electrolyte abnormalities. Underhydration may lead to shock. Large-volume fluid resuscitation

TABLE 12–3 **Electrolyte Compositions of Gastrointestinal Fluids**

Type	Na$^-$ (mEq/L)	K$^+$ (mEq/L)	Cl$^-$ (mEq/L)	HCO$_3^-$ (mEq/L)	Volume per Day (L)
Saliva	30	20	35	15	1.5
Gastric					
pH >3	100	10	100	—	2
pH 1–2	25	15	140	—	
Bile	140	5	60–120	30–50	1.5
Pancreatic	140	5	60–90	90–115	1
Small bowel					
Proximal	140	5	130	30	3.5
Distal	90	10	90	40	
Diarrhea	25–130	10–60	20–90	20–50	

should always be accompanied by adequate hemodynamic monitoring and frequent serum electrolyte determinations.

TYPES OF FLUID REPLACEMENT

Red Blood Cells

If the fluid deficit is due to ongoing blood loss, the correct fluid to replace is generally packed red blood cells (RBCs). Whole blood, which replaces plasma volume and RBCs, may not be available at all hospitals but may be reconstructed by the blood bank from packed RBCs and fresh frozen plasma. Always check with the resident before replacing blood or blood products.

Advantages

- Volume replacement
- Oxygen-carrying capacity (lower in banked blood than in fresh blood)

Disadvantages

- Preparation time: requires type and cross, except in cases of an emergency, such as trauma, in which uncrossmatched O type, Rh-negative blood may be used
- Infectious risks: HIV, hepatitis C, and cytomegalovirus (CMV), rarely bacteria
- Costly

Blood Products

These include fresh frozen plasma, cryoprecipitate, albumin, and platelets. They are used as a colloid source of volume expansion and may also replace or fulfill specific deficiencies such as specific blood coagulation factors or thrombocytopenia.

Advantages

- Volume replacement
- Replacement of osmotic pressure
- Concurrent replacement of clotting factors

Disadvantages

- Preparation time: some require special screening in the blood bank
- Infectious risk
- Costly

Colloid

These include dextran 40 or 70, and hetastarch. The goal of colloid administration is to replace fluid and osmotic elements to the intravascular space. Colloids serve to draw fluid from the interstitium by exerting osmotic pressure. They do not carry the risks of infection that blood products do and are more rapidly available. Some colloids are also used to enhance microcirculation by reducing blood viscosity, which may be desirable after revascularization procedures.

Advantages

- Volume replacement
- Replacement of osmotic pressure
- No risk of infection
- Reduction of blood viscosity

Disadvantages

- Preparation time: requires ordering from the pharmacy
- In settings of leaking capillaries, colloid will not remain in the vascular bed, resulting in peripheral or pulmonary edema
- No improvement in oxygen-carrying capacity
- Costly
- May interfere with coagulation

Crystalloid

Crystalloid is the most widely used option because it is available and inexpensive. Even if another fluid is ultimately desirable, it is often worth beginning the volume expansion with crystalloid until the other product becomes available. Because of its easy passage from the intravascular space into the extravascular space, crystalloid replacement tends to take four times the volume to achieve the same expansion of the intravascular space as does colloid. A list of available crystalloid products and their electrolyte compositions are presented in Table 12–4.

Advantages

- Volume replacement
- Inexpensive

TABLE 12–4 **Commonly Used Crystalloid Fluids**

Type	Glucose (g/L)	Na (mEq/L)	K (mEq/L)	Cl (mEq/L)	Ca (mEq/L)	Lactate (mEq/L)	Osm (mOsm/L)
D5W	50	—	—	—	—	—	252
D10W	100	—	—	—	—	—	505
D20W	200	—	—	—	—	—	1010
D50W	500	—	—	—	—	—	2525
NS	—	154	—	154	—	—	308
LR	—	130	4	109	3	28	272

D5W, 5% dextrose in water; D10W, 10% dextrose in water; D20W, 20% dextrose in water; D50W, 50% dextrose in water; NS, normal saline; LR, lactated Ringer's.

- Rapidly available
- No risk of infection

Disadvantages

- In settings of leaking capillaries, crystalloid will not remain in the vascular bed, resulting in peripheral or pulmonary edema
- Poor replacement of osmotic pressure
- No improvement in oxygen-carrying capacity

SPECIAL SURGICAL CONSIDERATIONS

Burn Patients

Adequate fluid resuscitation of patients with severe burn injuries is an important surgical consideration. Fluid losses are tremendous and are due to leakage across capillary membranes into the extravascular space (including into the lungs) and to surface evaporation. IV fluid replacement is indicated in those patients whose burn involves 15% or more of the body surface area (BSA) (10% in children).

There are a variety of resuscitation techniques, and most are based on the patient's body weight and the percentage of BSA involved in the burn. The major difference between the techniques is the timing of colloid administration. The goal of therapy is to supply daily fluid requirements and to replace ongoing losses, to maintain an adequate cardiac output.

A rapid estimation of BSA may be made by following the "rule of nines" (Fig. 12–3), in which body surfaces are roughly divided into 9% regions. Another simple technique is to remember that the palm is roughly 1% of the patient's BSA.

The fluid resuscitation is divided into two time frames, the acute phase (<48 hours) and the subacute phase (>48 hours). In the acute phase, fluid replacement is rapid (Table 12–5). LR solution is commonly used. Some centers advocate the addition of sodium bicarbonate (0.5 ampule/L) to the LR. The absolute volume (2 to 4 mL/kg/% of burned BSA) depends on which actual formula is used (2 to 3 mL/kg/% of BSA = Brooke's revised technique; 3 mL/kg/% of BSA = Duke University technique; 4 mL/kg/% of BSA = Baker and Parkland techniques). As most severe burn patients are initially behind in fluids, it is best to err on the high side (4 mL/kg/% of BSA) and decrease the rate later as UO dictates. Lightning strikes and severe electrical burns may require up to 7 mL/kg/% of BSA.

Deliver the first half of the replacement volume over the first 8 hours postburn (note that the clock starts at the time of the burn, not the time of admission). Deliver the second half of the fluid over the next 16 hours. Over the second 24 hours, attempt to reduce the fluid delivery rate. Do so slowly (25% drop in rate over 3 hours, as tolerated), until the rate equals a volume adequate to deliver maintenance fluids and replace ongoing losses. If the UO drops below

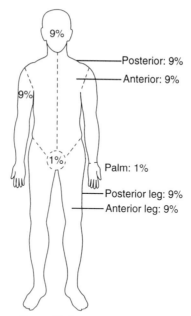

Figure 12–3 The "rule of nines."

30 mL/hour, return to the higher rate and bolus with crystalloid as necessary.

The adequacy of the fluid resuscitation must be closely monitored in the acute phase after a burn:

1. Measure hourly UO.
   - An indwelling urinary catheter is required for severe burns.
   - Maintain the UO at 30 to 50 mL/hour. Adjust the fluid rate based on the UO.
   - If the sodium delivery is too great, consider combining LR therapy with 5% dextrose in water (electrolyte free fluid) to maintain UO.
2. Measure daily body weights.
   - Expect an increase of 10% to 20% of the admission body weight in the first 48 hours after resuscitation. During the

TABLE 12–5 **Fluid Resuscitation Technique for Initial Treatment of Burn Patients During First 24 Hours**

Fluid	Volume	Rate of Administration
Lactated Ringer's	2–4 mL/kg/% BSA	½ over the 1st 8 hr (postburn, **not** postadmission) ½ over the next 16 hr

subacute phase, expect a loss of 1% to 2% of body weight per day for the next 7 to 10 days.

3. Measure pulmonary artery pressures with a Swan-Ganz catheter in selected patients, including the following:
   - Those who do not respond appropriately to initial attempts at resuscitation
   - Those with known cardiopulmonary disease
   - The elderly
4. Use electrolyte and hematologic laboratory data appropriately.
   - The hematocrit will vary due to surface blood loss, to the dilutional effects of the fluid resuscitation, and to the relative bone marrow aplasia due to acute illness; hematocrit is not a very accurate measurement of the adequacy of the fluid resuscitation.
   - Electrolytes should be checked at least every 6 hours during the acute phase of the burn.

Follow also the base deficit from the arterial blood gas (ABG) data. This is a reflection of the serum lactate level and is a good way to follow the efficacy of the resuscitation.

The subacute phase (>48 hours) of burn management still requires fluid replacement. This is due to the ongoing insensible surface losses. The volume of surface losses (in mL/hour) may be estimated by the following formula:

Total BSA (in m^2) × (25 + % of burned BSA). Continue to administer maintenance fluids in addition to replacement fluids for ongoing losses. Follow physiologic parameters of UO, end-organ perfusion, and serum electrolytes.

Colloid is generally withheld in the first 24 to 48 hours because of the severity of the capillary leak. This avoids extravasation of the osmotic agent into the extravascular space. When capillary leakage begins to abate, consider the addition of colloid to the fluid replacement:

1. Confirm that the serum albumin is less than 2.5 g/dL.
2. 50 g albumin/L of NS is equivalent to physiologic levels of protein (5 g/dL).
3. The rate of colloid delivery is also dependent on the severity of the burn; as follows:
   30 to 50% BSA = 0.3 mL/kg/% of BSA over 24 hours
   50 to 70% BSA = 0.4 mL/kg/% of BSA over 24 hours
   Greater than 70% BSA = 0.5 mL/kg/% of BSA over 24 hours.

Burn care is very difficult and requires appropriate initial management as well as complicated long-term therapies. Severe burns are best treated in specified burn units. Indications for referral to a burn facility include the following:

1. Adults with greater than 20% of BSA burns
2. Children with greater than 10% of BSA burns
3. Full-thickness burns of greater than 10% of BSA

4. Burns involving regions of great functional or cosmetic value (face, hands, feet, eyes, ears, and perineum)
5. High-voltage electrical injuries
6. Inhalation injuries
7. Burns associated with other trauma
8. Burns in patients with other severe medical conditions
9. Circumferential limb burns, which are at risk for compartmental syndrome

Remember

1. Rapid infusion of glucose-containing fluid will result in hyperglycemia and may cause an osmotic diuresis, which will be counterproductive to the resuscitative effort.
2. Rapid infusion of NS can result in hyperchloremic metabolic acidosis.
3. Fluid poured into a patient during a resuscitation effort will at some point need to be excreted during the resolution phase of the illness. Anticipate this shift, and be mindful that it may contribute to the cardiac complications of those patients who have marginal myocardial reserve.

COMMON ELECTROLYTE ABNORMALITIES

Sodium (Na⁺)

Normal range: 135 to 147 mmol/L

SODIUM METABOLISM

The serum concentration of sodium is not an indication of total body sodium; it is an indication of fluid status. Disturbances in water balance are evident by derangements in sodium levels. Hyponatremia is an indication of fluid overload, and hypernatremia, of fluid depletion. The signs and symptoms of sodium concentration derangements are more dependent on the rate of change of serum sodium levels than the actual level. Likewise, the rate of correction should be slow, unless severe symptoms are present.

Oral intake of sodium generally more than satisfies the needs of the body. Only about 30 mEq of sodium is lost through stool and sweat per day. The remainder is excreted through urine under the control of aldosterone. In settings of severe water deprivation, sodium is resorbed in exchange for potassium under the control of antidiuretic hormone (ADH). Free water is resorbed with the sodium. The physiologic stimulus for ADH secretion is increased serum osmolality.

Hypernatremia (>147 mmol/L)

Etiology

1. **Inadequate intake of water**
   a. Unconscious patient
   b. Hypothalamic disorder
2. Excessive water loss
   a. Renal losses of water
      (1) Diabetes insipidus (pituitary or renal origin) (UNa variable)
      (2) Osmotic diuresis (hyperglycemia, urea, and mannitol administration) (UNa >20 mEq/L)
   b. Extrarenal losses of water (UNa 10 mEq/L)
      (1) Vomiting and NG suction
      (2) Diarrhea
      (3) Insensible losses (sweating, open wounds, and respiration)
3. Excessive sodium gain (UNa >20 mEq/L)
   a. Iatrogenic (excessive sodium administration)
   b. Primary hyperaldosteronism
   c. Cushing syndrome
   d. Salt tablets
   e. Hypertonic dialysis

Selective Physical Examination

Symptoms of hypernatremia are the result of cellular dehydration in the brain. Other symptoms are secondary to extracellular fluid deficit (see The Fluid Depleted Patient section earlier).

MS:	Confusion, restlessness, irritability, and obtundation
Resp:	Respiratory paralysis
GU:	Polyuria and polydipsia
Neuro:	Muscular irritability, hyperreflexia, ataxia, and seizures

Additional tests:

1. Serum Na: Determine severity
2. Serum osmolality: Aids in diagnosis
3. Urine Na: Aids in diagnosis

Management

1. Determine the severity.
   The therapy is dependent on the patient's condition and symptoms and the results of laboratory studies listed above. Also the rate of development of hypernatremia must be taken into account. Serum osmolality may be measured in the laboratory or may be estimated from other laboratory data using the following formula:

Serum osmolality (mOsm) = 2[Na (mEq/L)]
+ [glucose (mg/dL)]/[18] + [BUN (mg/dL)]/[2.8]

Normal range: 280 to 295 mOsm.

In the absence of fluid deficit or other significant symptoms, and if the serum Na is less than 150 mEq/L, specific therapy may not be warranted.

2. Assess the patient's fluid status.

The effects of hypernatremia are due to cellular dehydration as water is drawn from the cell toward the high osmolality of the extracellular fluid. This is most likely due to an extracellular fluid deficit. An estimation of free water deficit in liters is given by the following formula:

Water deficit (L) =
[serum Na (observed) – serum Na (normal)] [0.6][Wt (kg)]/
[serum Na (normal)]

Assume serum Na (normal) = 140 mEq/L. The 0.6 represents the volume of distribution of sodium, which may be assumed to be the same volume as total body water. Another rapid key to determine fluid deficit is shown in Table 12–6.

3. Correct the fluid deficit.

The rate of fluid deficit replacement is dependent on the rate of development of the hypernatremia. Rapid onset with prominent symptoms should be corrected in several hours. A more chronic development of hypernatremia should be corrected no faster than 2 mOsm/hour to avoid formation of cerebral edema. The fluid of choice is NS until the patient is hemodynamically stable. Then reassess and switch to a more hypotonic solution, such as 5% dextrose in water + ½ NS, until the remainder of the extracellular volume depletion is corrected.

4. Correct the underlying cause.

In a very rare case, hypernatremia is noted in settings of fluid overload. In this case, a loop diuretic such as furosemide (Lasix) may be used to stimulate the excretion of both salt and water.

Special Surgical Considerations

Hypernatremia in surgical patients most likely results from underestimation of free water losses.

TABLE 12–6 **Estimation of Free Water Deficit in Settings of Hypernatremia**

Serum Na (Observed)	Estimated Free Water Deficit
150 mEq/L	50 mL/kg
160 mEq/L	90 mL/kg
170 mEq/L	140 mL/kg

Hyponatremia (>135 mmol/L)

Low serum sodium is a common postoperative problem. A normal physiologic response to surgery is the secretion of ADH from the pituitary gland. This occurs in the absence of hyperosmolar stimuli and may result in mild hemodilution due to the retention of water. This typically lasts for 3 to 5 days after an uncomplicated surgical procedure. This resolves without specific therapy with a physiologic diuresis. In settings of severe hyponatremia (<130 mEq/L), further diagnostic measures are warranted. The first step to diagnosis is to rule out spurious causes such as increased plasma glucose, proteins, or lipids.

Etiology

Hyponatremia may be present in either fluid excess or fluid deficit conditions.

1. Decreased extracellular volume
   a. Renal losses of sodium (UNa >20 mmol/L)
      (1) Diuretic medications
      (2) Mineralocorticoid deficiency
      (3) Salt-losing nephritis
      (4) Osmotic diuresis
      (5) Renal tubular acidosis
      (6) Metabolic acidosis
      (7) Ketonuria
      (8) Bartter syndrome
      (9) Diuretic phase of acute tubular necrosis
   b. Extrarenal losses of sodium (UNa <20 mmol/L)
      (1) GI losses (vomiting, diarrhea, and NG suctioning)
      (2) Sequestration (pancreatitis, peritonitis, and "third spacing")
      (3) Burns
      (4) Traumatized muscle
      (5) Sweating
2. Increased extracellular volume
   a. Acute and chronic renal failure (UNa >20 mmol/L)
   b. Other causes (UNa <20 mmol/L)
      (1) Nephrotic syndrome
      (2) Cirrhosis
      (3) Cardiac failure
3. Normal volume to moderate volume excess (UNa >20 mmol/L)
   a. Glucocorticoid deficiency
      (1) Addison disease
      (2) Inadequate steroid replacement in a steroid-dependent patient
   b. Hypothyroidism
   c. Pain
   d. Emotional stress

    e. Medications
    f. Syndrome of inappropriate ADH secretion (SIADH)
      (1) Tumors (small cell carcinoma of the lung, pancreatic carcinoma, and duodenal adenocarcinoma)
      (2) Central nervous system (CNS) disorders (tumor, trauma, meningitis, and encephalitis)
      (3) Pulmonary disorders (pneumonia and tuberculosis)
      (4) Medications (chlorpropamide, clofibrate, cyclophosphamide, vincristine, carbamazepine, narcotics, and tricyclic antidepressants)
    g. Pseudohyponatremia
      (1) With normal serum osmolality
        (a) Hyperlipidemia
        (b) Hyperproteinemia
      (2) With increased serum osmolality
        (a) Hyperglycemia
        (b) Urea
        (c) Mannitol administration
        (d) Alcohol (ethanol, methanol, and isopropyl alcohol)
        (e) Ethylene glycol

Major Threat to Life

It is the overly rapid correction of hyponatremia that is a threat to life. One response to hyponatremia is the export of solute from the cell to maintain volume. If the extracellular fluid in the brain becomes too hypertonic relative to the cells during correction, a net shift of fluid outward can cause cellular dehydration. The result can be central pontine myelinolysis. A slow correction is necessary to avoid cerebral damage. Do not exceed a rate of 2 mEq/L/hour.

Selective Physical Examination

MS: Lethargy, apathy, disorientation, agitation, and coma
Neuro: Weakness, decreased deep tendon reflexes (DTRs), and seizures

Additional tests:

1. Serum Na:	Determine severity
2. Serum osmolality:	Aids in diagnosis
3. Serum glucose:	Rule out pseudohyponatremia (Each increase in serum glucose of 100 mg/dL above normal decreases serum Na by 0.4 mEq/L.)
4. Serum protein:	Rule out pseudohyponatremia
5. Serum lipids:	Rule out pseudohyponatremia
6. Urine Na:	Aids in diagnosis

Management

1. Determine the severity.

The therapy is dependent on the patient's condition and symptoms and the results of laboratory studies are listed earlier. Also, the rate of development of hyponatremia must be taken into account. In the absence of fluid deficit or other significant symptoms, specific therapy may not be warranted.

2. Assess the patient's fluid status.
3. Correct fluid deficit (if present).

The rate of fluid deficit replacement is dependent on the rate of development of the hyponatremia. Initial correction of severe hyponatremia (<110 mEq/L) should not go beyond 120 to 125 mEq/L and should not exceed a correction rate of 2 mEq/L/hour to avoid cerebral dehydration and irreversible brain damage. The fluid of choice is NS until the patient is hemodynamically stable. If the patient is hyponatremic with a metabolic acidosis, consider replacement with sodium lactate (M/6 fluid). Then reassess and switch to a more hypotonic solution, such as 5% dextrose in water + ½ NS, until the remainder of the extracellular volume depletion is corrected.

4. Replace sodium if necessary.

Especially useful in settings of fluid deficit. Estimation of sodium deficit is calculated by the following formula:

[serum Na (desired) – serum Na (observed)] [0.6] [Wt (kg)]

Use 135 mEq/L as the serum Na (desired) as it represents the low end of normal serum sodium concentration. The method and rate of sodium replacement is dependent on the severity of the hyponatremia. In general, replace one-half of the deficit over 8 hours and the remaining one-half over the next 16 hours. Table 12–7 shows the sodium concentration of various preparations of saline. In rare cases, such as seizure associated with hyponatremia, it may be necessary to treat with hypertonic saline. Administer 3% saline at a rate of 2 mEq/L/hour until the serum sodium concentration is greater than 125 mEq/L or until the seizure activity stops.

5. Treat fluid excess (if necessary).

This may be accomplished with fluid restriction and the administration of diuretics. In settings of hyponatremia, a minimally salt wasting diuretic such as **spironolactone**

TABLE 12–7 **Sodium Concentrations in Various Saline Preparations**

Normal saline (0.9%)	157 mEq/L
Sodium lactate (M/6)	167 mEq/L
Lactated Ringer's	130 mEq/L
3% saline	500 mEq/L
5% saline	850 mEq/L

(Aldactone) is recommended. An initial dose of 100 mg is recommended, with daily doses ranging from 25 to 200 mg PO. The diuretic effects may be delayed by 2 to 3 days.
6. Correct the underlying cause.
    Specific disorders that require further treatment include SIADH and forms of pseudohyponatremia.

SIADH

This is a condition in which nonosmotic stimuli are responsible for the release of ADH. The possible causes are listed under the etiology of hyponatremia. The diagnosis is dependent on the following criteria:
1. Hyponatremia with low serum osmolality
2. Nonmaximal urine dilution despite serum hypo-osmolality
3. UNa >20 mmol/L
4. Normally functioning kidneys
5. Normally functioning thyroid
6. No diuretic therapy
Management measures include
1. Correction of the underlying cause
2. Water restriction to less than insensible losses (500 to 1000 mL/day)
3. In settings of severe hyponatremia (<115 mEq/L)
    Diuretic therapy with **furosemide (Lasix) 20 to 40 mg IV every 2 to 4 hours**
    Demeclocycline (Declomycin) 300 to 600 mg PO twice daily may be useful in patients with chronic SIADH/in which water restriction has not been effective.

Pseudohyponatremia

The many causes of pseudohyponatremia are listed under the etiologies of hyponatremia. The diagnosis is made by identifying the agent that is displacing sodium from the blood stream. As an example, an increase of 62 mg of glucose can cause a 1 mEq drop in plasma sodium. Pseudohyponatremia may be associated with a normal serum osmolality as with hyperproteinemia or hyperlipidemia; or it may be associated with an increased serum osmolality. Look for an "osmolar gap." Osmolar gap is the difference between the laboratory-measured osmolality and the osmolality calculated by hand using glucose and BUN concentrations (see page 129). If the osmolar gap is greater than 10 mmol/L, look for other osmotically active agents in the serum. Note that there may be an osmolar gap even if the serum osmolality is normal. The treatment of pseudohyponatremia depends on the underlying disease.

Of special note is hyperglycemia. In such cases, the true serum sodium concentration may be determined using the following formula:

$$\text{Actual serum Na} = [\text{glucose (observed)} - \text{glucose (normal)}]$$
$$[1.4]/[\text{glucose (normal)}] + \text{serum Na (observed)}$$

Correction of the hyperglycemia will tend to correct the hyponatremia.

Special Surgical Considerations

Surgical procedures that may be associated with postoperative hyponatremia include the following:

1. Spinal fusion surgery (20%)
2. Subtotal gastrectomy (67%)
3. Enterocutaneous biliary drainage (22%)
4. Mitral valve surgery (30%)
5. Trauma surgery (40%)

Potassium (K^+)

Normal range: 3.5 to 5 mmol/L. Daily requirement: 1 mEq/kg/day

POTASSIUM METABOLISM

Total stores of potassium are in the range of 50 to 55 mEq/kg; 98% of the potassium is intracellular. Intracellular concentrations are about 150 mEq/L, and extracellular concentrations are about 3.5 to 5 mEq/L with this gradient maintained by the Na^+/K^+-ATPase pump. Normal intake averages about 100 mEq/day with 95% excretion through the kidneys, and 5% loss through stool and sweat. Most of the potassium filtered through the glomerulus is resorbed in the proximal renal tubule. The site of potassium control is at the distal renal tubule where selective resorption and secretion takes place. Potassium excretion is under the control of aldosterone, plasma potassium levels, and glomerular filtration rates.

Acid–base imbalance also exerts a control on the ratios of intracellular and extracellular potassium. Alkalosis enhances excretion of potassium in exchange for resorption of H^+ and Na^+ ions in the distal renal tubule. Acidosis enhances renal conservation of K^+ in the distal tubule. High concentrations of H^+ ion also may displace intracellular K^+, causing an apparent hyperkalemia.

Hyperkalemia (>5 mmol/L)

Etiology

1. Excessive intake
   a. Iatrogenic supplementation (IV or PO)
   b. Salt substitutes
   c. High-dose potassium penicillin therapy
   d. Blood transfusions

2. Decreased excretion
   a. Renal failure (acute or chronic)
   b. Potassium-sparing diuretics (amiloride, spironolactone, and triamterene)
   c. Addison disease
   d. Hypoaldosteronism
   e. Distal tubular dysfunction
3. Fluid shifts of intracellular to extracellular
   a. Acidemia
   b. Insulin deficiency
   c. Tissue destruction (hemolysis, crush injuries, rhabdomyolysis, burns, and tumor lysis)
   d. Medications (arginine, beta-blockers, digoxin, and succinylcholine)
   e. Hyperkalemic periodic paralysis
4. Factitious
   a. Prolonged tourniquet application before blood draw
   b. Hemolysis of blood sample
   c. Leukocytosis
   d. Thrombocytosis

Major Threat to Life

Cardiac arrhythmias are the major threat to life.

Selective Physical Examination

CVS:	Fatal arrhythmias
Neuro:	Weakness, paresthesias, depressed DTRs
Additional tests:	
ECG:	The rhythm manifestations progress relative to the severity of the hyperkalemia (Fig. 12–4)
	Peaked T waves
	Depressed ST segments
	Decreased R wave amplitude
	Prolonged PR interval
	Small or absent P waves
	Wide QRS complexes
	Sine wave pattern

Management

1. Assess the severity.
   Perform a 12-lead electrocardiogram (ECG) and serum potassium level immediately. The degree of hyperkalemia dictates how aggressive the therapy should be.
2. Perform continuous cardiac monitoring.
   This should be continued for 24 hours after the resolution of the hyperkalemia. Fatal arrhythmias may occur at any time during therapy and at seemingly small increases in serum potassium.

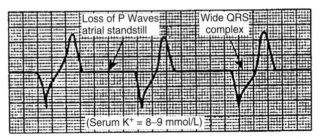

Figure 12–4 Progressive electrocardiographic manifestations of hyperkalemia.
(From Marshall SA, Ruedy J: On Call: Principles and Protocols, 2nd ed. Philadelphia, WB Saunders, 1993, p. 310.)

3. Correct the underlying cause, if known.
4. Remove potassium from IV fluids, if present.
   Discontinue or replace potassium-containing medications.
5. If the hyperkalemia is mild (<6.5 mEq/L)
   Consider continuous cardiac monitoring.
   Recheck the serum potassium every 4 to 6 hours until stabilized.
6. If the hyperkalemia is moderate (6.5 to 8 mEq/L)
   Perform continuous cardiac monitoring.
   Recheck the serum potassium every 1 to 2 hours until the serum potassium level stabilizes at less than 6.5 mEq/L.
   Administer one or more of the following:

a. **NaHCO$_3$, 1 ampule (44.6 mmol) IV**
    This shifts the potassium from the extracellular space into the intracellular space. The effect is immediate and lasts 1 to 2 hours.
b. Glucose and insulin
    50% dextrose in water, 50 mL IV, followed by **regular insulin 5 to 10 units IV.** This therapy shifts potassium from the extracellular space into the intracellular space. The effect is immediate and lasts 1 to 2 hours.
c. The glucose, insulin, and bicarbonate may be administered together as a cocktail.
    Add 3 ampules of NaHCO$_3$ and 20 units of regular insulin to 1000 mL 20% dextrose in water.
    Administer at 75 mL/hour as other therapies are being instituted.
d. **Sodium polystyrene sulfonate (Kayexalate)**
    15 to 30 g (4 to 8 tsp) in 50 to 100 mL of 20% sorbitol
    or
    20% dextrose in water administered PO every 3 to 4 hours, or 50 g in 200 mL 20% sorbitol or
    20% dextrose in water administered as a retention enema for 30 to 60 minutes every 4 hours. This is the only therapy that removes potassium from the body. The resin exchanges potassium for sodium.
7. If the hyperkalemia is severe (>8 mEq/L)
   • Perform continuous cardiac monitoring.
   • Notify your resident.
   • Recheck the serum potassium every 1 to 2 hours until the serum potassium level stabilizes at less than 6.5 mEq/L.
   Administer one or more of the following:
   a. NaHCO$_3$, **1 ampule (44.6 mmol) IV**
   b. Glucose and insulin
       50% dextrose in water 50 mL IV followed by **regular insulin 5 to 10 units IV.**
   c. Glucose, insulin, and bicarbonate cocktail
       Add **3 ampules of NaHCO$_3$** and 20 units of regular insulin to 1000 mL 20% dextrose in water. Administer at 75 mL/hour as other therapies are being instituted.
   d. **Sodium polystyrene sulfonate (Kayexalate) 15 to 30 g (4 to 8 tsp) in 50 to 100 mL of 20% sorbitol** or
       20% dextrose in water administered **PO every 3 to 4 hours,** or 50 g in 200 mL 20% sorbitol or
       20% dextrose in water administered as a retention enema for **30 to 60 minutes every 4 hours.**
   e. **Calcium gluconate 5 to 10 mL 10% solution IV over 2 minutes**
       This temporarily stabilizes the myocardial and neuromuscular effects of the hyperkalemia. Note that this therapy will not affect the serum potassium level. Hemodialysis

therapy is reserved for patients in renal failure or for whom the earlier measures have proved ineffective.

Hypokalemia (>3.5 mmol/L)

Because of fluid shifts associated with fluid resuscitation and surgical illness, hypokalemia is a common problem. The drop in the serum potassium level from 4 to 3 mEq/dL can represent a total body potassion deficit in the 100- to 200-mEq range. A drop from 3 to 2 mEq/dL represents an additional 200- to 400-mEq deficit.

Etiology

1. Renal losses (UK >20 mEq/day)
   a. Diuretic therapy
   b. Osmotic diuresis
   c. Antibiotic therapy (aminoglycosides, amphotericin, carbenicillin, nafcillin, and ticarcillin)
   d. Renal tubular acidosis (type I)
   e. Hyperaldosteronism
   f. Glucocorticoid excess
   g. Magnesium deficiency
   h. Chronic metabolic alkalosis
   i. Bartter syndrome
   j. Fanconi syndrome
   k. Ureterosigmoidostomy
   l. GI losses (vomiting and NG suctioning) due to the loss of hydrogen ions resulting in alkalosis
2. Extrarenal losses (UK <20 mEq/day)
   a. Diarrhea
   b. Intestinal fistulas
   c. Villous adenoma of the rectum
3. Inadequate potassium intake
4. Fluid shift from extracellular space to intracellular space
   a. Acute alkalosis (hyperventilation, GI losses, intestinal fistulas)
   b. Insulin therapy
   c. Vitamin B12 therapy
   d. Hypokalemic periodic paralysis
   e. Medications (lithium and salbutamol)

Major Threat to Life

Cardiac arrhythmias are the major threat to life.

Selective Physical Examination

CVS:	Premature atrial contractions (PACs) and premature ventricular contractions (PVCs); digoxin toxicity
Abd:	Paralytic ileus
Neuro:	Weakness, paresthesias, and depressed DTRs

Additional tests:

1. ECG:	The following findings may be present (Fig. 12–5): T wave flattening U waves Depression of ST waves
2. ABG:	Metabolic alkalosis
3. Serum Ca^{2+}:	Hypokalemia and hypocalcemia may coexist
4. Serum Mg^{2+}:	Hypokalemia and hypomagnesemia may coexist

Management

1. Assess the severity.

   Obtain a 12-lead ECG and a serum potassium level immediately.

2. Consider cardiac monitoring, especially if there is coexistent hypocalcemia.

3. Correct the underlying cause, if known.

   If the hypokalemia coexists with another electrolyte derangement, failure to correct the other deficiency will complicate the correction of the low serum potassium.

4. If the hypokalemia is mild (3.1 to 3.5 mEq/L, without severe cardiac arrhythmias)

   • Give oral potassium supplementation (see Table 12–8 for options).

   • Recheck serum potassium in the morning.

5. If the hypokalemia is moderate (<3 mEq/L, with PACs but infrequent PVCs)

   • Notify your resident.

   • Give oral potassium supplementation.

   • Give IV potassium supplementation.

   • Reserve this option for severe hypokalemia or for those patients who are unable to tolerate oral potassium.

   • Recheck serum potassium in the morning.

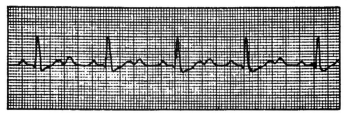

Figure 12–5 Electrocardiographic manifestations of hypokalemia. (From Marshall SA, Ruedy J: On Call: Principles and Protocols, 2nd ed. Philadelphia, WB Saunders, 1993, p. 313.)

TABLE 12–8 **Oral Potassium Supplements**

Slow-K	8 mEq/Tablet
Micro-K Extencaps	8 mEq/Tablet
Micro-K 10 Extencaps	10 mEq/Tablet
Kay Ciel liquid	20 mEq/15 mL
K-Lyte	25 mEq/packet
Banana	1 mEq/inch

6. If the hypokalemia is severe (<3 mEq/L, with frequent PVCs or digoxin toxicity)
   - Notify your resident.
   - Obtain continuous cardiac monitoring.
   - Give bolus IV potassium replacement.
     Give **10 mEq KCl in 100 mL 5% dextrose in water administered over 1 hour.** IV potassium in high concentrations is best delivered through central venous access, as severe burning and thrombophlebitis can occur if it is delivered through a peripheral vein.
   - Give continuous IV potassium replacement.
     KCl may be added to intravenous fluids (IVF) to final concentrations of **40 to 60 mEq/L, which may be delivered at rates up to 20 mEq/hour.**
   - Recheck serum potassium levels after every 20 to 30 mEq replaced and in the morning.
     Frequent monitoring is required to avoid iatrogenic hyperkalemia.

Calcium (Ca²⁺)

Normal range (total): 2.2 to 2.6 mmol/L
Normal range (ionized): 1.12 to 1.23 mmol/L

CALCIUM METABOLISM

Calcium is absorbed from the GI tract under control of vitamin D. Once absorbed, Ca^{2+} is deposited and resorbed from the bones under the control of vitamin D and parathyroid hormone (PTH).

Approximately 40% of serum calcium is bound by albumin. An additional 10% is bound as a complexing ion. The remaining 50% is free ionized Ca^{2+}, which is the physiologically available form. Hypoalbuminemia can result in factitious hypocalcemia if the **total** Ca^{2+} is measured. Measurement of **ionized** Ca^{2+} will circumvent this problem. To correct for aberrations in albumin level, use the following formula:

Add 0.2 mmol/L Ca^{2+} to the measured total Ca^{2+} value for every 1 g/L less than normal albumin (assume a normal albumin of 4 g/L).

Hypercalcemia (>2.6 mmol/L)

Etiology

1. Increased intake or absorption
   a. Vitamin D or A intoxication
   b. Excessive calcium supplementation
   c. Milk-alkali syndrome (excessive antacid ingestion)
   d. Sarcoidosis or other granulomatous disease
2. Increased mobilization from bone
   a. Primary hyperthyroidism
   b. Severe secondary hyperthyroidism associated with renal failure
   c. Neoplasm
      (1) Bony metastasis (prostate, breast, thyroid, kidney, and lung)
      (2) PTH-like substance secreted by tumor (lung, kidney, ovary, and colon)
      (3) Increased bony resorption mediated by prostaglandin E2
      (4) Osteoclast-stimulating factor (due to multiple myeloma and lymphoproliferative disorders)
   d. Paget's disease
   e. Long-term immobilization
   f. Hyperthyroidism
   g. Adrenal insufficiency
   h. Acromegaly
   i. Sarcoidosis; in addition to increased absorption from the GI tract, sarcoidosis increases conversion of 25-(OH) vitamin D to 1,25-$(OH)_2$ vitamin D
   j. Chronic lithium use
3. Decreased excretion
   a. Thiazide diuretics
   b. Familial hypocalciuric hypercalcemia.

Major Threat to Life

Bradycardia and complete heart block are the major threats to life.

Selective Physical Examination

VS:	Bradycardia
MS:	Insomnia, restlessness, delirium, dementia, lethargy, and coma
HEENT:	Corneal calcification
CVS:	Bradycardia, dysrhythmias, hypertension, and digoxin sensitivity
Abd:	GI upset, anorexia, nausea, vomiting, constipation, and pancreatitis
GU:	Polyuria, polydipsia, and nephrolithiasis
Neuro:	Muscle weakness, hyporeflexia, bone pain, and pathologic fractures

Additional tests:

1. ECG: Shortened QT interval and prolonged PR interval (Fig. 12–6)
2. ABG: May show hyperchlorhydric metabolic acidosis
3. PTH: If no known malignancy is found, a serum PTH should be drawn. A high PTH is indicative of hyperparathyroidism; a low PTH requires workup for occult malignancy.

Management

1. Determine the severity.

   Treatment is determined by the absolute calcium level. Severe symptoms generally appear above total Ca^{2+} levels of 3.2 mmol/L. Be mindful of recent trends or symptoms. A rapid or continuous rise in Ca^{2+} will require immediate treatment, as will a symptomatic patient.

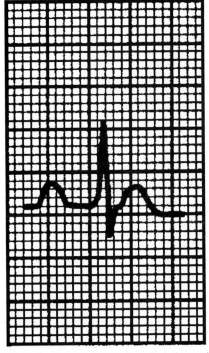

Figure 12–6 Hypercalcemia (short QT interval, prolonged PR interval). (From Marshall SA, Ruedy J: On Call: Principles and Protocols, 2nd ed. Philadelphia, WB Saunders, 1993, p. 287.)

2. If the hypercalcemia is mild (2.6 to 2.9 mmol/L)
   - Expand volume.
   - Administer a **500-mL NS bolus IV** as rapidly as possible. Expansion of the intravascular space will bring the Ca^{2+} level down by hemodilution. Further fluid boluses may be given depending on the patient's fluid status.
   - Take care in rehydrating a patient with a history of CHF.
   - Recheck the serum calcium in the morning.
3. If the hypercalcemia is moderate (2.9 to 3.2 mmol/L)
   - Expand volume.
   - Induce diuresis (UO of >2500 mL/day is sufficient).
   - **Furosemide (Lasix)** in doses of **20 to 40 mg IV every 2 to 4 hours** should be sufficient to ensure that UO should be greater than 2500 mL/day. Continue to maintain volume expansion during the diuresis; do not get behind in fluid administration. Furosemide has the additional advantage of inhibiting calcium absorption in the renal tubule.
   - Thiazide diuretics are not desirable, as they will elevate serum calcium levels.
   - Closely follow serum K^+ and Mg^{2+} levels.
   - Recheck serum calcium in 4 to 6 hours and in the morning.
4. If the hypercalcemia is severe (>3.2 mmol/L, or if the patient is symptomatic)
   - Expand volume.
   - Induce diuresis.
   - Perform dialysis, useful for severe hypercalcemia (>4.5 mmol/L).
   - Give medications.

   One or more of the following medications are useful in the treatment of severe hypercalcemia:
   a. **Disodium etidronate** (EHDP) **(Biphosphonate)** inhibits bone resorption of Ca^{2+} **(5 to 10 mg/kg/day IV over 2 hours for 3 days)**, followed by a repeat course in 7 days if necessary; longer term therapy may be maintained with **20 mg/kg/day PO for 30 days.**
   b. **Plicamycin (Mithracin)** inhibits bone resorption of Ca^{2+} **(15 to 25 mcg/kg in 1 L NS over 3 to 6 hours).** (This is not an acute acting medication; the onset of action is delayed by 48 hours. Calcium nadir is expected at 60 hours, and the effects may last days to weeks.)
   c. **Phosphate (Fleet Phospho-Soda)** causes Ca^{2+} to be removed from the blood and deposited in extravascular tissues; it should be given to any patient whose serum PO_4^- is less than 1 mmol/L, and whose kidneys are working well **(5 mL PO 3 to 4 times daily** until serum PO_4^- is 1.6 mmol/L).
   d. **Prednisone** decreases Ca^{2+} absorption in malignancy and may have antitumor effects **(10 to 25 mg PO every 6 hours).**

(This is not an acute acting medication; effects are noted in 2 to 3 days.)

e. **Calcitonin** decreases bone resorption **(4 U/kg IV followed by 4 U/kg SC every 12 hours).** (Not effective in 25% of patients.)

f. **Indomethacin (Indocin)** is used for hypercalcemia associated with malignancy, and it inhibits the synthesis of prostaglandin E_2 **(50 mg PO every 8 hours).**

Recheck serum Ca^{2+} and PO_4^- levels as well as other appropriate laboratory studies to monitor hydration.

Hypocalcemia (>2.2 mmol/L)

Etiology

1. Decreased intake or absorption
   a. Malabsorption
   b. Intestinal bypass surgery
   c. Short bowel syndrome
   d. Vitamin D deficiency
2. Decreased production or mobilization from bone
   a. Hypoparathyroidism (after subtotal thyroidectomy or parathyroidectomy)
   b. Pseudohypoparathyroidism
   c. Vitamin D deficiency (decreased production of 25-(OH) vitamin D or 1,25-(OH)$_2$ vitamin D)
   d. Acute hyperphosphatemia (tumor lysis syndrome, acute renal failure, and rhabdomyolysis)
   e. Acute pancreatitis
   f. Hypomagnesemia
   g. Alkalosis (hyperventilation, GI losses, and intestinal fistulas)
   h. Neoplasm
      (1) Paradoxical hypocalcemia associated with osteoblastic metastases from lung, breast, or prostate cancer
      (2) Medullary carcinoma of the thyroid (calcitonin-producing tumor)
      (3) Tumor lysis syndrome
3. Increased excretion
   a. Chronic renal failure
   b. Medications (aminoglycosides and loop diuretics)

Major Threat to Life

Fatal arrhythmia is the major threat to life.

Selective Physical Examination

MS: Confusion, irritability, and depression
HEENT: Papilledema and diplopia

Stridor (laryngospasm)	Abdominal cramping
Abd:	
Neuro:	Paresthesias of the fingers and toes
Special examinations:	Increased DTRs, carpopedal spasm tetany, and seizures

1. *Chvostek's sign:* Facial muscle spasm elicited by light tapping on the facial nerve at the angle of the jaw; may be a normal finding in about 10% of the population despite normal calcium levels.
2. *Trousseau's sign:* Carpal spasm elicited by placement of a blood pressure cuff on the arm and inflation to above SBP for 3 to 5 minutes. (This is often a painful test for the patient.)

Additional tests:
1. ECG: Prolonged QT interval without U waves (Fig. 12–7).

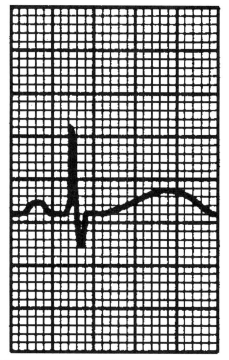

Figure 12–7 Hypocalcemia (long QT interval).
(From Marshall SA, Ruedy J: On Call: Principles and Protocols, 2nd ed. Philadelphia, WB Saunders, 1993, p. 290.)

Management

1. Assess the severity.

    Measure serum calcium and albumin levels. Correct for low albumin as earlier. Asymptomatic patients do not require aggressive therapy.

2. Measure the serum phosphate level.

    If the level is severely elevated (>6 mmol/L), correct the hyperphosphatemia with glucose and insulin therapy, as described with hyperkalemia above, before replacing calcium. The calcium and phosphate in the blood stream can ionically bind and deposit into tissues. This is most often associated with renal failure, and nephrology service consultation may be required.

3. If the hypocalcemia is mild (total calcium = 1.9 to 2.2 mmol/L)
    - Give oral replacement of calcium with 1000 to 1500 mg/day PO.
    - Recheck serum calcium at daily to weekly intervals.

4. If the hypocalcemia is moderate (total calcium = 1.5 to 1.9 mmol/L)
    - Give oral replacement of calcium with 1000 to 1500 mg/day PO.
    - Recheck serum calcium at daily to weekly intervals.
    - Evaluate further as warranted.

5. If the hypocalcemia is severe (total calcium <1.5 mmol/L, or if the patient is symptomatic)
    - Perform continuous cardiac monitoring.
    - Special caution is required for patients taking digoxin as calcium will potentiate its effects.
    - Contact your resident.
    - Confirm a normal to low serum PO_4^-.
    - Give bolus IV replacement of calcium.
    - Give calcium gluconate (10 to 20 mL of 10% solution [1 to 2 g] in 100 mL 5% dextrose in water given IV over 30 minutes). This dose may be given without dilution as rapidly as over 2 minutes if symptoms of tetany or laryngospasm are apparent.
    - Perform continuous IV replacement of calcium.
    - If the serum calcium level is still <1.9 mmol/L after 6 hours, start a continuous drip with **calcium gluconate (10 mL of a 10% solution [1 g] diluted into 500 mL 5% dextrose in water, infused IV over 6 hours).**
    - If the serum calcium has not normalized after 6 hours of the continuous infusion, **add 15 mL of the 10% solution (1.5 g) to the next 500 mL 5% dextrose in water and infuse IV over 6 hours.**
    - Give oral replacement of calcium.

- Give **200 mg elemental calcium PO every 2 hours for 4 doses.** This may be started at the same time as the bolus IV injection.
- Recheck serum calcium levels every 6 hours.

Special Surgical Considerations

The patient who has undergone subtotal thyroidectomy or parathyroidectomy may require replacement of **1 to 1.5 g calcium gluconate/hour. This may be achieved by continuous drip of calcium gluconate. Add 100 mL of a 10% solution (10 g) to 500 mL 5% dextrose in water and run at 50 mL/hour (1 g/hour).**

Often thyroidectomy patients can manage their own mild postoperative hypocalcemia by taking an oral supplement made available at the bedside (such as 1 or 2 chewable Tums) when they notice symptoms of circumoral or fingertip tingling. Make sure to have the bedside caregiver monitor the quantity of calcium consumed. Long-term calcium supplementation is rarely required.

Magnesium (Mg^{2+})

Normal range: 1.3 to 2.1 mEq/L (65% to 70% is in the ionized state).

MAGNESIUM METABOLISM

Magnesium is required for proper function of many cellular mechanisms including the Na^+/K^+-ATPase pump. Derangements in magnesium levels should be sought in conditions associated with abnormalities in potassium or calcium concentrations.

Hypermagnesemia (>2.1 mEq/L)

Etiology

1. Medications
   a. Lithium
   b. Magnesium-containing drugs in settings of renal failure
2. Tumor metastases to bone
3. Hypothyroidism
4. Viral hepatitis
5. Acidosis

Major Threat to Life

Respiratory depression is the major threat to life.

Selective Physical Examination

Symptoms generally do not become apparent until the level is greater than 4 mEq/L.

VS:	Bradycardia
CVS:	Hypotension
Resp:	Respiratory depression
Abd:	Nausea and vomiting
Skin:	Flushing
Neuro:	Loss of DTRs, and muscular paralysis

Management

1. Identify and eliminate the magnesium source.
2. Give **calcium gluconate (or CaCl$_2$) (100 to 200 mg IV over 5 to 10 minutes).** Effects are immediate but transient.
3. Provide dialysis for cases of severe hypermagnesemia, especially in settings of renal failure.
4. Avoid magnesium in the future.

Hypomagnesemia (<1.3 mEq/L)

Etiology

Hypomagnesemia is most commonly due to urinary or GI losses.
1. Diminished PO intake
   a. Malabsorption
   b. Malnutrition (prolonged IV therapy and alcoholism)
2. GI losses
   a. Chronic diarrhea (laxative abuse, gastroenteritis, and inflammatory bowel disease)
   b. High outputs from fistulas and NG drainage
   c. Emesis
3. Medications that increase urinary losses
   a. Cisplatin
   b. Digoxin
   c. Aminoglycosides
   d. Amphotericin B
   e. Diuretics (loop, thiazide)
   f. Cyclosporine

Major Threat to Life

Ventricular arrhythmia is the major threat to life.

Selective Physical Examination

MS:	Confusion, mood alteration, psychosis, and coma
HEENT:	Nystagmus
CVS:	Arrhythmias and digoxin toxicity
Abd:	Anorexia, vomiting, and difficulty in swallowing
Neuro:	Paresthesias, tremors, weakness, vertigo, ataxia, and seizures

Management

1. Treat acute magnesium deficiencies.
   Give **magnesium sulfate 2 g (8 mEq/g as a 20% solution) IV over 2 to 5 minutes, followed by 10 g IV over the next 24 hours, followed by 4 to 6 g/day IV or PO for the next 4 to 5 days.** Kidneys must be functioning normally.
2. Treat chronic magnesium deficiencies.
   Give **magnesium sulfate 3 to 6 g/day IV or PO for the next 3 days.** Kidneys must be functioning normally.
3. Provide prophylactic therapy.
   Magnesium sulfate 1 to 2 g/day may be added to IV fluids. Kidneys must be functioning normally.

COMMON ACID–BASE ABNORMALITIES

The normal buffering systems of the body (bicarbonate, hemoglobin, phosphate, and protein) are frequently overwhelmed by disease states. Excess acid (acidosis) or insufficient acid (alkalosis) in the blood stream may have metabolic or respiratory etiologies. The differentiation of respiratory causes from metabolic causes is often easily achieved by proper interpretation of the arterial blood gas (ABG) data. Recall that the bicarbonate data on an ABG are calculated values derived from the Henderson–Hasselbach equation (Table 12–9). If an accurate diagnosis is desired, a serum bicarbonate level should be sent to the laboratory in addition to the ABG.

Acid–base abnormalities may occur singly or in combination (mixed disorders). An algorithm describing the common findings in various simple acid–base states is detailed in Table 12–10. For each primary aberration (change in partial pressure of carbon dioxide [PCO_2] or bicarbonate [HCO_3^-] concentration) there is a compensatory response by the body, which abates the effects of pH. Rapid responses occur in the lung with modulation of the respiratory rate (RR); slower responses occur in the kidney with alterations in the absorption or excretion of bicarbonate.

ACIDOSIS (pH <7.35)

A small volume of acid (approximately 70 mEq) is added to the body daily. This is generally excreted by the kidney. The major load

TABLE 12–9 **The Henderson-Hasselbach Equation**

pH = 6.1 + log [HCO_3^- (mEq/L)/0.03 × PCO_2 (mm Hg)]

TABLE 12–10 **Blood Gas Data in Various Simple Acid–Base Abnormalities**

	Initial Finding	Compensatory Finding	Resultant pH
Acidosis (pH ≤7.35)			
Metabolic	↓ [HCO$_3$]	↓ PCO$_2$	↑
Respiratory	↑ PCO$_2$	↑ [HCO$_3$]	↑
Alkalosis (pH ≥7.45)			
Metabolic	↑ [HCO$_3$]	↑ PCO$_2$	↓
Respiratory	↓ PCO$_2$	↓ [HCO$_3$]	↓

of total body acid is the result of oxidative metabolism (approximately 22,000 mEq/day) and is excreted as CO_2 by the lungs. An additional 50 to 100 mEq soluble acid/day is created as H_3PO_4 and H_2SO_4 during protein catabolism. Conversion of the soluble acid to volatile acid is according to the following equation:

$$CO_2 + H_2O \leftrightarrow H_2CO_3 \leftrightarrow H^+ + HCO_3^-$$

Acidosis is defined as arterial pH of lesser than 7.35. Causes include respiratory etiologies such as hypoventilation and metabolic etiologies such as excess acid or decreased bicarbonate in the serum. Rapid compensation to acidosis is respiratory with an increased respiratory rate. More chronic compensation occurs in the kidneys where bicarbonate is synthesized. The renal response takes 12 hours to become apparent and is maximum at 3 to 5 days.

Respiratory Acidosis

Etiology

Respiratory acidosis results from the accumulation of CO_2 in the blood stream due to hypoventilation. Etiologies include the following:

1. CNS depression
    a. Medications (residual anesthesia, narcotics, and benzodiazepines)
    b. Primary brain lesions in the respiratory centers
2. Neuromuscular disorders
    a. Medications (paralytics)
    b. Primary muscular disease
    c. Hypokalemia and hypophosphatemia
    d. Primary neuropathies
3. Respiratory disorders
    a. Acute airway obstruction (sleep apnea or aspiration)
    b. Severe lung parenchymal disease (especially with oxygen delivery, which may inhibit respiratory drive)
    c. Pleural effusion
    d. Pneumothorax

e. Pulmonary edema
f. Aspiration
g. Limitation of inspiration motion (i.e., due to postoperative pain)
4. Cardiac arrest

Major Threat to Life

- Ventricular arrhythmias
- Hypotension

Selective Physical Examination

Signs and symptoms are generally nonspecific. Acidemia is generally associated with hypoxia.

VS:	Decreased RR
MS:	Drowsiness and confusion
HEENT:	Papilledema
Neuro:	Asterixis
Blood gas:	The pH will be lesser than 7.35. PCO_2 will be elevated, $[HCO_3^-]$ will be normal to elevated. The expected increase in $[HCO_3^-]$ in response to a pure acute respiratory acidosis is 0.1 mEq for each elevation of 1 mm Hg in pCO_2. In a chronic condition the increase in $[HCO_3^-]$ is 0.4 mEq for each elevation of 1 mm Hg in pCO_2. If the increase is less, suspect a mixed disorder.

Management

1. Assess the severity.

Mild	pH = 7.30 to 7.35
Moderate	pH = 7.20 to 7.29
Severe	pH <7.20

2. Treat reversible causes.
   Mild acidemia may be observed cautiously. Moderate to severe acidemia requires intervention to avoid respiratory arrest.
3. Notify your resident if acidemia is moderate or severe.
   If hypoventilation is present, consider intubation of the patient and transfer to the intensive care unit (ICU)/cardiac care unit (CCU) for cardiac monitoring.
4. Monitor serial blood gases to follow therapy.

Special Surgical Considerations

A common cause of respiratory failure in postoperative patients is overmedication with narcotic pain relievers or benzodiazepines. Look at the pupils, which will be pin point with narcotic overdose. Review the medication delivery logs. Reverse narcosis with **naloxone (Narcan) 0.4 to 2 mg IM or IV every 2 to 3 minutes to a maximum dose of 10 mg.** Reverse benzodiazepine overdose with **flumazenil (Romazicon) 0.2 mg IV every 30 to 60 seconds to a maximum dose of 3 mg.**

Metabolic Acidosis

Etiology

Metabolic acidoses are caused by accumulation of acids in the serum. These fall into two categories: normal anion gap (or hyperchloremic) acidosis or increased anion gap (or normochloremic) acidosis.

The anion gap is defined by the following equation:

$$\text{Anion gap} = (Na + K) - (Cl + HCO_3)$$

Normal values range from 10 to 12 mEq/L and reflect the unmeasured anionic role of plasma proteins. Hypoalbuminemia must be corrected for in this equation by adding 4 mEq/L to the calculated anion gap for each decrease in albumin of 1 g/dL. (Assume a normal of 4 g/dL.)

1. Normal anionic gap acidosis
   a. Loss of HCO_3
      (1) Diarrhea, paralytic ileus, and intestinal fistula
      (2) High-output ileostomy
      (3) Renal tubular acidosis
      (4) Carbonic anhydrase inhibitors
      (5) Ureterosigmoidostomy
   b. Addition of acid
      (1) NH_4Cl
      (2) HCl (as with administration of arginine or lysine as HCl salts in total parenteral nutrition)
      (3) Rapid or high volume NaCl administration
      (4) Blood transfusions
2. Increased anionic gap acidosis
   a. Lactic acidosis
   b. Ketoacidosis (diabetes mellitus, starvation, or alcohol)
   c. Renal failure
   d. Medications (aspirin, ethylene glycol, methanol, and paraldehyde)
   e. Rhabdomyolysis

Major Threat to Life

- Ventricular arrhythmias
- Hypotension

Selective Physical Examination

Signs and symptoms are generally nonspecific.

VS:	Increased RR
MS:	Confusion, stupor, and coma
CVS:	Decreased cardiac contractility; peripheral vasodilation leading to hypotension
Neuro:	Fatigue

Blood gas: The pH will be less than 7.35. PCO_2 will be normal to decreased, $[HCO_3^-]$ will be decreased. The expected decrease in PCO_2 in response to a pure acute metabolic acidosis is 1 to 1.5 mm Hg for each decrease of 1 mEq in $[HCO_3^-]$. If the decrease is less, suspect a mixed disorder.

Management

1. Assess the severity.

Mild	pH = 7.30 to 7.35
Moderate	pH = 7.20 to 7.29
Severe	pH <7.20

2. Treat reversible causes.

Mild acidemia may be observed cautiously. Moderate to severe acidemia requires intervention to avoid respiratory arrest.

3. Notify your resident if acidemia is severe.

If hypoventilation is present, consider intubation of the patient and transfer to the ICU/CCU.

4. Monitor serial blood gases to follow therapy.

5. $NaHCO_3$.

IV sodium bicarbonate should be reserved for patients who are in acute, severe acidemia. At HCO_3 levels of less than 10 mEq/L, and pH of less than 7.1, the buffering capacity of bicarbonate is exhausted and hydrogen ion builds up rapidly in the serum.

The amount of bicarbonate to replace may be calculated by the following formula:

$$HCO_3 \text{ to be replaced (in mEq)} = Wt \text{ (in kg)} \times (0.4)$$
$$(15 - \text{measured bicarbonate})$$

or

$$HCO_3 \text{ to be replaced (in mEq)} = \text{(base deficit) (Wt in kg) (0.4)}/2$$

The goal of therapy is not to normalize bicarbonate levels, but to bring the pH to greater than 7.2 and the bicarbonate to about 15 mEq/L. The rate of replacement depends on the severity of the acidemia.

In general, a slower approach is preferred to avoid complication of fluid overload or overshoot alkalemia (e.g., over 8 to 12 hours). In cases of severe, life-threatening acidemia, i.e., pH of less than 7, it may be necessary to administer a rapid bolus of 150 mEq $NaHCO_3$ by IV push.

Unless given in a code situation, always dilute bicarbonate in a large volume of fluid (such as 50 to 150 mEq/L of 5% dextrose in water); rapid infusion can cause cardiac dysrhythmias.

Renal tubular acidosis responds well to oral administration of bicarbonate; consult a nephrologist for appropriate care of these disorders.

Complications of bicarbonate administration include:
a. Fluid overload
b. Hypernatremia
c. Shift of potassium ion to intracellular, causing hypokalemia
d. Drop in ionized calcium, leading to tetany
e. Cardiac dysrhythmias with rapid infusion

Special Surgical Considerations

After a large operation or severe trauma, inadequate fluid resuscitation can exacerbate metabolic acidosis. Be sure to adequately replace fluid losses.

ALKALOSIS (pH >7.45)

Alkalosis is defined as arterial pH of >7.45. Causes include respiratory etiologies such as hyperventilation and metabolic etiologies such as loss of acid or increased bicarbonate in the serum. Common surgical causes include prolonged nasogastric suction or vomiting. Rapid compensation to alkalosis is respiratory with a decreased RR. This compensatory response is limited by the hypoxic drive to ventilation. More chronic compensation occurs in the kidneys where bicarbonate is actively excreted. This causes a measurable drop in serum bicarbonate. The drop in bicarbonate is greater in metabolic alkalosis (0.6 mEq/L) when compared with respiratory alkalosis (0.2 to 0.4 mEq/L). The renal response takes 12 hours to become apparent and is maximum at 3 to 5 days.

Respiratory Alkalosis

Etiology

Respiratory alkalosis results from decreased CO_2 in the blood stream due to hyperventilation. Etiologies include the following:
1. Physiologic oxygen need (pregnancy or high altitude)
2. Hypoxia
3. CNS states or disorders (anxiety, pain, fever, tumor, trauma, and infection)
4. Medications (aspirin, nicotine, and progesterone)
5. Respiratory disorders
   a. CHF
   b. Pulmonary embolism
   c. Asthma
   d. Pneumonia
6. Hepatic failure
7. Hyperthyroidism
8. Sepsis or other hypermetabolic states

Major Threat to Life

Major threat to life depends on the underlying cause.

Selective Physical Examination

Signs and symptoms are generally nonspecific.

MS:	Confusion and lightheadedness
Neuro:	Numbness, tingling, and perioral or acral paresthesias; tetany, in severe cases
Blood Gas:	The pH will be greater than 7.45. PCO_2 will be decreased, $[HCO_3^-]$ will be normal to decreased. The expected decrease in $[HCO_3^-]$ in response to an acute respiratory alkalosis is 0.1 to 0.3 mEq for each fall of 1 mm Hg in pCO_2. In a chronic condition the decrease in $[HCO_3^-]$ is 0.2 to 0.5 mEq for each decrease of 1 mm Hg in pCO_2. If the decrease is less, suspect a mixed disorder. The $[HCO_3^-]$ will rarely drop below 14 mEq/L.

Management

1. Assess the severity.

Mild	pH = 7.45 to 7.55
Moderate	pH = 7.56 to 7.69
Severe	pH >7.7

2. Treat reversible causes.

   Mild alkalemia may be observed cautiously. Moderate to severe alkalemia may require intervention. Symptomatic treatment, such as antipyretics for fever, or anxiolytics for agitation may be all that is required. Moderate alkalemia with symptoms of tetany may be treated with a rebreathing bag, which will recirculate exhaled CO_2. Take care in correcting chronic alkalemia in this fashion, as increasing CO_2 may precipitate as acidemia.

3. Notify your resident if alkalemia is severe.
4. Monitor serial blood gases to follow therapy.

Metabolic Alkalosis

Etiology

Metabolic alkalosis results from a loss of acid from the serum or an accumulation of base. The etiologies may be divided into chloride-responsive alkalemia and chloride-resistant alkalemia.

1. Chloride responsive (UCl <20 mEq/L)
   a. GI losses (NG suction and emesis)
   b. Chloride deficiency (diuretics and villous adenoma of the colon)
   c. Posthypercapnea

    d. Contraction alkalosis due to fluid depletion or diuretic use

    e. Excessive $NaHCO_3$ administration, or administration of agents that are metabolized to bicarbonate, such as citrate (in blood products), lactate, or acetate

    f. Medications (penicillin, carbenicillin, and ticarcillin)

2. Chloride resistant (UCl >20 mEq/L)

    a. Severe K^+ deficiency (K^+ <2 mEq/L)

    b. Magnesium deficiency

    c. Mineralocorticoid excess

       i. Primary aldosteronism

       ii. Cushing syndrome

       iii. Exogenous steroid replacement

       iv. Licorice ingestion

       v. Renal artery stenosis

    d. Bartter syndrome

    e. Poststarvation feeding

    f. Alkali ingestion

Major Threat to Life

Major threat to life depends on the underlying causes.

Selective Physical Examination

Signs and symptoms are generally nonspecific.

MS:	Apathy, confusion, and stupor
Blood Gas:	The pH will be greater than 7.45. PCO_2 will be normal to increased, $[HCO_3^-]$ will be increased. The expected increase in PCO_2 in response to a pure acute metabolic alkalosis is 0.25 to 1 mm Hg for each increase of 1 mEq in $[HCO_3^-]$. If the increase is less, suspect a mixed disorder.

Management

1. **Assess the severity.**

Mild	pH = 7.45 to 7.55
Moderate	pH = 7.56 to 7.69
Severe	pH > 7.7

2. **Treat reversible causes.**

    Mild alkalemia may be observed cautiously. Moderate to severe alkalemia may require intervention.

3. **Notify your resident if alkalemia is severe.**

4. **Monitor serial blood gases to follow therapy.**

5. **Administer fluids.**

    Chloride-responsive alkaloses generally are associated with fluid deficit and respond well to replacement using NS with supplemental KCl.

    Chloride-resistant alkaloses are associated with a concurrent deficiency in K^+ and therefore do not respond to NaCl replacement. Usually the underlying cause must be corrected.

6. **Provide histamine H2 blockade or proton pump inhibition.**

    If gastric losses are the cause of alkalosis, diminishing the production of acid in the stomach may decrease the net loss of chloride.

7. **Administer acid therapy.**

    This is reserved for cases of severe alkalemia. Notify your resident before administration of any of these agents.

    ARGININE HCL (50 MEQ HCL/100 ML)

    Use this therapy with caution as arginine can move to the intracellular space. This displaces intracellular potassium, and life-threatening hyperkalemia can result.

    NH_4CL

    Ammonium chloride must be converted to H^+ and NH_3 in the liver and is therefore contraindicated in patients with liver disease.

    0.1 M HCL

    This is the safest of current options. Still, it is best administered through central venous access over 8 to 12 hours.

8. **Acetazolamide (Diamox) 250 to 500 mg PO or IV every 8 hours may be useful to decrease excess fluid in cases of fluid overload.**

    This diuretic also enhances renal excretion of bicarbonate.

9. **Bartter syndrome is usually treated with additional alkali as needed with supplementation of KCl-replacement and indomethacin.**

MIXED ACID–BASE DISORDERS

Many disorders of acid–base status are combinations of simple situations. These may be identified by noting that the magnitude of biochemical derangement is greater than expected from a simple abnormality alone (a simple acid–base disorder will never overcompensate). A breakdown in the normal relationship between PCO_2, pH, and HCO_3 (as in the Henderson–Hasselbach equation) suggests a mixed disorder. See Figure 12–8 for a graphic depiction of various pH value and PCO_2 relationships in various simple acid–base disorders. Frequently encountered examples include the following:

Chronic Respiratory Acidosis Plus Metabolic Alkalosis

This is encountered in patients with chronic obstructive pulmonary disease (COPD) who are concurrently treated with gastric suction, diuretics, or a low-salt diet. The blood pH may be normal, but the PCO_2 and HCO_3 will be abnormal or changed from the patient's baseline. The goal of therapy is to normalize the pH and not the PCO_2.

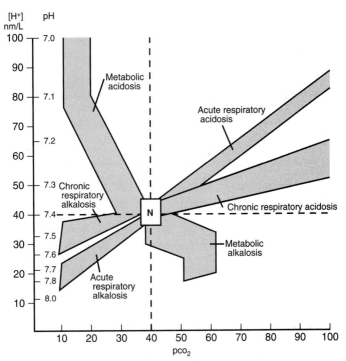

Figure 12–8 Acid–base map determination of usual compensatory responses to primary acid–base disturbances.

Acute Respiratory Acidosis Superimposed on Chronic Respiratory Acidosis

In severe COPD patients who retain CO_2, a pulmonary decompensation such as pneumonia, sedative medication, or oxygen administration may lead to this finding.

Acute Respiratory Acidosis Superimposed on Metabolic Acidosis

This is often seen after cardiac arrest, where there is accumulation of lactic acid from hypoperfusion and accumulation of CO_2 due to hypoventilation. The acidemias may be additive and may be very dangerous.

Respiratory Alkalosis Plus Metabolic Alkalosis

This finding is characteristic of early sepsis and aspirin intoxication.

13

Gastrointestinal Bleeding

Gastrointestinal (GI) bleeding is a stressful on-call problem to manage. It is common in hospitalized patients, and it includes a broad spectrum of disorders. GI bleeding can represent a minor problem or a life-threatening emergency. Initial management involves resuscitation and stabilization. History taking, evaluation, and definitive treatment should follow in rapid sequence.

PHONE CALL

Questions

1. **Where is the blood coming from, and what does it look like?**

   It is important to have the RN describe to you what the bleeding looks like. This will help you better delineate what type of GI bleeding the patient may have. Melena (passage of black or tarry stools) indicates blood entering the GI tract at any point from the mouth to the cecum. The dark color is the result of oxidation of heme by bacterial and digestive enzymes. Hematochezia is the passage of bright-red blood from the rectum. It usually indicates bleeding from the colon, the rectum, or the anus. Hematemesis, or vomiting of bright-red or dark blood, usually indicates a bleeding source proximal to the ligament of Treitz.

2. **How much blood has been lost?**

   Ask the RN to estimate the amount of blood loss. This will give you an idea as to whether the GI bleeding represents a life-threatening problem. Remember that rapid GI bleeding is an emergency.

3. **What are the vital signs?**

   Rapid GI hemorrhaging may be associated with hypotension and tachycardia.

4. **Did the patient have surgery, and if so, what was the operation and when did it occur?**

   The stress of surgery may precipitate acute GI bleeding. Stress gastritis in the perioperative period may occur in patients undergoing major surgery. In addition, patients undergoing surgery on the GI tract may develop GI bleeding if a suture line has broken down or if a major blood vessel has ruptured.

159

5. **What are the major medical problems?**
   Some conditions such as liver disease, esophageal varices, coagulopathies, and gastric or duodenal ulcer predispose patients to either more frequent or more serious GI bleeding.
6. **Is the patient taking ulcerogenic medications, anticoagulants, or thrombolytic agents?**
   Patients taking nonsteroidal anti-inflammatory drugs (NSAIDs) or steroids are more likely to develop gastric ulcers and GI bleeds. Patients taking anticoagulants such as warfarin (Coumadin), aspirin, and heparin may develop severe GI bleeding refractory to conventional treatment. Often, anticoagulant medications must be discontinued or reversed if severe bleeding occurs. Thrombolytic agents such as streptokinase or urokinase may require discontinuation in an actively bleeding patient.

Orders

For any significant GI bleed:
1. Ask the RN to stay at the bedside with the patient and to get help from additional nursing staff.
2. Order immediate placement of two large-bore intravenous (IV) lines with 14- to 16-gauge catheters in large peripheral veins. Antecubital veins are preferred if available. Large peripheral lines are preferred to central lines.
3. Ask the RN to draw an immediate hematocrit, prothrombin time (PT), partial thromboplastin time (PTT), and platelet count, at the time of IV placement if possible. If not already done, have the RN also draw an immediate type and cross-match. Always have 4 to 6 units of packed red blood cells (PRBCs) available in a major GI bleed (stay ahead by 4 units).
4. Once the hematocrit is drawn, start rapid infusion of isotonic saline, lactated Ringer solution (LR). The rate of volume infusion should correlate with the patient's condition and the volume of blood lost.
5. If a massive upper GI bleeder is suspected, order an Ewald nasogastric (NG) tube (32 to 36 Fr) or a Minnesota tube (if esophageal variceal bleeding) to the bedside.
6. Ask the RN to have the patient's chart at the bedside.

Inform RN

Will arrive at the bedside in . . . minutes.
   Significant upper or lower GI bleeding or bleeding associated with changes in vital signs (hypotension or tachycardia) requires immediate evaluation of the patient.

ELEVATOR THOUGHTS

What causes GI bleeding?
   Upper GI bleed

1. Peptic ulcer
   Duodenal ulcer
   Gastric ulcer
2. Esophageal varices
3. Esophagitis
4. Gastritis
5. Duodenitis
6. Mallory–Weiss tear
7. Upper GI neoplasm

Lower GI bleed

1. Hemorrhoids
2. Rectal fissures
3. Polyps
4. Lower GI neoplasms
5. Ulcerative or infectious colitis
6. Ischemic colitis
7. Dead bowel
8. Diverticulosis
9. Meckel's diverticulum
10. Angiodysplasia

In one study of one hundred patients with GI bleeding, over half were attributable to acid-related disease. But nearly 40% were associated with cancerous or pre-cancerous lesions. In any patient, GI bleeding can be caused or exacerbated by coagulopathy.

MAJOR THREAT TO LIFE

Hypovolemic Shock/Exsanguination

Patients with rapid GI hemorrhaging will quickly deplete their intravascular volume and become hypotensive. Sympathetic activation (tachycardia and vasoconstriction) occurs in an attempt to maintain blood pressure (BP). Continued GI bleeding rapidly overcomes the body's attempts to maintain BP, and hypovolemic shock ensues. Shock can be prevented by aggressive fluid resuscitation using adequate IV access. The rate of fluid resuscitation should be dictated by the amount and the rapidity of blood loss. Crystalloid (normal saline [NS] or LR) should be used until blood products are available. If ongoing massive GI hemorrhaging occurs and there is a significant delay in obtaining crossmatched blood, consider replacement of crystalloid infusion for O-negative blood. The best way to prevent shock in GI bleeding patients is to restore intravascular volume. See Chapter 17.

Always notify your resident if you are considering transfusion of blood products. The mortality of lower GI bleeding can be as high as 10% to 15%.

BEDSIDE

Quick Look Test

Does the patient look well (comfortable), sick (uncomfortable or distressed), or critical (about to die)?

Patients with minor GI bleeding look comfortable and well perfused. Patients with significant GI bleeding are often pale, uncomfortable, tachycardic, tremulous, and apprehensive.

Airway and Vital Signs

Airway

It is imperative that the airway be protected in patients with upper GI bleeding. It is common for a debilitated patient to aspirate during ongoing upper GI bleeding. Consider endotracheal intubation in the presence of shock, diminished mental status, hepatic encephalopathy, massive hematemesis, or active variceal hemorrhage.

Vital Signs

Assess the BP and the heart rate (HR) carefully. Hypotension and tachycardia while the patient is in the supine position signal severe hypovolemia. In patients with GI bleeding and less pronounced vital sign changes, check orthostatics. Start by measuring the HR and BP with the patient in the supine position, and then compare those measurements with the HR and the BP while the patient sits with legs dangling off the side of the bed. If there are no significant changes with this positional change, measure the BP and the HR with the patient standing. A fall in systolic blood pressure (SBP) by greater than 15 mm Hg or an increase in HR of greater than 15 beats/minute or any decrease in diastolic pressure indicates orthostatic change and significant hypovolemia.

Selective Physical Examination I

The initial evaluation is for assessing the patient for evidence of hypovolemia or shock.

VS:	Repeat now; pay particular attention to BP and HR
CVS:	Assess perfusion; note skin color and temperature
Neuro:	Note level of consciousness and mental status

Patients who demonstrate inadequate tissue perfusion in the presence of GI bleeding may be in shock. These patients generally have an SBP of less than 90 mm Hg and a urine output (UO) of less than 20 mL/hour or 250 mL/8-hour-shift. As BP falls in the presence of significant GI bleeding, cerebral perfusion decreases. Patients with hypovolemia from GI bleeding may become lethargic, somnolent, delirious, or unconscious.

INITIAL MANAGEMENT

1. Control the airway, if necessary
2. Fluid resuscitation with crystalloid
3. Placement of Foley catheter
4. Close monitoring of vital signs
5. Transfusion of PRBCs, fresh frozen plasma (FFP), and platelets as necessary
6. Monitor O_2 saturation with pulse oximetry
7. Hold any heparin or other anticoagulant as appropriate

An important step in management is to replenish intravascular volume. For a patient with significant GI bleeding associated with hypovolemia and hypotension, give a 500- to 1000-L bolus of NS or LR through large-bore peripheral IVs. Watch the effect that the fluid challenge has on the BP. For massive bleeds, consider repeating the bolus two or three times to maintain normotensive BPs. Patients with congestive heart failure or pulmonary disease may develop cardiopulmonary complications of rapid fluid resuscitation. Such complications may worsen heart failure and cause pulmonary edema. If the patient remains hypotensive despite two or three crystalloid boluses, consider switching to blood or blood product replacement.

Fluid status is best managed with a Foley catheter. UO is a sensitive measure of end-organ perfusion. While crystalloid boluses are being given, check on the availability of PRBCs. If at least 4 units of PBRCs are not available, send for a type and crossmatch immediately. You must always stay ahead of a significant bleed by at least 4 units of PRBCs. If blood is deemed necessary before the crossmatch is completed, order O^- uncrossmatched blood to be given.

It may also be useful to see if the hematocrit sent earlier is available. Remember that hematocrit results in the presence of acute GI bleeding may be a relatively unreliable indicator of the extent of blood loss. This is because it takes time for the acute changes in intravascular space to equilibrate with fluid from the extravascular space. Remember this when evaluating hematocrit results obtained during periods of acute bleeding.

Crystalloid is useful and expands the intravascular compartment, but it does not raise the oxygen-carrying capacity of blood. With continued crystalloid administration, blood cells become diluted. Patients who have significant blood loss should be resuscitated initially with crystalloid and, when available, transfused with appropriate volumes of blood. There is not a 'magic' number to aim for with respect to post-transfusion hematocrit, and as the knowledge of the side effects of massive transfusion becomes more clear, the absolute number is decreasing. Maintain a hematocrit of at least 25 to 28 in elderly patients or in patients with heart disease. Young, otherwise healthy patients can easily tolerate hematocrit values of less than 20 to 25 without transfusion, unless there is risk of rebleeding. Use good judgment in determining what hematocrit is satisfactory. Your goal is to transfuse to avoid shock, to provide adequate perfusion of tissues, and to keep the patient from becoming symptomatic (orthostatic). If there is a significant likelihood of rebleeding, it is a good idea to resuscitate the patient adequately, such that he or she has a reserve if acute rebleeding occurs.

Remember to record BP, pulse, central venous pressure (if central line is present), hematocrit, and UO hourly. You must document the need for blood transfusions in the medical record.

Check the results of coagulation studies. If a patient with significant GI bleeding has significant coagulopathy from elevated PT or PTT, consider transfusion with FFP. Two units of FFP are usually required for any significant clinical effect on bleeding. For many patients, 2 to 4 units of FFP are required to correct coagulopathy to the extent that clotting is significantly enhanced.

Low platelet count or platelet dysfunction may cause or worsen GI bleeding. Patients with thrombocytopenia may develop spontaneous upper GI bleeding. GI bleeding associated with platelet counts of less than $40,000/\text{mm}^3$ requires platelet transfusion. A patient with a normal platelet count may develop severe GI bleeding, or existing bleeding may be exacerbated if significant platelet dysfunction is present. Uremia, von Willebrand's disease, recent ingestion of NSAIDs, and other conditions may prolong bleeding time and result in bleeding that is difficult to control without platelet transfusion. Consider platelet transfusion if bleeding is uncontrollable and the patient has a significant risk for platelet dysfunction. If time allows, an Ivy bleeding time test will provide evidence of bleeding dysfunction. A bleeding time of greater than 7 minutes indicates abnormal platelet function.

Platelet dysfunction due to uremia also may be responsive to DDAVP.

Remember that massive blood loss will be associated with deficiency in all blood components simultaneously. Many institutions have 'massive transfusion' policies which give guidelines as to when FFP and platelets ought to be considered while replacing pRBCs.

Selective History and Chart Review

Once the patient is stabilized, review the history and medications as indicated in the medical record. If the patient is able to converse, ask about previous bleeds, medications, and known diagnoses that may cause GI bleeding. These data will help you diagnose the likely cause of bleeding and help with management.

Has the patient had an episode of GI bleeding during this admission or at any time recently?

Is there a known condition that predisposes the patient to GI bleeding?

Is the patient taking any medications that predispose to bleeding?

The following common medications are known to interfere with normal coagulation function: heparin, fractionated and low molecular weight heparin, warfarin (Coumadin), NSAIDs, and some antibiotics.

Selective Physical Examination II

This examination focuses on identifying whether the bleeding is from the upper or the lower GI tract. If possible, the site of bleeding is identified.

VS:	Repeat now.
HEENT:	Look for nosebleed.
Abd:	When melena or coffee-ground emesis is present, pass NG tube into stomach. Perform gastric aspiration.
	Evaluate for epigastric tenderness (bleeding gastric or duodenal ulcer).
	Look for left lower quadrant tenderness (diverticulitis, ischemic bowel, angiodysplasia, or bleeding colon cancer).
Rectal:	Note hematochezia, melena, and hemorrhoids.

DEFINITIVE MANAGEMENT

The goal of the second stage of management is to maintain adequate fluid resuscitation and oxygen-carrying capacity (hemoglobin), to slow or stop the bleeding if possible, and to identify the lesion responsible for the bleeding.

It is important to understand the differences in management between upper and lower GI bleeding.

Upper GI Bleeding

1. Peptic ulcer, acute gastritis, esophageal varices, and Mallory–Weiss tear account for more than 90% of upper GI bleeds.

   These sources are proximal to the ligament of Treitz. They generally present with hematemesis, coffee-ground emesis, and/or melena.

2. Insert a large-bore NG tube (16 Fr or greater).

   Perform gastric aspiration to determine if bleeding is from the stomach. An Ewald tube may be needed if large amounts of clot are present. Most gastric bleeds and greater than 75% of bleeding duodenal ulcers will give positive gastric aspirates for blood.

3. Lavage the stomach free of blood and clots.

   Irrigate the stomach with a large syringe and several liters of iced saline. Continue lavage until blood no longer returns. Iced saline is very effective at slowing or stopping small-to-moderate GI bleeds.

4. If bleeding continues or if the patient becomes hemodynamically unstable despite fluid and blood replacement, urgent esophagogastroduodenoscopy (EGD) is indicated.

Contact the GI fellow or the attending gastroenterologist to perform the EGD. Sclerosis of varices, banding, electrocoagulation, or epinephrine injections can be performed through the scope to stop bleeding. Stabilized patients who stop bleeding may benefit from elective EGD 24 hours after the bleeding episode.

5. Management for particular lesions

Esophageal varices

For esophageal varices, **IV octreotide (Sandostatin): 25- to 50-μg bolus** followed with **a drip of 25 to 50 μg/hour, or IV vasopressin infusion (100 U in 250 mL 5% dextrose in water)** may help slow bleeding while awaiting EGD.

Start infusion at 0.4 U/minute (60 mL/hour). If life-threatening bleeding occurs from known esophageal varices, insertion of a Sengstaken–Blakemore tube or a Minnesota tube may be helpful until the medications are available (Fig. 13–1). Although these tubes may balloon tamponade bleeding varices, they also carry the risk of causing airway obstruction, aspiration, and esophageal rupture.

Ulcers

Ulcers may be treated with antacids via NG tube every 1 to 2 hours. Ulcer rebleeding may be minimized with H2-receptor blockade:

Cimetidine (Tagamet) 300 mg IV every 6 hours, or
Ranitidine (Zantac) 50 mg IV every 8 hours, or
Famotidine (Pepcid) 20 mg IV every 8 hours

Or a proton pump inhibitor (PPI) may be used:

Pantoprazole (Protonix) 80 mg IV push followed by 8 mg/hour continuous infusion

Other PPIs are in oral form, and are appropriate for those patients able to tolerate PO, but may not be useful during a massive upper GI bleed:

Omeprazole (Prilosec) 20 mg PO each day, or
Lasoprazole (Zoton) 15 mg PO each day, or
Rabeprazole (Pariet) 20 mg PO each day, or
Pantoprazole (Protonix) 40 mg PO each day

Mallory–Weiss tears

Mallory–Weiss tears are often self-limited and respond to conservative therapy. However, if life-threatening bleeding occurs, angiographic embolization may be indicated. It is appropriate to treat with one of the antacids noted above.

Stress gastritis

Likewise, stress gastritis often responds to antacids as above.

6. Treat patients for *H. pylori*, if positive.

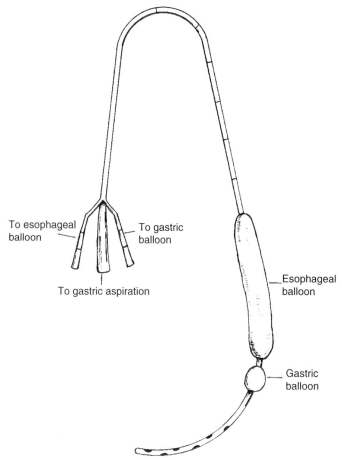

To esophageal balloon

To gastric balloon

To gastric aspiration

Esophageal balloon

Gastric balloon

Figure 13–1 The Sengstaken–Blakemore tube. The Minnesota tube is similar; it has an additional port for esophageal aspiration.
(From Marshall SA, Ruedy J: On Call: Principles and Protocols, 2nd ed. Philadelphia, WB Saunders, 1993, p. 102.)

7. Consider surgery for any patient with greater than 6 units of blood loss in a day or any patient with uncontrollable bleeding despite other therapeutic maneuvers.

Other lesions frequently requiring surgery include ulcers with visible large vessels at the ulcer base and ulcers that rebleed significantly during the same hospital stay. Obtain surgical consultation early. It is helpful to have the surgical team following the patient.

Lower GI Bleeding

1. Lower GI bleeds are associated with dark to bright-red blood from the rectum.

    The color of the blood is associated with the length of time in the GI tract. These bleeds occur distal to the ligament of Treitz. Bright-red blood from the rectum can be associated with a proximal lesion, such as a duodenal bleed, if the transit time through the gut is short.

2. Perform digital rectal examination, anoscopy, or sigmoidoscopy.

    Treat any bleeding lesion noted on examination (e.g., bleeding hemorrhoid).

3. Insert an NG tube and check aspirate.

    Gross blood, coffee-ground blood, and occult blood should be noted. Blood in the stomach indicates an upper GI bleed. EGD should be performed.

4. If EGD is negative and sigmoidoscopy and anoscopy show that bleeding is coming from above the sigmoid colon, consider the following steps:

    a. Perform radionuclide scanning

    If the radionuclide scan is positive for bleeding, consider colonoscopy or angiography; if the radionuclide scan is negative, consider colonoscopy.

    b. Proceed immediately with colonoscopy if EGD is negative and sigmoidoscopy suggests colonic bleeding.

    In addition to potentially localizing the lesion, colonoscopy by an expert endoscopist may allow electrocoagulation or other treatment of the bleeding lesion.

    c. Angiography

    Angiography may be diagnostic and potentially therapeutic if the bleeding site can be localized.

    The limitations of both nuclear medicine scans and angiography is that there has to be active bleeding at the time of the study, and the rate has to be sufficient to allow detection (usually in excess of 0.5 to 1.0 cm^3/minute for angiography, and 0.1 to 0.5 cm^3/minute for radionuclide scanning).

5. Surgical treatment is reserved for those patients in whom bleeding persists despite all conservative measures.

    If the bleeding site is known, segmental resection is indicated. In cases where no bleeding site has been identified, it may be necessary to perform a total abdominal colectomy.

Glucose Management and Surgical Nutrition

This chapter covers briefly the nutritional needs of surgical patients. They differ from other patients in the hospital in that in addition to basal metabolic demands and the increased nutritional requirements of disease and immune defense, surgical patients also have demands that result from the surgical procedure and wound healing. In many cases the normal enteral route of feeding is not available.

BASIC METABOLIC REQUIREMENTS

The average (70-kg) resting patient has a basal requirement of 1800 to 2000 kcal/day. Those calories must include approximately 180 g of glucose to supply the needs of obligate glucose-requiring tissues such as brain, red blood cells (RBCs), white blood cells (WBCs), and renal medulla. The fasting patient will generally have sufficient stores in muscle and adipose tissues to maintain protein and glucose needs for a short time perioperatively. Unless the patient is severely malnourished or is expected to be fasting for a long period of time, only glucose and crystalloid fluids are replaced routinely. This is generally accomplished with sufficient maintenance fluid volumes of 5% dextrose in water.

Various disease states will increase caloric requirements well above the basal state. These are summarized in Table 14–1. In addition, the patient's activity level will affect the caloric requirements. A patient undergoing physical therapy will use more energy than one restricted to bed rest.

TABLE 14–1 **Metabolic Rates of Various Disease States**

Basal metabolic rate	100%
Elective surgery	124%
Skeletal trauma	132%
40% burn	134%
Head trauma (with steroid use)	161%
Sepsis	179%

Patients known to be at risk for requiring supplemental enteral or parenteral nutrition are those patients undergoing major bowel resection, severely ill patients, and patients identified as malnourished preoperatively (15% documented weight loss or albumin level of less than 3.0 mg/dL).

CHANGES IN METABOLIC NEEDS RELATED TO SURGERY

Patients after serious injury or a major surgical procedure are in a "stress state" of metabolism. This state differs from simple starvation. The metabolic needs increase well above the basal requirements, and there are changes in the origin and consumption of proteins, lipids, and carbohydrates. A variety of neuroendocrine influences affect substrate availability and utilization. These are summarized briefly in Tables 14–2 and 14–3. The sum total of responses depends on the severity of the injury or illness and the general health and nutrition of the patient. Wound healing occurs as a "priority" even in severely injured or ill individuals, but additional stress (which may include malnutrition or concomitant injury elsewhere) will delay or abrogate normal wound healing. If you have a question regarding the nutritional status of a patient, a nutritional consultation may be obtained, but this is generally not an on-call issue.

TABLE 14–2 **Hormones Affecting Metabolism**

Anabolic	Catabolic
Insulin	Cortisol
Growth hormone (early)	Epinephrine
	Glucagon
	Growth hormone (late)
	Vasopressin
	Somatostatin

TABLE 14–3 **Factors Influencing Neuroendocrine Effects on Metabolism**

Changes in tissue levels of oxygen, hydrogen ion, and carbon dioxide
Changes in circulating blood volume
Changes in substrate availability
Changes in tissue levels of oxygen, hydrogen ion, and carbon dioxide
Changes in body temperature
Pain
Infection
Emotional state

Other high-metabolic stress states to be mindful of include major burns, sepsis (and other sources of fever), polytrauma, and frequent seizure activity.

Protein

After major stress, patients are in an obligate protein catabolic state in which nitrogen excretion increases from a basal level of 5 to 7 g/day to a level of 8 to 11 g/day. Negative nitrogen balance occurs despite adequate delivery of glucose and amino acids. Protein wasting lasts until the wounds are closed, adequate circulating volume has been established, pain is well controlled, and infection is eliminated. This may take several days to several weeks. Some energy needs during stress are met through gluconeogenesis with a net catabolism of 300 to 500 g of lean body mass/day. Most energy in a stress situation is derived from fat, and replacement of amino acids is needed to minimize the negative nitrogen balance. In general, 10% to 15% of the daily calories should be delivered as protein (optimally, 1.5 to 2.5 g/kg/day). The most efficient use of protein occurs when a ratio of 150 to 250 nonprotein calories (carbohydrates and fats) for each protein calorie is given. This may increase to a ratio of 400 to 500 to 1 in settings of severe illness or hepatic or renal decompensation.

Nitrogen balance is defined by the following formula:

$$\text{N balance} = \text{24-hour protein intake}/6.25 - [(\text{24-hour UUN}) + (4)]$$

where 24-hour UUN is urinary urea nitrogen excretion (in g/day), 4 is obligatory loss (in g/day), and 6.25 is the number of grams of protein that yield 1 g N_2. The goal of therapy is +4 g/day balance.

Lipid

Recovery from injury is fueled mostly by fats. There is net increased lipolysis despite increased insulin concentrations. In the liver there is increased free fatty acid synthesis. The fatty acids are used primarily for oxidation. Ketogenesis is increased in minor injury or stress, but it is nearly absent in major injury or stress. The high fat content of the average American diet makes it unnecessary to supplement fats routinely, but for prolonged nutritional replacement, fats are the most concentrated source of calories. Replacement of lipids is indicated to supply calories and to avoid depletion of essential fatty acids.

Carbohydrate

One of the hallmarks of injury or stress is hyperglycemia. This sets stress apart from fasting or starvation. Blood sugar rises in response to catabolic neuroendocrine hormones. Initially, the hyperglycemia is due to decreased circulating insulin secondary to beta-cell insensitivity to glucose. Soon, insulin levels become normal or elevated, and persistent hyperglycemia is probably due in part to peripheral resistance to insulin. Despite the insulin resistance, the increased glucose in the blood stream allows greater uptake of glucose into the tissues during stress. Healing wounds must be thought of as obligate glucose-requiring tissues like brain and RBCs. This requirement may be due to the large number of infiltrating WBCs in the wound.

MEANS OF DELIVERING CALORIES

Simple replacement of maintenance fluids, salt, and glucose is the most frequent and the most simple of approaches. When it is determined that a patient does need supplemental calories, there are a variety of avenues available for use, depending on the needs and constraints of the particular patient.

Enteral

If the patient has adequate bowel function, the enteral route is best. It allows physiologic use of the bowel, decreases bacterial translocation across the bowel wall (which may be a significant source of sepsis) and allows normal glucose use. The delivery of enteral feeds depends on the patient.

ORAL

The oral route is available to awake, alert patients whose gastrointestinal (GI) continuity is intact. Patients who have had esophageal or gastric procedures, or those with fresh anastomoses in the proximal GI tract, may not be the best candidates for the oral approach.

FEEDING TUBES

Feeding tubes are useful for patients who are not able to take food by mouth or for those in whom an anastomosis must be protected. Feeding tubes may be temporarily placed through the oral or the nasal passageway or may be surgically or endoscopically placed. Either the stomach (gastrostomy) or the proximal small intestine (jejunostomy) may be used. If the jejunum is used, bolus feedings are not possible.

Parenteral

In patients in whom the bowel is not functioning properly or in whom the absorptive surface is insufficient to maintain adequate nutrition, enteral feeds may be supplemented with or replaced by parenteral delivery of nutrition. This may be delivered as complete nutritional replacement, in which case it is termed total parenteral nutrition (TPN). TPN uses a hypertonic solution delivered through a central venous catheter. TPN consists of adequate glucose, protein, and lipid replacement to facilitate wound healing and anabolism (Table 14–4). Another approach does not require central venous

TABLE 14–4 **Caloric Content of TPN Constituents**

Dextrose (10% solution)	0.34 kcal/mL
Lipid (10% solution)	1.1 kcal/mL
Amino acids	3.33 kcal/g

6.25 g amino acids = 1 g nitrogen; TPN, total parenteral nutrition.

access and is termed peripheral parenteral nutrition (PPN). The fluids used in PPN are of a low enough osmolarity to allow delivery through peripheral veins, but they will not deliver adequate calories when used alone. They must be coupled with enteral feeds or with body stores of nutrients. Each hospital has specific guidelines as to safe and effective delivery of parenteral nutrition. The concentrations of glucose and lipid must be increased slowly to avoid complications of hyperglycemia and hyperlipidemia; the electrolytes and the blood glucose concentrations must be followed closely; and the central access must be well protected from infection, as the nutrients delivered make this site more vulnerable to bacterial and yeast infection. There are often printed TPN delivery orders that may be followed. Consult with your resident, the pharmacy, or the specific dietary department before starting or stopping TPN.

When adequate calories are delivered with TPN, the concentration of glucose is high, and the pancreas becomes acclimated to the rate of glucose delivery. The maximum rate can reach 5 to 8 mg/kg/minute. This puts a patient at risk for hypoglycemia if the TPN infusion is discontinued abruptly. If a central line becomes unusable, a peripheral line may be used for concentrations as high as 10% dextrose in water for a short period of time. Periodic glucose checks must be made to ensure adequate blood sugar levels. When TPN is no longer needed, the infusion is reduced slowly over 1 to 2 days, and care is taken to make sure that adequate blood sugar levels are maintained.

Vitamins and trace elements should be provided as directed by the TPN guidelines in your institution. In general, an ampule of multivitamins should be added to the formulation per day. Additional vitamin K (10 to 20 mg) should be administered to the patient, intramuscularly (IM) or subcutaneously (SC) once per week. Additional vitamin and mineral supplementation is outlined in Table 14–5.

Electrolyte administration will vary with each patient; reasonable guidelines are listed in Table 14–6. The patient must be followed closely with daily electrolyte, phosphorus, and glucose levels until the administration of TPN has stabilized (usually 1 to 2 weeks) and then 3 times per week thereafter. Weekly liver function tests and triglyceride levels should be monitored.

Complications of TPN delivery are common and can be severe. They are divided into physical, metabolic, and infectious complications. The physical complications are related to placement and

TABLE 14–5 **Vitamin and Mineral Supplementation to Support Wound Healing in Patients with Chronic Steroid Use**

Vitamin A	50,000 IU PO/IV every day
Vitamin C	1000 mg PO every day
Zinc sulfate	220 mg (50 mg elemental Zn) PO every day or 10 mg IV every day

PO, by mouth; IV, intravenously.

TABLE 14–6 **Guidelines for Daily Electrolyte Replacements in TPN**

Sodium	75–100 mEq/d
Potassium	75–100 mEq/d
Calcium	10–20 mEq/d
Magnesium	10–20 mEq/d
Phosphate	5–40 mEq/d

TPN, total parenteral nutrition.

maintenance of the central line. The metabolic complications are influenced by the formulation of the TPN solution, the rate of delivery, and the underlying biochemistry of the patient. The infectious risks are nearly inevitable with long-term administration but can be minimized by close adherence to sterile technique during placement and by following the TPN line protocols of your institution. A summary of complications is listed in Table 14–7.

SPECIAL SURGICAL CONSIDERATIONS

Normal Return of Bowel Function After Abdominal Procedures

The loss of function of the intestines after surgery is a physiologic protective measure termed paralytic ileus. Paralytic ileus is poorly understood and most likely multifactorial. Influences include anticholinergic medications, pain medications, and irritation of the peritoneum. It is prolonged with major surgery, infection, or electrolyte or acid–base abnormalities. Consider starting TPN by the second postoperative day if there is a lesser than 50% chance of normal bowel function by the fifth postoperative day.

The uncomplicated return of bowel function occurs in stages as summarized in Table 14–8. It is not a synchronous event. First to return is the small bowel function, which generally occurs in 5 to 8 hours; often the small bowel is seen to undergo peristalsis during return of the bowels to the abdomen following a surgical procedure.

TABLE 14–7 **Potential Complications of TPN Administration**

Physical	Metabolic	Infectious
Pneumothorax	Hyperglycemia	Insertion site infection
Hemothorax	Hypoglycemia	
Hemomediastinum	Electrolyte derangement	Phlebitis
Arterial injury	Vitamin deficiency	Systemic infection
Venous injury	Mineral deficiency	Bacterial
Thoracic duct injury	Essential fatty acid deficiency	Yeast
		Line sepsis
Brachial plexus injury	Hyperlipidemia	
Venous thrombosis	Metabolic acidosis	
Superior vena cava syndrome	Respiratory failure	
	Hepatic disorders	
Air embolism	Anemia	
Pulmonary embolism	Bone demineralization	
Catheter embolism		
Catheter malposition		
Horner syndrome		

TPN, total parenteral nutrition.

TABLE 14–8 **Timing of Uncomplicated Return of Bowel Function**

Structure	Timing	Hallmark
Small intestine	5–8 hr	Bowel tones
Stomach	24 hr	Decreased nasogastric tube output, abdominal bloating
Large intestine	24–60 hr	Passage of flatus, stool

Bowel tones are present with small bowel function. Next to return is gastric motility, which occurs in 24 hours. A decrease in nasogastric tube output, mild abdominal bloating, or a subjective increase in patient belching may be noted. The last to return is colonic motility. This normalizes in 24 to 60 hours and is preceded by the passage of flatus. It is safe to wait for the passage of gas before the introduction of oral food. The introduction of oral food may be further delayed by the creation of a new anastomosis or a major loss of absorptive surface, as with extensive bowel resections.

THE DIABETIC PATIENT

Patients with diabetes have a higher risk of coronary disease, renal insufficiency, and peripheral vascular disease. These patients also require surgical therapy more frequently than nondiabetics. Poor diabetic control will predispose a patient to a higher risk of bacterial and fungal infections and poor wound healing.

The stress of surgery or infection will exacerbate insulin insensitivity of non-insulin-dependent (type II) diabetes and may increase the insulin requirement of insulin-dependent (type I) diabetes. Remember that hyperglycemia is a normal physiologic response to surgical stress. The goal of postoperative glucose control is not normal glucose levels but the avoidance of extreme hyperglycemia. In general, maintenance of serum glucose levels of less than 250 mg/dL is sufficient. It is important to remember that the real risk of diabetic treatment is hypoglycemia resulting from overzealous treatment.

Peripheral insulin resistance will wane as a patient improves. It is useful to treat changes in the diabetic patient's response to insulin with an insulin "sliding scale" or "rainbow" approach. This is a range of insulin doses given in response to the patient's glucose levels. An example of a sliding scale order is given in Table 14–9. It must be emphasized that the sliding scale not only must be initially individualized to the patient's routine insulin needs, but must be frequently monitored and amended to maintain normal to slightly increased glucose levels. When the patient is taking food by mouth well, the preoperative insulin regimen can be reinstated and the sliding scale continued as necessary. Diabetic patients will require insulin despite decreased or suspended oral food intake.

Insulin requirements of an insulin-dependent diabetic range from 0.5 to 1.2 U/kg/day. This is usually delivered in divided SC doses 2 to 3 times per day in patients who are taking meals. In patients who are on continuous TPN, the insulin may be added to the bag for continuous IV infusion. There has been a recent proliferation of insulin types and combinations. The times of onset and duration of various insulin preparations are listed in Table 14–10.

PERIOPERATIVE INSULIN MANAGEMENT

Preoperative

The preoperative diabetic patient will usually require insulin on the morning of surgery.

1. Start routine 5% dextrose in water + ½ NS + 20 mEq/L KCl the evening before surgery at a rate of 75 to 100 mL/hour.
2. Give the patient nothing by mouth after midnight.
3. The morning of surgery, obtain a finger stick glucose reading.
4. For type II patients, administer 5 units of regular insulin SC.
5. For type I patients, administer about one-half the routine morning dose of regular insulin.
6. Do not administer NPH insulin.

TABLE 14–9 **Example of Insulin Sliding Scale Order**

1. Glucose finger stick every 6 hr and as needed	
2. For glucose:	
<80 mg/dL	Call house officer, have 1 ampule of 50% dextrose at bedside
	If the patient is able to take PO, give 5–10 oz of orange juice
	Recheck blood glucose in 30 min
80–200 mg/dL	No treatment
201–250 mg/dL	4 U regular insulin SC
251–300 mg/dL	6 U regular insulin SC
301–350 mg/dL	8 U regular insulin SC
351–400 mg/dL	10 U regular insulin SC, and call house officer
>400 mg/dL	12 U regular insulin SC, and call house officer

TABLE 14–10 **Onset and Duration of Action of Various Insulin Preparations Delivered SC**

Preparation	Onset (hr)	Peak Action (hr)	Duration (hr)
Rapid Acting			
Insulin lispro (Humalog)	0.15–0.5	0.5–2.5	3–4
Insulin aspart (NovoLog)	0.25	0.5–1	1–3
Short Acting			
Regular insulin (Humulin R, Novolin R, and others)	0.5–1	2–5	3–8
Intermediate Acting			
Lente insulin* (Humulin L)	1–4	4–10	12–18
NPH^{œ} (Humulin N)	1–4	4–10	10–16
Long Acting			
Ultralente insulin	6–10	10–16	8–20
Glargine insulin	2–4	None	24
Combinations			
50% NPH/50% regular	0.5–1	Dual	10–16
70% NPH/30% regular	0.5–1	Dual	10–16
75% NPH/25% lispeo	<0.25	Dual	10–16

*Lente is a mixture of 30% Semilente insulin and Ultralente insulin.
^{œ}NPH, neutral protamine Hagedorn.

Postoperative

The goal is to maintain blood sugars at less than 200 mg/dL.

1. Obtain an immediate blood glucose level in the recovery room.

2. Continue 5% dextrose in water + one-half NS + 20 mEq/L KCl at a rate of 75 to 100 mL/hour.
3. Obtain glucose finger sticks every 6 hours, and administer regular insulin by a sliding scale.

The management of hyperglycemia and hypoglycemia are outlined below. The principles are applicable for both diabetic and non-diabetic patients.

HYPERGLYCEMIA

Etiology

1. Poor control of diabetes mellitus, or new-onset disease
2. Stress (surgery, infection, and injury)
3. Medications (corticosteroids and thiazide diuretics)
4. Administration of TPN or other glucose-containing solution

Major Threat to Life

Dehydration
Diabetic ketoacidosis

Selective Physical Examination

The symptoms of hyperglycemia vary, depending on severity.
Mild hyperglycemia
Polyuria and polydipsia
Moderate hyperglycemia
Fluid depletion
Polyuria and polydipsia
Severe hyperglycemia

VS:	Tachycardia, rapid respiratory rate, and hypotension
MS:	Obtundation, delirium, and coma
HEENT:	"Fruity" breath (ketones)
	Flat neck veins
Resp:	Kussmaul's respiration
Abd:	Anorexia, ileus, and gastric dilation
	Abdominal pain that may mimic an acute abdomen
GU:	Polyuria and polydipsia
Neuro:	Hyporeflexia and hypotonia
ABG:	Acidosis

Management

1. General concepts
   If a finger stick value is too high or too low, or simply does not make sense, confirm that there are no glucose-containing fluids being administered IV and send a confirmatory serum glucose to the laboratory. A new diagnosis of diabetes should be confirmed with a glucose tolerance test and with serum insulin levels.

Note: A new diagnosis of diabetes cannot be made in settings of severe surgical, infectious, or other hypermetabolic stress.

The normal control of blood glucose is a balance of the following three elements:

a. Exercise (which tends to lower blood sugar)

b. Calorie sources such as food and intravenous fluids (IVFs) (which increase blood sugar)

c. Insulin (which lowers blood sugar)

Look for alterations in any of these components when trying to decipher changes in blood sugar trends.

2. Assess the severity.

This includes a fluid volume status evaluation and laboratory analysis. In addition to finger stick glucose values, frequent blood glucose samples should be sent to the laboratory along with serum electrolytes.

3. Administer fluid resuscitation, if necessary.

Follow the guidelines listed in Chapter 12 until hemodynamic stability is maintained. The fluid of choice is normal saline (NS). Do not administer glucose-containing fluids initially, as the extra glucose will exacerbate the osmotic diuresis. Care should be used with fluid administration in the elderly and in those patients with a history of congestive heart failure (CHF).

4. Order insulin administration.

The goal of ongoing insulin administration is the maintenance of serum blood glucose levels of less than 250 mg/dL.

The regimen of delivery depends on the severity of the hyperglycemia and on the severity of the illness.

Examine the pattern of blood sugars relative to recent insulin doses and make appropriate adjustments.

Use Table 14–10 as a guide to which insulin type to use and when to time its administration.

MILD HYPERGLYCEMIA

This condition is often asymptomatic and does not require urgent treatment.

1. Confirm an abnormal finger stick reading with a serum glucose level sent to the laboratory.

2. Monitor glucose finger sticks every 6 hours and as necessary.

3. Monitor serum glucose level and electrolytes every morning.

4. Monitor urine by dipstick for reducing sugars and acetate.

5. Limit glucose-containing IVFs.

6. Administer routine IV insulin doses.

In the diabetic patient who takes no food orally, administer regular insulin IV as required in doses every 6 hours and cover with a sliding scale. Adjust routine insulin doses as finger stick levels dictate.

7. Give SC bolus insulin.

In the diabetic patient who is able to take regular meals by mouth, administer routine regular and longer-acting insulin SC doses and cover with a sliding scale. Adjust routine insulin doses as finger stick levels dictate.

MODERATE HYPERGLYCEMIA

1. If the patient is already receiving insulin therapy, an adjustment may be required.
2. Confirm an abnormal finger stick reading with a serum glucose level determined by a laboratory.
3. Monitor glucose finger sticks every 2 to 4 hours and as necessary.
4. Monitor serum glucose level and electrolytes every morning.
5. Monitor urine by dipstick for reducing sugars and acetate.
6. Give IV bolus insulin.

About 5 to 10 units may be given initially. For rapid response, the use of regular insulin, administered IV, is desirable.
7. Administer routine IV insulin doses.

Follow the initial bolus with routine regular insulin IV doses every 6 hours as required, and cover with a sliding scale.
8. Advance to SC administration of regular and long-acting insulin as the patient improves and begins to tolerate meals by mouth.
9. Determine the cause of poor blood glucose control.
   a. Change in diet
   b. Change in infusion rate of glucose-containing IVFs
   c. Increased metabolic stress
   d. Inadequate insulin dosages
   e. Medications
   f. Pancreatitis

SEVERE HYPERGLYCEMIAS

Diabetic Ketoacidosis

Diabetic ketoacidosis is a severe medical disease. It is seen most commonly in patients with type I diabetes and represents a prolonged lack of insulin. If severe hyperglycemia is present with evidence of acidosis and hypotension, immediate care is required.

1. Contact your resident.
2. Prepare the patient for transfer to the intensive care unit (ICU).
3. Consult the appropriate medical team.
4. Give fluid resuscitation.

Follow the guidelines listed in Chapter 12 until hemodynamic stability is maintained. The fluid of choice is NS. Do not administer glucose-containing fluids initially, as the extra glucose will exacerbate the osmotic diuresis. Care should be taken with fluid administration in the elderly and in those patients with a history of CHF.

5. Send a baseline serum glucose to the laboratory.
   Also send baseline arterial blood gas (ABG), blood urea nitrogen (BUN), creatinine, serum insulin level, and electrolytes.

6. Monitor glucose finger sticks every 1 hour and as necessary.

7. Monitor serum glucose, electrolytes, and ABGs every 2 to 4 hours.

8. Monitor urine by dipstick for reducing sugars and acetate.

9. Give initial insulin bolus.
   5 to 10 units regular insulin IV.

10. Give continuous infusion of regular insulin.
    Start with a rate of 0.1 U/kg/hour and adjust as necessary. Continue the infusion until the blood sugars stabilize at 150 to 200 mg/dL. The rate of blood sugar drop should be about 20 to 30 mg/dL/hour (2 mmol/L/hour). As the blood sugar falls it will be necessary to slow the insulin infusion to 0.025 to 0.05 U/kg/hour.

11. Hold SC insulin doses and oral hypoglycemics.
    When blood sugars have stabilized, SC insulin doses may be added to the regimen. Remember to continue the continuous IV infusion until the SC insulin has taken effect (1 to 2 hours).

12. Add the glucose to IVFs by switching from NS to 5% dextrose in water when the serum glucose level falls below 250 to 300 mg/dL.

13. Correct other electrolyte and acid–base abnormalities.
    Common problems include acidemia and hypokalemia. These generally resolve with hydration and insulin therapy. Consider treating a pH of less than 7.2 with additional $NaHCO_3$. Initial hypokalemia may be treated by addition of KCl to the IVF.

14. Determine the cause of poor blood glucose control.
    a. Dietary indiscretion
    b. Dehydration
    c. Increased metabolic stress (infection and illness)
    d. Inadequate insulin dosages
    e. Medications
    f. Pancreatitis

Hyperosmolar Nonketotic Coma

This complication is most commonly seen in patients with poorly controlled type II diabetes. It is the result of prolonged glucose-driven diuresis leading to profound dehydration. The hyperglycemia may be severe, but ketoacidosis is absent.

1. Contact your resident.
2. Prepare the patient for transfer to the ICU.
3. Consult the appropriate medical team.
4. Give fluid resuscitation.

   Follow the guidelines listed in Chapter 12 until hemodynamic stability is maintained. The fluid of choice is NS. Do not administer glucose-containing fluids initially, as the extra glucose will exacerbate the osmotic diuresis. Care should be taken with fluid administration in the elderly and in those patients with a history of CHF. Start with administration of 500 mL of NS over 2 hours. When the patient is hemodynamically stable, replace fluids as the patient's condition dictates based on a reassessment of fluid status and serum sodium levels. Change to hypotonic fluids, such as ½ NS, at this time.
5. Send a baseline serum glucose to the laboratory.

   Also send baseline ABG, BUN, creatinine, serum insulin level, and electrolytes.
6. Monitor glucose finger sticks every 1 hour and as necessary.
7. Monitor serum glucose, electrolytes, and ABGs every 2 to 4 hours.
8. Monitor urine by dipstick for reducing sugars and acetate.
9. Give initial insulin bolus.

   5 to 10 units regular insulin IV.
10. Give continuous infusion of regular insulin.

    Patients with hyperosmolar nonketotic hyperglycemia require less insulin than those with ketoacidosis.
    Start in the range of 0.025 to 0.05 U/kg/hour and adjust as necessary. Continue insulin therapy as described in the discussion of ketoacidosis earlier.
11. Determine the cause of poor blood glucose control.
    a. Infection
    b. Dehydration
    c. Other increased metabolic stress (myocardial infarction and stroke)

HYPOGLYCEMIA

Etiology

1. Excessive exogenous insulin or oral hypoglycemics
2. Decreased calorie intake (missed meals or snacks)
3. Increased exercise
4. Medications (alcohol, pentamidine, disopyramide, and monoamine oxidase inhibitors)

5. Hepatic failure (impaired gluconeogenesis)
6. Adrenal insufficiency
7. Too rapid a withdrawal from high-glucose concentration IV fluids

Major Threat to Life

Brain Hypoglycemia

The brain is an obligate glucose user, and acute drops in blood glucose may severely and permanently damage brain functioning.

Selective Physical Examination

The symptoms are divided into two groupings, the more acute adrenergic responses, which are due to catecholamine release, and a more indolent central nervous system response, which may take 1 to 3 days to develop. Patients treated with oral hypoglycemia medications may not exhibit the adrenergic responses.

VS:	Tachycardia
MS:	Anxiety, confusion, and coma
HEENT:	Diplopia
CVS:	Palpitations
Skin:	Diaphoresis
Neuro:	Headache, perioral and fingertip numbness, focal neurologic abnormalities, tremulousness, seizures, or coma

Management

1. Assess the severity.
    Symptomatic patients require treatment; this may be safely started while the hypoglycemia is being confirmed.
2. Draw blood before treatment for laboratory studies.
    These may include serum glucose, insulin, and C-peptide levels.
3. Give oral glucose.
    If the patient is awake and able to take food by mouth, administer sweetened fruit juice.
4. Give IV glucose.
    If the patient is not able to take food by mouth, administer 50 mL of 50% dextrose in water by slow IV push.
5. Give glucagon 0.5 to 1 mg SC or IM.
    This is reserved for patients who have no IV access.
6. Give continuous IV fluids containing glucose.
    This is especially important for the patient who is unable to tolerate food by mouth or for whom hypoglycemia is an expected long-term problem.
7. Recheck finger stick glucose levels in 1 hour and every 2 to 4 hours thereafter until stable.
8. Seek a cause of hypoglycemia.

Nutrition and Wound Healing

A surgical wound has nutritional requirements as does any other tissue. Aberrations in the nutrition status of the patient will have profound effects on the normal progression of wound healing. Collagen synthesis and cross-linking is impaired by protein malnutrition; infiltrating WBCs require adequate tissue levels of glucose; and various vitamins and cofactors should be available or supplemented to effect normal healing. Vitamins A and C and the mineral zinc are of particular importance. A multivitamin is generally enough to supplement these factors.

Patients who are taking high-dose corticosteroids will have delayed wound healing. This is because of decreased inflammatory response, diminished protein synthesis, and inhibition of fibroblast proliferation. This may be reversed in part by administration of a vitamin cocktail outlined in Table 14–5. This should be continued until the wound is well healed.

Headache

While on call, you will be asked to evaluate and treat patients with headache. Postsurgical patients may develop headache as a sequela of anesthesia, stress, sleep disturbance, drug reaction, increased intracranial pressure (ICP), and other causes. Other patients may have a history of recurrent, chronic headache. Usually, a slow-onset, chronic headache is associated with a relatively benign process. Rapid-onset headache associated with fever or a change in neurologic status is more concerning as a potentially serious process.

PHONE CALL

Questions

1. **How serious is the headache?**

   A serious headache is more likely to represent a concerning problem.

2. **Are there any neurologic changes?**

   When neurologic changes are associated with headache, there is a high likelihood of a serious process. Although some transient neurologic changes can be associated with headache (e.g., migraine headache and visual changes).

3. **Was the headache of sudden onset or gradual onset?**

   Sudden-onset headaches are frequently of vascular origin and include migraine headaches, cluster headaches, subarachnoid hemorrhage, and intracerebral hemorrhage.

4. **What are the vital signs?**

   Hypertension and headache may indicate increased ICP. Make sure you ask about the patient's temperature. Infectious processes of the central nervous system, including bacterial meningitis, may present with fever and headache.

5. **Does the patient have a history of headache? Any medical problems?**

   An easy way to diagnose and treat headache is to know if a patient has a history of chronic, recurrent headache. Ask the RN to ascertain if the headache is a typical chronic headache. If it is a typical headache, find out the medication from which the patient obtains relief.

6. **Did the patient have surgery and is there a ventriculoperitoneal (VP) shunt?**

A severe headache after neurologic surgery may represent cerebral edema or intracranial bleeding. A history of VP shunt and headache may indicate shunt malfunction or infection.

Orders

1. Ask the RN to take a full set of vital signs and to assess the neurologic status if not previously done.

   Although this may seem unnecessary in most patients, it will be useful in the occasional patient who may have an impending serious process.

2. If the patient has a gradual-onset, mild headache without neurologic changes, prescribing an analgesic agent such as **acetaminophen 650 mg orally (PO)** (for adults) is appropriate. The pediatric dose of **acetaminophen** is **10 mg/kg/dose PO or PR**.

   Instruct the RN to call you back if the headache does not improve in 1 to 2 hours.

3. If the headache is associated with a deteriorating level of consciousness, ask the nurse to insert an intravenous (IV) line and place the patient on O_2.

Inform RN

Will arrive at the bedside in . . . minutes.

Headaches associated with altered mental status, change in level of consciousness, fever, or vomiting require you to assess the patient immediately. These signs frequently represent serious intracranial processes such as bleeding, swelling, or infection. Failure to recognize and treat serious intracranial problems may result in permanent neurologic dysfunction or death. If a patient who was treated for a mild headache obtains no relief or develops worsening pain, a bedside evaluation is appropriate.

ELEVATOR THOUGHTS

What causes headaches?

Slow-Onset or Chronic Headache

1. Migraine headache
2. Cluster headache
3. Temporomandibular joint (TMJ) disorder
4. Drugs (e.g., nitrates and calcium channel blockers)
5. Tension headache
6. Cervical osteoarthritis
7. Referred pain

Acute Headache

Infectious Causes

1. Meningitis
2. Encephalitis
3. VP shunt infection
4. Subdural abscess
5. Brain abscess
6. Craniotomy wound infection
7. Headache associated with viral syndrome or flu

Vascular Causes

1. Arteriovenous malformation (AVM)
2. Subarachnoid hemorrhage
3. Intracerebral hemorrhage
4. Intracranial aneurysm
5. Malignant hypertension

Increased Intracranial Pressure Causes

1. Cerebral edema
2. Hydrocephalus
3. Tumors
4. Space-occupying fluid collections (blood and abscess)

Local Causes

1. Postcraniotomy or postsurgical pain
2. Temporal arteritis
3. Visual process (acute-angle glaucoma)

MAJOR THREAT TO LIFE

- Herniation syndromes
- Meningitis
- Subarachnoid hemorrhage

Brain herniation refers to a process in which increased ICP forces a vital portion of the brain to be displaced under a rigid intracranial supporting structure. This leads to compression and loss of function of the displaced area of brain. The three rigid areas that tend to entrap brain tissue are the foramen magnum, tentorial edge, and falx cerebri. Patients with increased ICP and impending brain herniation are usually unconscious. They demonstrate a deteriorating neurologic examination and are at high risk for death. Tables 15–1 and 15–2 give the main types of herniation syndromes and the classic signs. Meningitis may be caused by a range of factors including bacterial, fungal, or viral infection. Patients with bacterial meningitis often present with a rapidly deteriorating course and must be treated with intravenous antibiotics early. Subarachnoid hemorrhage, most

TABLE 15–1 **Major Herniation Syndromes**

Type	Regions Involved
Uncal herniation	Lateral mass displaces uncus of temporal lobe medially over tentorial edge
Central herniation	Downward displacement of brainstem through foramen magnum
Cerebellar herniation	Cerebellum herniates downward through foramen magnum
Subfulcine herniation	Cingulate gyrus is displaced below falx cerebri

TABLE 15–2 **Typical Presenting Signs of Major Herniation Syndromes**

Stage of Herniation	Sign
Early	Ipsilateral pupillary dilation
	Progressive decrease in mental status
	Respiratory pattern changes (Cheyne–Stokes)
Progressing	Decreasing level of consciousness
	Hyperventilation
	Contralateral hemiplegia
	Decerebrate posturing
	Pupillary constriction
Advanced	Bilateral decerebrate rigidity (uncal herniation)
	Irregular respiration
	Flaccidity (central herniation)
	Death

frequently caused by trauma, ruptured berry aneurysms, and AVMs, must be recognized and treated rapidly.

BEDSIDE

Quick Look Test

Does the patient look well (only mildly uncomfortable), sick (very uncomfortable or distressed), or critical (about to die)?

Patients with processes causing increased ICP look sick. They frequently have either an altered mental status or a deteriorating neurologic examination. On the other hand, patients with chronic headaches are often mildly uncomfortable but do not appear sick.

Airway and Vital Signs

What is the patient's blood pressure (BP) and heart rate (HR)?

Headache may be caused by severe hypertension with systolic blood pressure (SBP) of greater than 190 mm Hg or diastolic blood pressure (DBP) of greater than 110 mm Hg. Hypertension in comatose patients with head injury or increased ICP may be due to herniation. In the advanced stages of herniation or near death, hypotension may occur. Bradycardia associated with hypertension may occur with increased ICP.

What is the patient's temperature?
   Fever and headache may indicate meningitis, subdural empyema, brain abscess, or shunt infection.

Selective Physical Examination I

Does the patient have increased ICP or meningitis?
   VS: Assess BP, HR, respiratory rate, and temperature
   HEENT: Look for signs of head injury
                 Nuchal rigidity (most common with subarach-
                 noid hemorrhage or meningitis)
                 Papilledema (sign of increased ICP) (Fig. 15–1)
                 Check for presence of a VP shunt

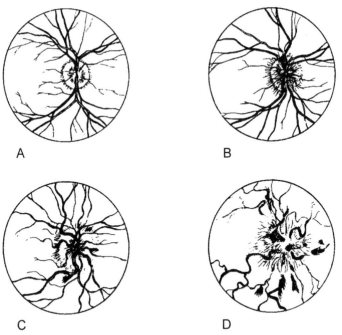

A   B

C   D

Figure 15–1 Disk changes seen in papilledema. *A*, Normal. *B*, Early papilledema. C, Moderate papilledema with early hemorrhage. *D*, Severe papilledema with extensive hemorrhage.
(From Marshall SA, Ruedy J: On Call: Principles and Protocols, 2nd ed. Philadelphia, WB Saunders, 1993, p. 107.)

	Check for craniotomy wound infection
Neuro:	Mental status examination: evaluate for acute changes (Table 15–3)
Pupillary examination:	Note size, reactivity, and symmetry of the pupils
	Brudzinski's sign and Kernig's sign (Fig. 15–2)
	Brief motor examination (Table 15–4)
	If there are signs of nuchal rigidity, acute mental status changes, motor changes, or papilledema, a full and detailed neurologic examination is indicated.

Initial Management

Headache Associated with Increased Intracranial Pressure

1. Elevate head of the bed.
2. Order computed tomographic (CT) scan immediately.
3. Obtain neurosurgical consultation.
4. If the ICP is greatly elevated, hyperventilate the patient if intubated (e.g., trauma patient); lower the arterial partial pressure of carbon dioxide ($PaCO_2$) to 25 to 30 mm Hg.

   Most patients with greatly elevated ICP are unconscious, are unstable, and require intubation. Those patients who are still conscious may need elective intubation if the need to lower the ICP is emergent.
5. Consider the use of diuretics.

   Mannitol is a good osmotic diuretic and may be given up to **1 g/kg IV every 3 hours.** Hold for serum osmolarity of greater than 305.

TABLE 15–3 **The Mental Status Examination**

Response to External Stimuli
Assess if patient is awake and alert
Assess response to verbal commands
If patient does not respond to verbal commands, evaluate response to pain (localization, withdrawing to painful stimuli, and posturing in response to pain)
Response to Cognitive Testing
Test orientation to person, place, and time
Memory testing
Months of the year in reverse order
Serial 7s
Naming three objects in 5 min (short-term memory)
Naming of past presidents and major past events
Simple calculations
Evaluate speech
Fluency
Rate

Figure 15–2 *A, Brudzinski's sign.* The test result is positive when the patient flexes his or her hips and knees in response to passive neck flexion by the examiner. *B, Kernig's sign.* The test result is positive when pain or resistance is elicited by passive knee extension, from the 90-degree hip/knee flexion position.
(From Marshall SA, Ruedy J: On Call: Principles and Protocols, 2nd ed. Philadelphia, WB Saunders, 1993, p. 109.)

TABLE 15–4 **Brief Motor Examination**

Muscle tone and bulk (fasciculation and atrophy indicate lower motor neuron disorder, increased tone and spasticity indicate upper motor neuron disorder)
Muscle strength (grades 0–5)
Muscle symmetry (look for unilateral weakness)
Reflex testing (hyporeflexia, upper motor neuron; hyperreflexia, lower motor neuron)
Gait (if possible)

6. Steroids are useful stabilizers of the blood–brain barrier.

     Consider **dexamethasone (Decadron) 10 to 50 mg IV once, then 2 to 5 mg IV/IM every 6 hours.**

     Place the patient on a histamine H_2 blocker to decrease the risk of a peptic ulcer.

7. Consider loading with **phenytoin (Dilantin)** to reduce the risk of seizure.

     Load with **18 mg/kg IV at a maximum rate of 25 mg/minute. Maintain at 100 mg IV every 8 hours.**

     Check serum phenytoin levels.

Headache Associated with Nuchal Rigidity and No Sign of Increased Intracranial Pressure

1. If bacterial meningitis is suspected (by history or presence of fever), establish IV access.
2. Order CT scan of the head immediately if possible.
3. Order the kit to perform a lumbar puncture (LP) immediately.

     Note: Do not perform LP if there is evidence of increased ICP (risk of herniation). Obtain a CT scan first.

     Measure the opening pressure and note the appearance of the cerebrospinal fluid (CSF). Also obtain cell counts, bacterial and fungal cultures, Gram stain, and India ink stain. Bacterial meningitis is most often associated with cloudy CSF, increased white blood cell (WBC) count and protein, and decreased glucose.

     Viral meningitis may be associated with turbid fluid, increased WBCs, slightly elevated protein, and normal glucose. A subarachnoid hemorrhage usually presents with bloody CSF, about 1 WBC for every 100 red blood cells, increased protein, and normal glucose.

4. Start IV antibiotics immediately if LP suggests meningitis.
5. Consider phenytoin prophylaxis.

Headache with Nuchal Rigidity and Signs of Increased Intracranial Pressure

1. Do not perform LP (risk of herniation).
2. Order CT scan immediately. An LP may be performed after CT rules out signs of increased intracranial pressure.
3. Start empirical IV antibiotics.
4. Consider brain abscess of subdural empyema.
5. Obtain neurosurgical consultation for mass lesions.
6. Consider phenytoin prophylaxis.

Selective History and Chart Review

Once emergent management is taken for life-threatening processes associated with headache, a more detailed evaluation may be performed. If the patient has an isolated headache and does not require aggressive initial management, a carefully taken history will often clarify the best management.

Does the patient have a history of headaches?

Frequently, patients suffer from recurrent headaches and can describe the form of treatment that best relieves the symptoms. Patients with a history of migraine or cluster headaches may also describe the form of drug therapy that is effective for relief of the symptoms.

Does head position affect headache severity?

Patients with headaches sensitive to vertical positioning of the head may have an increased ICP.

Does the patient have TMJ syndrome or referred headache pain?

Patients with TMJ syndrome frequently develop headaches as a result of muscle spasm. These patients clench and grind their teeth while asleep and then awaken with a headache. They may be helped with non-narcotic analgesics such as nonsteroidal anti-inflammatory drugs (NSAIDs) and muscle relaxants (e.g., *Flexeril*). Ask the patient what type of therapy has worked best in the past. Ultimately, many of these patients will need dental treatment and a mouth guard to wear while sleeping, to prevent clenching and grinding.

Is there a history of head trauma in the recent or remote past?

Epidural hematomas are caused by a collection of blood between the calvaria and the dura and are usually seen associated with a skull fracture. Subdural hematomas are usually caused by brain surface bleeding or bleeding from venous structures near the brain surface. Subdural hematomas may be acute (symptoms within 72 hours of injury), subacute (3 to 20 days after injury), or chronic (3 weeks or longer after injury). Mass effect and an abnormal neurologic examination usually require craniotomy and removal of the clot.

Are there any prodromal or visual changes?

Visual auras may occur before migraine headaches and include blurred vision and scintillations. Remember that visual changes may also be associated with transient ischemic attacks.

Does the patient have a fever and a ventriculoperitoneal (VP) shunt?

VP shunts have a 5% to 10% infection rate; organisms causing infection include *Staphylococcus aureus, S. epidermidis,* and gram-negative rods. Shunt culture (sterilely obtaining fluid from the reservoir) is indicated. IV and intrathecal antibiotics are indicated for shunt infections; infected shunts may ultimately need to be removed and replaced at a different site. Consult with a neurosurgeon for shunt problems.

What drugs is the patient receiving?

Nitrates, calcium channel blockers, and other drugs may cause headaches.

Has the patient had a recent lumbar puncture or spinal anesthesia?

Removal of small amounts of CSF can cause headache, especially when the patient is upright. Treatment is bed rest.

Selective Physical Examination II

VS:	Repeat now
HEENT:	Scalp lacerations and depressed skull fractures
	Hemotympanum (blood medial to tympanic membrane) or raccoon eyes (basilar skull fracture)
	CSF otorrhea or rhinorrhea (dural tear and possible basilar skull fracture)
	Red eye (narrow-angle glaucoma)
	Eyelid ptosis (cranial nerve 3 dysfunction or levator disinsertion)
	Retinal hemorrhages (hypertension or trauma)
	Tender, enlarged temporal arteries (temporal arteritis)
	Tenderness over the frontal or maxillary sinuses (sinusitis)
	Crepitus and tenderness over the TMJ; possible restricted mouth opening (TMJ syndrome)
Neuro:	Perform a complete neurologic examination
	Mental status (if not already tested): evaluate the level of consciousness and look for new-onset somnolence
Cranial nerves:	Look for asymmetries
	Motor examination including gait and reflexes: look for asymmetries, weakness, and abnormal reflexes
	Sensory examination

Definitive Management

Evidence of Head Trauma

A patient who has had head trauma with a loss of consciousness should have a head CT scan. The other alternative is to admit the patient for close neurologic observation. The head CT scan is advantageous because it may be a less costly and a more efficient way to screen for head injury. Any significant intracranial mass or brain injury discovered on head CT scanning requires evaluation by neurosurgery.

Posttraumatic Headache

If a patient has suffered head trauma without a loss of consciousness, it is important to be able to follow this patient's neurologic examination in the immediate posttraumatic period. Care must be taken to not sedate the patient with an analgesic. It is best to use acetaminophen for mild headache. For more severe pain, use **codeine 30 mg intramuscularly (IM).** Do not use drugs that thin the blood inhibit platelet function (e.g., NSAIDs).

Pseudotumor Cerebri

This condition, also known as benign intracranial hypertension, presents as headache and increased ICP (papilledema), without obvious intracranial mass on CT scanning. This condition does not require emergent management at night, and referral to a neurologist may be made during normal working hours.

Migraine Headache

Migraines may present in a variety of ways, although they are often lateralized and throbbing. Many patients have a short prodromal period, or "aura," before the severe migraine pain begins. Migraine headaches may be associated with blurring of vision, visual field defects, visual hallucinations, aphasia, numbness, paresthesias, or transient focal weakness. Triggering factors include sleep deprivation, emotional distress, reactions to food, and certain drugs (e.g., oral contraceptives). Treatment for mild pain includes aspirin or acetaminophen. If a more severe migraine begins and is still in its prodromal stage, treatment with a 5-HT receptor agonist may be helpful (**sumatriptan, rizatriptan,** and others). **Sumatriptan (Imitrex)** comes in injectable, oral, and nasal spray formulations.

The oral dose is **25 mg PO with additional doses of 25 to 50 mg PO every 2 hours to a maximum of 200 to 300 mg/day.** Avoid the use of 5-HT receptor agonists in the setting of known coronary artery disease, uncontrolled hypertension, or concomitantly with ergot compounds.

If no response is noted with the 5-HT receptor agonists, **Cafergot,** a combination of ergotamine tartrate and caffeine, may be helpful. The patient should take **2 tablets** (1 tablet = 1 mg ergotamine + 100 mg caffeine) **at the onset of the headache or the prodrome.** If the symptoms have not subsided **at 20 minutes,** the patient should be given **1 more tablet every 30 minutes, up to 6 tablets/24 hours.** If the patient vomits during the migraine headache, **ergotamine IM (0.25 to 0.5 mg)** can be given. Frequently, a narcotic analgesic such as **meperidine (Demerol) 75 to 100 mg** IM is required for adequate analgesia. Avoid the use of ergotamine-containing preparations in patients who are pregnant or who have a history of unstable angina or poorly controlled hypertension.

Cluster Headache

These headaches are most common in middle-aged men. Pain begins as an episode of unilateral periorbital pain that lasts about 1 hour. Pain generally occurs daily for several weeks. Pain is accompanied by eye tearing, rhinorrhea or nasal congestion, or Horner syndrome. Adequate treatment is difficult. Ergotamine tartrate aerosol or **inhalation of 100% oxygen for 15 to 20 minutes** is usually helpful. The use of narcotic analgesics, such as meperidine, is also useful.

Tension Headache

These headaches are extremely common. They usually present as vise-like, generalized pain. The posterior neck muscles are frequently involved and are often tender. Headache may be exacerbated by stress, noise, or fatigue. Treatment involves aspirin or acetaminophen, and relaxation techniques. Hot baths and massage are also useful. Avoid the use of benzodiazepines chronically in these patients.

Temporal Arteritis

This condition involves inflammation of the temporal arteries, which may become thrombosed. In addition to temporal arteries, vertebral and ophthalmic arteries may also be involved. Clinical examination reveals tenderness of the superficial temporal artery over the scalp. Temporal arteritis must be treated immediately, because untreated disease can lead to blindness. If the diagnosis is suspected, start the patient on **prednisone 60 mg PO every day,** obtain an erythrocyte sedimentation rate (ESR) (look for ESR of greater than 60 mm/hour), and arrange for a temporal artery biopsy.

Malignant Hypertension

Uncontrolled sustained hypertension, with diastolic pressures of greater than 130 mm Hg, leads to widespread arteriolar damage. This is manifested by headache, retinal hemorrhages, papilledema, renal failure, myocardial infarction, and stroke. Refer to Chapter 16 for the treatment of malignant hypertension.

Meningitis

The most frequent causative agents for community-acquired meningitis are *S. pneumonia, Neisseria meningitides,* and *Listeria monocytogenes.* Follow the guidelines listed above under the heading of Headache with nuchal rigidity. Empiric antibiotics may include:

> **Cefotaxime 2 gm IV every 6 hours,** or **ceftriaxone 2 gm IV every 12 hours, WITH**
>
> **Ampicillin 2 gm IV every 4 hours** (in the elderly to cover Listeria sp.), **AND**
>
> **Vancomycin 15 mg/kg IV every 12 hours** +/- **rifampin 20 mg/kg PO each day** in divided doses if your institution has a significant population of penicillin-resistant pneumococci species.
>
> **Dexamethasone 10 mg PO every 6 hours for 4 days** starting before or with the first dose of antibiotics.

Hypertension

The goal on-call is to treat hypertensive episodes that are symptomatic or that put the patient at risk for myocardial infarction (MI), stroke, or bleeding. As the on-call physician, it is best to leave the fine-tuning of a patient's blood pressure (BP) to the primary team caring for the patient.

PHONE CALL

Questions

What is the BP?

Always evaluate the magnitude of the BP elevation. A mild BP elevation is not serious. However, an episode of malignant hypertension may result in sudden death.

Why is the patient in the hospital? Did the patient have surgery? If so, what was the operation and when was it performed?

It is important to ascertain why the patient is in the hospital and whether the patient is postoperative. For example, a diagnosis of pheochromocytoma would explain elevated BP.

Is the patient in pain or anxious?

Pain and anxiety result in sympathetic stimulation and elevation of BP.

Is there a history of hypertension? If so, is the patient taking any antihypertensive medications?

Patients with a history of hypertension are likely to have BP control problems while in the hospital.

Patients taking antihypertensive medications frequently miss doses of medication just before admission.

Sometimes, hypertensive patients are not placed on their BP medications on admission.

Are there any symptoms of a hypertensive emergency, such as chest pain, back pain, shortness of breath (SOB), headache, neck stiffness, vomiting, or seizures?

MI or aortic dissection may cause chest pain or back pain. SOB may be caused by MI or pulmonary edema secondary to severe hypertension. Headache, neck stiffness, vomiting, and seizures may be related to subarachnoid hemorrhage or stroke.

Orders

If asked to treat a patient with mildly symptomatic elevation in BP, ask the RN if the patient is currently taking antihypertensive drugs. If the patient is not currently on drug therapy for hypertension and is otherwise healthy and not pregnant, consider ordering **nifedipine 10 mg orally (PO) or sublingually (SL).** A patient currently on anti-hypertensive therapy may benefit from an additional incremental dose of the current medication.

In the event of a hypertensive emergency (diastolic BP greater than 120 mm Hg), a functional intravenous (IV) line should be available. If an IV is not in place, order an IV placed immediately. Run crystalloid to keep the vein open.

Inform RN

Will be at the bedside in . . . minutes.

Mild BP elevation is not an emergency, and it can usually be handled over the phone. However, hypertensive emergencies require your immediate evaluation and treatment of the patient.

These hypertensive emergencies include the following conditions:
1. Preeclampsia and eclampsia
2. Aortic dissection
3. Hypertensive crisis
4. Hypertensive withdrawal syndromes (e.g., cocaine and alcohol)
5. Coronary ischemia or infarction
6. Catecholamine crisis
7. Hypertensive encephalopathy
8. Pulmonary edema

ELEVATOR THOUGHTS

What causes hypertension?
- Essential hypertension
- Renal disease
- Preeclampsia and eclampsia
- Pain
- Fear or emotional stress
- Fluid overload
- Increased intracranial pressure (ICP) (e.g., intracranial tumor or bleed)

- Cushing syndrome
- Pheochromocytoma
- Coarctation of the aorta
- Hypoxia
- Drugs of abuse (e.g., cocaine or amphetamine toxicity)
- Drug interactions (e.g., monoamine oxidase [MAO] inhibitors and tricyclics)
- Drug withdrawal

There are many causes of hypertension. Essential hypertension is the most common form of high BP and accounts for more than 90% of chronic hypertension cases. The cause of essential hypertension is not known.

Preeclampsia is a condition associated with pregnancy and is manifest by hypertension, proteinuria, generalized edema, and sporadic liver function abnormalities (including coagulopathy). Eclampsia includes the findings of preeclampsia but also includes generalized seizures. Hypertension in the setting of pregnancy is dangerous for both the fetus and the mother. Special care must be used in treating these conditions, because some antihypertensive agents have adverse effects on fetal development.

Pain is a common cause of hypertension in postsurgical and trauma patients. Ascertain that postoperative patients have appropriate pain control. Inadequate sedation of intubated patients may lead to hypertension. Emotional states such as anxiety and fear also contribute to elevated BPs.

Increased ICP may be a cause of hypertension in neurosurgical and trauma patients. Tumors, subdural or epidural hematomas, or diffuse brain swelling may all cause increased ICP.

Endocrine disorders may be associated with hypertension. Cushing disease associated with adenoma or exogenous steroid use may cause significant hypertension. Pheochromocytoma may cause a malignant hypertensive crisis through overproduction and release of large quantities of epinephrine and norepinephrine.

Cocaine and amphetamines block reuptake of norepinephrine in nerve synapses. These drugs may cause severe hypertension when taken in overdose amounts. MAO inhibitors and tricyclic antidepressants may also cause hypertension and toxicity when taken in overdose amounts. These drugs may cause serious interactions when taken with indirect-acting (tyramine) or direct-acting (epinephrine) catecholamines.

Withdrawal from alcohol and drugs can lead to hypertension and severe sympathetic overactivity. Alcohol withdrawal is associated with significant morbidity and mortality. Withdrawal of cocaine or other sympathomimetic drugs can produce hypertension after chronic use. Narcotic withdrawal may cause tremulousness, hypertension, and tachycardia.

MAJOR THREAT TO LIFE

The following conditions, associated with hypertension, are either directly life threatening or may lead to complications that are life threatening:

1. Malignant hypertension
2. Cerebrovascular accident (CVA, stroke)
3. MI
4. Pulmonary edema
5. Aortic dissection
6. Eclampsia
7. Drug withdrawal
8. Hypertensive encephalopathy

BEDSIDE

Quick Look Test

Does the patient look well (comfortable), sick (uncomfortable or distressed), or critical (about to die)?

Most patients with mild elevations in BP are asymptomatic and look comfortable. Most patients with signs and symptoms of chest pain, SOB, or pain in the chest or back associated with hypertension will look distressed.

Airway and Vital Signs

Is the airway adequate?

Hypertension may be seen in a patient with airway obstruction or hypoxia. In both intubated and nonintubated patients, assess that ventilation and oxygenation are adequate.

What is the BP?

Take the BP in both arms. If the readings are not within 5 mm Hg of each other, repeat both pressures. Recall that coarctation of the aorta and aortic dissection may produce different BP readings in the two extremities.

What is the heart rate?

Hypertension and tachycardia are seen in states of catecholamine excess. This is commonly found in hypertensive crisis, drug overdose, and drug withdrawal. If the patient is hypertensive and bradycardic, look for signs of increased ICP. Beware that beta-blockers may produce bradycardia in a patient with hypertension.

Selective History and Chart Review

Does the patient have a history of hypertension?

Was the patient taking any medications outside the hospital?

Is the patient being continued on antihypertensive medications while in the hospital?

Patients who take antihypertensive medications frequently do not have these medications continued on admission to the hospital. This is usually an oversight at the time of admission. Discontinuation of antihypertensive therapy may be responsible for poor BP control.

Does the patient have any symptoms suggestive of a hypertensive emergency?

Ask the patient about the following symptoms:
1. Chest pain (MI or aortic dissection)
2. Back pain (aortic dissection)
3. SOB (pulmonary edema)
4. Headache (increased ICP or hypertensive encephalopathy)
5. Unilateral weakness or paresis (CVA)

Selective Physical Examination

The physical examination should be directed at looking for evidence of hypertensive crisis.

VS:	Repeat now; be sure to perform BP readings on both arms if not already done.
HEENT:	Fundoscopy: first look for papilledema, which is evidence of malignant hypertension; evidence of more chronic hypertensive changes, such as arteriolar narrowing, hemorrhages, or exudates, should also be noted.
Resp:	Note crackles or rales (pulmonary edema) and evidence of pleural effusions (congestive heart failure [CHF]).
CVS:	Listen for S_3 (CHF); look for evidence of elevated jugular venous distention.
Neuro:	Look for focal weakness or paresis (CVA); also note changes in mental status, including level of agitation, and confusion (increased ICP or hypertensive encephalopathy).

MANAGEMENT

Hypertensive Crisis

This state is defined when the diastolic BP is greater than 120 mm Hg. The severity of the crisis depends on both the absolute BP and the rapidity with which the BP elevation occurs. Hypertension associated with target organ damage (TOD) is an emergency, and it must be treated immediately. Common examples of TOD are shown in Table 16–1.

Hypertensive crisis with associated TOD changes should be treated with IV drug therapy. For patients in an intensive care unit

TABLE 16–1 **Target Organ Damage Associated with Hypertensive Crisis**

Target Organ/System	Associated Changes
Cardiac/respiratory	Myocardial ischemia
	Infarction
	Pulmonary edema
Renal	Hematuria
	Azotemia
Central nervous system	Mental status changes
	Seizures
	Coma
Retina	Papilledema
	Hemorrhages
	Exudates

(ICU) environment and with an arterial line, **sodium nitroprusside** is the first-line drug to reduce severe hypertension. Sodium nitroprusside is rapid acting and is easily titratable. Its action is short-lived when infusion is discontinued. Start therapy with a **0.5 mcg/kg/minute IV drip** and titrate the dosing as tolerated. Patients with renal failure should be started at **0.25 mcg/kg/minute.** Most patients will respond to doses of less than 2 mcg/kg/minute. Dosing should never be greater than 10 mcg/kg/minute. Sodium nitroprusside is light sensitive and is associated with thiocyanate toxicity and methemoglobinemia when given in high doses (>2 to 3 mcg/kg/ minute) or for prolonged duration. Patients with renal dysfunction are also at increased risk for thiocyanate toxicity. Toxicity is associated with acidosis, dyspnea, vomiting, and dizziness. Thiocyanate levels should be checked every 2 to 3 days.

If sodium nitroprusside is not readily available or if intra-arterial monitoring has not been established, other IV agents may be useful. IV bolus therapy may be initiated with metoprolol, labetalol, diazoxide, and hydralazine. These drugs allow rapid BP reduction. Continuous IV infusion can be continued with labetalol and diazoxide. The effects of these drugs are not as easy to control as those of sodium nitroprusside, due to longer duration of action. Table 16–2 provides a list of common IV antihypertensive agents and their onsets, durations, dosages, and commonly occurring adverse effects.

AORTIC DISSECTION

Patients with aortic dissection will often present with a history of sudden, severe chest pain with radiation to the back, the abdomen, and the extremities. Shock usually occurs with the later stages of the process. More than 60% of dissections occur in the ascending aorta,

TABLE 16–2 An Overview of Common Intravenous Antihypertensive Agents

Drug	Route/Onset	Mechanism/Duration	Dose	Considerations
Sodium nitroprusside	IV infusion immediate	Smooth muscle relaxant, 3 min	0.5 mcg/kg/min starting dose, titrate to achieve desired effect up to 10 mcg/kg/min as tolerated; consider 0.25 mcg/kg/min in renal failure	Hypotension, nausea, vomiting, thiocyanate toxicity; check thiocyanate levels
Nitroglycerin	IV infusion immediate	Preload and afterload reduction, venous dilatation, 15 min	5–20 mcg/min, titrate to achieve desired effect	Useful for moderate hypertension in patients with myocardial ischemia; watch for excessive preload reduction in patients with right-sided heart failure
Labetalol	IV bolus 5 min IV infusion	Alpha and beta blockade, 3–5 hr	10–80 mg every 5 min, up to 1300 mg 5–100 mcg/min	Beware of inducing heart failure and hypotension; very effective agent
Metoprolol	IV bolus 5–15 min IV PO	Selective beta-1 blockade, Dose dependent	5 mg IV q 2 min, up to a maximum dose of 15 mg 100–200 mg PO each day in divided doses	Monitor in settings of diabetes and liver failure
Diazoxide	IV bolus 1–3 min	Direct arterial dilatation, 6–10 hr	50–100 mg every 5 min, up to 500 mg 10–30 mg/min	Causes reflex tachycardia; avoid use in acute MI or in dissecting aortic aneurysm
Hydralazine	IV infusion IV bolus 10 min	Vasodilation, 3–5 hr 3–5 hr	5–10 mg every 10 min	Tachycardia, hypotension; consider different agent if no significant effect after 20–30 mg
Esmolol	IV infusion 1–3 min	Selective beta-blocker, 10 min	200–400 mcg/kg/min for first 1–3 min, then 50–200 mcg/kg/min	Watch for heart block, hypotension, and bronchospasm

IV, intravenous; MI, myocardial infarction.

whereas 20% occur in the distal arch, and 20% in the descending thoracic or abdominal aorta. Mediastinal widening may be visible on chest x-ray. Computed tomographic scanning with contrast provides a noninvasive diagnostic tool. Aortography is diagnostic.

Aortic dissections that involve the ascending aorta are known as type A. These dissections mandate emergent surgery due to the high likelihood of aortic rupture and cardiac tamponade. Type B dissections begin at the subclavian artery, and surgical therapy is often deferred. Control of the process is attempted with antihypertensive therapy. Severe pain, inability to control BP, compromise of blood flow to end-organs, or high risk of rupture are complications of type B dissections that mandate surgery (see Fig. 7–1).

The mainstay of treatment includes bed rest and antihypertensive therapy. The goal of antihypertensive therapy is to achieve a systolic BP of 100 to 120 mm Hg or the lowest possible BP that allows adequate organ perfusion. For BP control, a sodium nitroprusside drip is the treatment of choice because of the ability to titrate the BP finely without tachyphylaxis. A beta-blocker must be used concurrently with sodium nitroprusside, because sodium nitroprusside alone causes an increase in left ventricular dv/dt and subsequent arterial shearing forces. **Propranolol** may be used at **0.5 mg IV followed by 1 mg IV every 5 minutes until the pulse pressure is reduced to 60 mm Hg or to a total dose of 0.15 mg/kg in any 4-hour period.** Esmolol may be more convenient to use, since it is a cardioselective beta-blocker and is less likely to cause problems in asthmatics or patients with chronic obstructive pulmonary disease. Consider **200 to 400 mcg/kg/minute esmolol** for the first 1 to 3 minutes followed by 50 to 200 mcg/kg/minute. When using beta-blockers concurrently with sodium nitroprusside, be careful to avoid hypotension and heart block.

Second-choice therapy in treating aortic dissection is **labetalol.** It can be used successfully as a single agent, but it should be reserved for situations in which sodium nitroprusside cannot be tolerated or when it is not available. Start with **labetalol 20 to 80 mg IV bolus, up to 250 mg. Begin continuous infusion at 0.5 to 2 mg/minute**.

PREECLAMPSIA AND ECLAMPSIA

Managing hypertensive pregnant patients is difficult and should be done only with the consultation of an obstetrician. Attempt to contact the patient's obstetrician if possible. Treatment for hypertension in pregnant patients should be considered when the diastolic BP is greater than 100 mm Hg. The treatment of choice when the mother is near term is magnesium sulfate given as an IV infusion. Magnesium sulfate does not decrease BP, but it decreases fetal and maternal morbidity until delivery can be induced or cesarean section performed. Ask the obstetrician to order and manage the magnesium sulfate drip.

If antihypertensive therapy is required for a pregnant patient, **methyldopa 250 to 500 mg IV bolus** is the recommended first-line therapy. An alternative drug is **hydralazine 5 to 10 mg IV every 10 minutes,** followed by oral maintenance therapy (Table 16–3). Some antihypertensive agents have been associated with perinatal morbidity and mortality. Angiotensin-converting enzyme inhibitors are toxic to the fetus. Beta-blockers such as propranolol have been shown to alter uterine contractility; calcium channel blockers also alter uterine contractility. Diuretic use in pregnant patients has been shown to cause neonatal toxicity and maternal dehydration.

HYPERTENSIVE ENCEPHALOPATHY

In this condition, severe hypertension is accompanied by drowsiness, confusion, headache, nausea, and deteriorating mental status. A greatly elevated BP, often greater than 250/150 mm Hg, is characteristic. Common findings include papilledema, retinal hemorrhages, and exudates. There are usually no focal neurologic deficits found early in the progression of the disease. However, if focal neurologic deficits are present, a concurrent CVA may have occurred.

Treatment requires transfer to an ICU for electrocardiographic (ECG) and BP monitoring. A single **5- to 10-mg PO dose of nifedipine** can gently bring down BP while ICU transfer is taking place. Once the patient is in the ICU, an arterial line should be placed. First-line drug therapy is sodium nitroprusside, as outlined in Table 16–2. In patients with known or suspected atherothrombotic cerebrovascular disease, remember to bring down the BP slowly. These patients are at increased risk of CVA if blood pressure is reduced too quickly. It is reasonable to attempt to reduce the mean arterial BP by about 25% over the first several hours of therapy. Slowly titrate the infusion of nitroprusside to gradually decrease the BP.

There are other options for treating the hypertension associated with hypertensive encephalopathy. Diazoxide and labetalol may be used as outlined in Table 16–2. Once BP control is achieved through parenteral means, an appropriate oral regimen can be selected for maintenance (see Table 16–3).

HYPERTENSION ASSOCIATED WITH MYOCARDIAL ISCHEMIA OR PULMONARY EDEMA

Patients with hypertension and myocardial ischemia/infarction or pulmonary edema should be transferred to the ICU immediately. Consider **SL nitroglycerin 0.3 mg** to control chest pain during the transfer. Once in the ICU, begin **nitroglycerin infusion at 5** mcg/minute, and **titrate** the dose to **20 mcg/minute** to attempt to

TABLE 16-3 **An Overview of Common Antihypertensive Agents Available by Oral, Sublingual, and Transcutaneous Routes**

Drug	Route Available	Mechanism	Initial Dosage
Nifedipine	PO/sublingual	Calcium channel blocker	10 mg 3 times per day, may repeat sublingual dosing once
Nifedipine XL	PO	Calcium channel blocker	30 mg every day
Verapamil	PO	Calcium channel blocker	80 mg 3 times
Verapamil XL	PO	Calcium channel blocker	120 mg PO every day
Atenolol	PO	Selective beta antagonist	50 mg PO every day
Metoprolol	PO	Selective beta antagonist	50 mg PO 2 times per day
Propranolol	PO	Nonselective beta antagonist	40 mg PO 2 times per day
Labetalol	PO	Alpha and beta antagonist	100 mg PO 2 times per day
Captopril	PO	ACE inhibitor	10 mg PO every day
Enalapril	PO	ACE inhibitor	5 mg PO every day
Lisinopril	PO	ACE inhibitor	10 mg PO every day
Clonidine	PO	Centrally acting agent	0.1 mg PO 2 times per day
Clonidine patch	Trans-cutaneous	Centrally acting agent	TTS 1/wk
Chlorothiazide	PO	Thiazide diuretic	500 mg PO every day
HCTZ	PO	Thiazide diuretic	25 mg PO every day
Furosemide	PO (or IV)	Loop diuretic	20 mg PO every day
Spironolactone	PO	Potassium-sparing diuretic	50 mg PO every day

PO, by mouth; HCTZ, hydrochlorothiazide; IV, intravenous; ACE, angiotensin-converting enzyme; TTS, transdermal therapeutic system.

control both the hypertension and the chest pain. Nitroglycerin reduces the myocardial demand for oxygen while reducing both pre-load and afterload. Nitroprusside is not the first-line drug therapy in hypertensive patients with myocardial ischemia because nitroprusside may cause a coronary steal phenomenon and increase the area of myocardial ischemia. Treat pulmonary edema from congestive heart failure as outlined in Chapter 28.

CATECHOLAMINE CRISIS

There are many conditions that greatly increase catecholamine or catecholamine-like activity. Cocaine and amphetamine toxicity, anti-hypertensive drug withdrawal, alcohol withdrawal, and food or drug interactions with MAO inhibitors can lead to hypertensive crisis. Taking a good history is important in delineating what substances may be involved.

Pheochromocytomas may release dopamine, epinephrine, norep-inephrine, and vasoactive peptides, resulting in severe hypertension. Classic symptoms include episodic hypertension associated with pal-lor and subsequent flushing, palpitations, headache, nervousness, excessive perspiration, and anxiety. In about one-half the cases, hypertension is sustained. Elevated levels of urinary vanillylmandelic acid and metanephrine are suggestive; direct measurement of ele-vated urinary or serum epinephrine or norepinephrine is diagnostic.

A patient with malignant hypertension and catecholamine crisis should be transferred to the ICU. ECG and intra-arterial BP monitor-ing is appropriate. Drug therapy is as follows:

1. Cocaine and amphetamine toxicity
   Propranolol 1 to 3 mg every 2 to 5 minutes IV to a max-imum of 8 mg. Attempt to control both BP and tachycardia. Sedation may be helpful to reduce anxiety.
2. Pheochromocytoma
   The alpha-adrenergic blocking drugs are the treatment of choice. **Phenoxybenzamine hydrochloride** may be given **at an initial dose of 10 mg IV every 8 hours**. Phenoxy-benzamine is a selective alpha blocker with a long duration of action. The dosage may be increased until all signs of cate-cholamine toxicity have resolved.
   Watch for postural hypotension with use of alpha-blocking drugs. Propranolol may be useful when cardiac dysrhythmias and severe tachycardia present. However, use propranolol only after alpha blockade has been performed (hypertensive crisis can ensue if alpha blockade is not performed and beta blockade is given).

Hypotension and Shock

Hypotension is a common and serious complication of a patient's hospital course. In mild and early stages there are many compensatory responses that can support tissue perfusion. If it worsens, circulatory collapse can ensue, resulting in shock. Shock is the extreme form of hypotension and refers to the condition of inadequate end-organ tissue perfusion. With a small amount of information and knowledge of a patient's trends over time, the early warning signs of hypotension may be detected and appropriately treated. Shock may not always be avoided, but the patient can receive the benefits of improved circulation throughout the hypotensive episode.

The phone call will usually deal with a blood pressure (BP) number. Although this is of value, it is important to remember that there is no absolute systolic or diastolic number that defines hypotension. It is different in each patient. Look at the body's response, that is, the pulse relative to the BP, orthostatic BPs, and tissue perfusion (especially skin, kidneys, and brain) before assuming that a particular BP is inadequate.

PHONE CALL

Questions

What is the BP, and is this number a change in the BP trends?
How was the BP measured?
Consistency is the key. BPs will vary somewhat depending on the size of the BP cuff used, the limb used, and whether the value was derived from a normally functioning arterial line.

What is the pulse?
Be especially mindful of orthostatic BPs with pulses. Is there a change in pulse trends?

Are there changes in end-organ perfusion?
Is the patient conscious (brain)? What is the urine output (UO) (kidney)? Are the distal extremities warm (skin)?

Has the patient undergone a surgical procedure, and if so, how long ago?
Is the patient having a surgically related loss of fluid such as postoperative bleeding or sequestration into a third space?

Are there any other symptoms such as chest pain, respiratory distress, or rash?

Are there any changes in vital signs?
Be especially mindful of fever. Fever with hypotension is evidence of impending septic shock.

Orders

1. Order intravenous (IV) access.
   For rapid fluid replacement, a large-bore (16 gauge) peripheral IV is best. This will allow more rapid vascular space volume expansion than will central venous access. Begin fluid resuscitation through any existing line while another appropriate line is started. More than one line may be used and may be desirable.
2. Begin volume expansion.
   Rapid fluid replacement begins with crystalloid. This is the cheapest and most readily available fluid. Start with a **bolus of normal saline (NS) 500 mL IV** and repeat as necessary until the BP improves. If massive blood loss is the cause of the hypotension, consider, in addition, replacement with O type, Rh-negative uncrossmatched blood.
3. Support cerebral perfusion.
   Place the patient in 15° Trendelenburg's position with the feet elevated.
4. Support oxygenation.
   Have a pulse oximeter placed on the patient, and deliver O_2 by mask to keep the saturation at greater than 93%. If tissue perfusion is poor, the pulse oximeter may not be effective. Deliver O_2 at 4 to 10 L/minute by mask.
5. If the patient is anaphylactic (hives, hypotension, and respiratory distress), have epinephrine available for administration, as follows:
   Epinephrine (1:1000) 0.5 mL (0.5 mg) subcutaneously (SC) or
   Epinephrine (1:10,000) 5 mL (0.5 mg) IV.
   (Label these carefully by their route of administration, so no mistake is made. Either may be necessary, depending on the severity of the reaction.)
6. Send laboratory studies. The following should be sent immediately:
   - Complete blood count (CBC)
     Remember that the hemoglobin may be initially normal (or unchanged) in settings of acute hemorrhage.

- Arterial blood gas (ABG)

    This will give information on acid–base status and oxygenation.

    Pay special attention to the base deficit. This is a good initial indication of the severity of the hypoperfusion and may be followed sequentially to assess the efficacy of the resuscitation.
- Baseline serum chemistries

    Rapid fluid expansion will require frequent assessment of serum Na^+, K^+, Cl^-, blood urea nitrogen, and creatinine.
- Baseline urine chemistries

    End points of fluid resuscitation include normal urine output (UO) and normal specific gravity (1.01).

    Consider an immediate type and crossmatch for blood if acute hemorrhage is the cause of hypotension.
7. Consider other studies, as follows:
   - Portable chest x-ray immediately to assess for pneumothorax or pulmonary infection
   - 12-lead electrocardiogram (ECG).

Degree of Urgency

The patient must be evaluated immediately.

ELEVATOR THOUGHTS

What causes shock?

Remember that shock is inadequate for end-organ perfusion. Perfusion is based on appropriate cardiac function, blood volume, and peripheral vascular tone in relationships described by the following formulas:

Cardiac output (CO) = heart rate (HR) × stroke volume (SV)
BP = CO × systemic vascular resistance (SVR)

Factors that cause shock act at one or more of the elements that contribute to BP (CO or SVR):
1. Cardiogenic
   - Pump malfunction (inadequate HR or SV)
   - Occlusion of the outflow tract (inadequate CO)
2. Hypovolemic (inadequate SV)
3. Septic (inadequate SVR)
4. Anaphylactic (inadequate SVR)
5. Neurogenic (inadequate SVR)

MAJOR THREAT TO LIFE

1. Shock
2. Complications of inadequate perfusion
   - Myocardial infarction (MI)
   - Stroke
   - Multiple organ failure

BEDSIDE

Quick Look Test

A hypotensive patient who is not yet in shock will appear well to mildly ill. A patient who is in shock will appear ill or moribund.

Airway and Vital Signs

1. Maintain the airway.

   If the patient is unconscious, place the patient in a supine position. Remove dentures and other foreign objects. Make sure the airway is patent and clear. An oral airway may be necessary. If the patient is very ill, consider endotracheal (ET) intubation. If patients cannot protect their own airways (history of aspiration or absent gag reflex), intubation is required to decrease the risk of aspiration pneumonia. Place the patient in the left lateral decubitus position until intubation is performed. Contact the intensive care unit (ICU)/cardiac care unit (CCU) for immediate transfer of the patient. Contact your resident.

2. Maintain respirations.

   If the patient is breathing spontaneously, maintaining the airway may be sufficient. Note the respirations, however; rapid, sonorous respirations are indicative of acidosis, which will require treatment. In addition, the work of breathing may be more effort than the patient can maintain, and ET intubation will be required to save the patient's energy.

3. Maximize oxygenation.

   The definition of shock is poor delivery of oxygen to the tissues. Oxygen delivery to the patient should be optimized to take advantage of what little perfusion is available.

4. Assess blood pressure.

   This should be done continuously during fluid resuscitation. In the ICU/CCU this may be done by continuous arterial line monitoring (see Chapter 19 for placement information). On the ward, serial BPs may be taken, or a mechanical BP device may be left on the patient during the resuscitative effort.

   Orthostatic BPs can help determine the intravascular volume status. Orthostatics are HR and BP taken while the patient is lying flat, while the patient is sitting, and while the patient is standing.

   If possible, allow 1 or 2 minutes to pass between each change in position so the patient may equilibrate. A rise in HR of 15 beats/minute or a drop in systolic blood pressure of 15 mm Hg or any drop in diastolic blood pressure with a change in position is evidence of a significant intravascular deficit.

The absolute number of systolic pressure must be considered with the state of tissue perfusion. The three organs that give the most readily available information are the skin, the kidney, and the brain. Confirm the following:

- The skin is warm and moist.

  One response to hypotension is to decrease perfusion of the peripheral vascular beds. Skin that is poorly perfused is cool, blue, and dry. A capillary refill time of greater than 1.5 seconds is highly suggestive of hypovolemia.

- The UO is adequate.

  Normal UO is usually considered greater than 20 mL/hour. A smaller urine volume is considered oliguria and may be due to hypotension.

- The patient is mentating well or at least at the baseline level

  Decreased tissue perfusion causes delirium, lethargy, and confusion. Extreme cases cause coma.

  If the patient has evidence of decreased tissue perfusion, this is the clinical definition of shock.

5. Assess the HR.

   Hypotension can have primary cardiac causes. Noting the timing and the quality of the pulse and analyzing the ECG can give vital information, as follows:

Bradycardia

Defined as lesser than 50 beats/minute, bradycardia has many etiologies including the following:

a. Autonomic dysfunction: The most common dysfunction is iatrogenic; beta blockade or calcium channel blockers, at normal or overdose levels, can cause an inability of the body to adequately respond to a hypotensive challenge; remember that the normal response to hypotension is a compensatory tachycardia; without the compensatory increase in HR, tissue perfusion can be in peril. Other causes include sick sinus syndrome or primary autonomic neuropathy.

b. Heart block: Usually as the result of acute MI, complete block is readily apparent on ECG (Fig. 17–1); see Chapter 9 for a complete discussion of the diagnosis and treatment of arrhythmias.

c. Vasovagal reaction: This is generally a response to pain, change in position, or straining; if present, the hypotension is generally short-lived.

Tachycardia

Sinus tachycardia is the expected response to hypotension. This includes HRs from 80 to 150 beats/minute. Greater than this number is indicative of a tachyarrhythmia, which may require treatment. A rapid HR is not always associated with adequate stroke volume, as

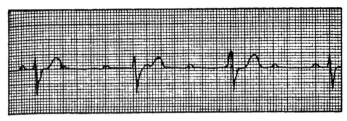

Figure 17–1 Bradycardia; third-degree atrioventricular block.
(From Marshall SA, Ruedy J: On Call: Principles and Protocols, 2nd ed.
Philadelphia, WB Saunders, 1993, p. 131.)

Figure 17–2 Atrial fibrillation with rapid ventricular response.
(From Marshall SA, Ruedy J: On Call: Principles and Protocols, 2nd ed.
Philadelphia, WB Saunders, 1993, p. 154.)

the heart may not have sufficient time for filling after each beat.
Significant tachyarrhythmias include the following:

  a. Atrial fibrillation: The ventricular response rate varies but may
     be as rapid as 240 beats/minute (Fig. 17–2). Note the absence
     of *p* waves.
  b. Supraventricular tachycardia (Fig. 17–3): The QRS complex
     may be narrow or wide.
  c. Ventricular tachycardia (Fig. 17–4): Note the wide QRS complex.
     Any of these tachyarrhythmias are life threatening. Notify
     your resident immediately and institute advanced cardiac life
     support (ACLS) protocols as necessary.
  • Asystole
     This lack of rhythm would obviously result in hypoten-
     sion. ACLS protocols should be instituted immediately.
  • Pulseless electrical activity (PEA)
     Pulseless electrical activity (PEA) is an uncoupling of the
     electrical stimulation of the heart as seen on ECG from the
     mechanical action of pumping. Whenever a rhythm is noted
     on cardiac monitoring, confirm that the rhythm actually
     corresponds to a palpable pulse. PEA is also a medical emer-
     gency and requires institution of ACLS protocols.

Figure 17–3 Supraventricular tachycardia.
(From Marshall SA, Ruedy J: On Call: Principles and Protocols, 2nd ed. Philadelphia, WB Saunders, 1993, p. 154.)

Figure 17–4 Ventricular tachycardia.
(From Marshall SA, Ruedy J: On Call: Principles and Protocols, 2nd ed. Philadelphia, WB Saunders, 1993, p. 155.)

Initial Management

In addition to the measures started in the orders section earlier,

1. If the patient is bradycardic, give **atropine 0.5 mg IV**; may repeat every 15 minutes to a total dose of 2 mg.
2. If the patient has a tachyarrhythmia, refer to Chapter 9 for a complete discussion on treatment.

Selective Physical Examination

Look for clues as to the cause of the hypotension. This may be done while resuscitative efforts are under way. Examination of the patient does not preclude initiation of fluid replacement.

Fluid status:	Perform a rapid fluid status assessment (see Chapter 12)
VS:	Repeat frequently during the resuscitative effort
MS:	Declining mental status, delirium, confusion, or coma (decreased tissue perfusion)
HEENT:	Elevated jugular venous distention (JVD) (congestive heart failure [CHF]); flat neck veins (hypovolemia)
CVS:	S_3 (CHF); arrhythmia
Resp:	Wheezes (anaphylaxis and CHF); crackles (CHF)

GU:	Oliguria (decreased tissue perfusion)
Skin:	Cyanosis, cool, and clammy (decreased tissue perfusion); hives with urticaria (anaphylaxis)
Extrem:	Ankle, pretibial or sacral edema (CHF)
Additional tests:	As outlined earlier in the orders

MANAGEMENT

Normalize Intravascular Volume

The goal of this treatment is to optimize cardiac preload. Look quickly at the neck veins of the patient. If the veins are distended, then preload may be high, and it is the pump that is not working well. The finding of rales and peripheral edema will also support the diagnosis of CHF. This is cardiogenic shock and is treated with fluid restriction and preload reduction (see Chapter 28 for the treatment of CHF).

If the neck veins are flat, then preload may be inadequate. All forms of shock other than cardiogenic are treated initially with fluid. The fluid of choice is crystalloid. The absolute volume required is patient dependent and may be large. Repeat boluses of NS or lactated Ringer's in volumes of 200 to 500 mL are sufficient. These are given until tissue perfusion returns.

Fluid resuscitation will require frequent monitoring of fluid and electrolyte status.

1. Send baseline electrolytes, urinalysis, and CBC.

    Repeat electrolytes every 6 to 8 hours during rapid fluid replacement until the patient stabilizes, then reduce as is reasonable.

2. Send baseline ABG for a base deficit.

    Base deficit is a reasonable reflection of serum lactate levels. This is a good screening test of the severity of the initial hypoperfusion and may be followed hourly to assess the resuscitation. As perfusion improves, base deficit will return to normal.

3. Place a Foley catheter to monitor UO.

    Adequate UO (>20 mL/hour) is a good end point to use to judge hydration.

4. Place the patient on cardiac monitoring, especially if the patient is at risk for MI or CHF.

5. If necessary, gain central venous access to monitor central venous pressure (CVP) (see Chapter 19 for techniques to gain access to the central venous system).

    Normal CVP is 0 to 6 cm H_2O (this corresponds to a JVD of 2-3 cm). For some patients it may be necessary to maintain a CVP in the 7 to 10 cm H_2O range to ensure adequate preload. A CVP of greater than 15 cm H_2O is an indication of left ventricular dysfunction. For patients with a history of cardiac events or for very ill patients, a Swan-Ganz catheter may be necessary to give adequate cardiac data. Swan-Ganz catheterization is best left for ICU/CCU management and is not used in patients on the ward.

Give Inotropic Agents

Further support cardiac output and perfusion with vasopressor agents as necessary. **Inotropic support should not be given without first optimizing the intravascular fluid volume.** The action of these agents results from interaction at the various adrenergic receptors:

1. Alpha: Located on vascular smooth muscle; effects include vasoconstriction, resulting in increased SVR.
2. $Beta_1$: Effects are inotropic and chronotropic, resulting in increased CO.
3. $Beta_2$: Effects include dilation of smooth muscles, resulting in decreased SVR.

These agents generally require central venous access and ICU/CCU transfer. Commonly used drip preparations are summarized in Table 17–1. The physiologic effects are summarized in Table 17–2. Because increasing SVR will ultimately diminish the blood flow to some organs, watch carefully for changes in UO or other end-organ dysfunction when administering alpha-adrenergic agents.

- Correct hypoxia.

    Part of maintaining adequate tissue perfusion is optimizing the oxygen delivered to the end-organs. If the patient is in shock, distal extremity perfusion may not be adequate for a pulse oximeter to give reliable data.

    Rely on ABG data. Deliver O_2 by mask to maintain arterial partial pressure of O_2 (PaO_2) of greater than 60 mm Hg.

    Monitor ABG data as needed. Consider transfusions of packed red blood cells for a hematocrit of less than 25%.

- Correct acidosis.

    Poor tissue perfusion results in tissue hypoxia. The conversion to anaerobic metabolism is associated with the buildup of lactic acid and metabolic acidosis. Monitor this with ABGs and base deficits. Acidosis secondary to hypoperfusion is generally treated by improving the peripheral circulation. The administration of sodium bicarbonate is reserved for code situations. In some cases, correction of pH of less than 7.2 with bicarbonate is desirable. See Chapter 12 for a complete discussion of acidosis.

    Give additional treatment based on underlying etiology, as follows:

TABLE 17–1 Common Intravenous Drip Inotropic Agents

Name	Action	Indication	Dose Range	Comments
Amrinone	Nonadrenergic	Cardiogenic shock	5–20 mcg/kg/min	Long half-life (6 hr)
Dobutamine	β_1-adrenergic	Cardiogenic shock	2.5–10 mcg/kg/min	Titrate to desired BP
Dopamine	Dopaminergic	Renal perfusion	1–2 mcg/kg/min	
	α, β_1-adrenergic	Cardiogenic shock	2–10 mcg/kg/min	Titrate to desired BP
	α-adrenergic	Hypotension	10–20 mcg/kg/min	Titrate to desired BP
Epinephrine	α, β-adrenergic	Hypotension, low SVR	0.025–0.1 mcg/kg/min	Titrate to desired BP, increases myocardial O_2 req't
Isoproterenol	β-adrenergic	Bradycardia, septic shock	0.05–0.5 mcg/kg/min	Titrate to desired BP, increases myocardial O_2 req't
Norepinephrine	α, β-adrenergic	Hypotension, low SVR	0.05–0.5 mcg/kg/min	Titrate to desired BP, increases myocardial O_2 req't
Vasopressin	Nonadrenergic	Vasodilatory shock	5–15 U bolus, then 0.01–0.04 U/min	Titrate to desired BP

BP, blood pressure; SVR, systemic vascular resistance.

TABLE 17–2 **Physiologic Effects of Inotropic Agents**

Name	CO	PCWP	SVR	MAP	HR	CVP	PVR
Amrinone	↑	↓	↓	↔	↑	↓	↓
Dobutamine	↑	↓	↓	↑	↑	↓	↓
Dopamine							
1–6 mcg/kg/min	↑	↑	↑	↑	↑	↑	↔
7–20 mcg/kg/min	↑	↑ ↑	↑ ↑	↑ ↑	↑	↑ ↑	↑
Epinephrine	↑	↑	↑	↑	↑	↑	↑
Isoproterenol	↑	↓	↓	↓	↑	↓	↓
Norepinephrine	↑	↑	↑	↑	↔	↑	↑
Vasopressin	↑	↑	↑	↔			

CO, cardiac output; PCWP, pulmonary capillary wedge pressure; SVR, systemic vascular resistance; MAP, mean arterial pressure; HR, heart rate; CVP, central venous pressure; PVR, pulmonary vascular resistance; ↑, increased; ↓, decreased; ↔, unchanged.

CARDIOGENIC SHOCK

Hypotension and Elevated JVD

The causes of cardiogenic shock are essentially the causes of CHF. MI heads the list. The treatment for CHF is described in Chapter 28. It is important to confirm that the patient is in CHF. Other causes of hypotension associated with elevated JVD include the following (each is an emergent situation and necessitates contacting the resident):

1. Tamponade

    Look for Beck's triad of hypotension, elevated JVD, and muffled heart tones. Pulsus paradoxus of greater than 10 mm Hg also suggests this diagnosis. Use an ultrasound to confirm the diagnosis. It is treated by emergent pericardiocentesis as described in Chapter 28.

2. Pulmonary embolus

    Cyanosis and marked hypoxia may suggest this diagnosis. Look also for evidence of right-sided heart failure, i.e., enlarged liver, peripheral edema, right ventricular heave, tricuspid murmur, and increased pulmonary heart sound.

3. Superior vena cava obstruction

    Look for swelling that is limited to the face and upper extremities. Also, collateral venous return may be prominent.

4. Tension pneumothorax

    Respiratory distress and hypoxia associated with hyper-resonance of a hemithorax. The trachea may be deviated away from the side of the pneumothorax. It is initially treated with placement of a 16-gauge angiocatheter into the thorax at the midclavicular line between the first and second ribs. This will confirm the diagnosis and allow a venting of built-up pressure. A tube thoracostomy must then be placed (see Chapter 30).

HYPOVOLEMIC SHOCK

Hypotension with Fluid Loss or Redistribution

The source of intravascular fluid loss may not be readily apparent.

1. Postoperative or acute gastrointestinal blood loss should be evaluated and treated as described in Chapters 26 and 13, respectively.
2. Excess fluid loss or sequestration should be treated with NS replacement; sequestration, as with acute pancreatitis, may require massive fluid replacement.
3. Inotropic agents are used to maintain perfusion unresponsive to fluid resuscitation alone.
   Use of most vasopressor agents requires placement of central venous access and ICU/CCU transfer. Occasionally, **dopamine administration in doses of 2 to 5 mcg/kg/minute** are used in patients to facilitate renal perfusion.
4. Certain medications may contribute to poor perfusion by their effects on the heart or the circulatory system.
     Among the more common offenders are
   a. Opiates
   b. Nitroglycerin
   c. Beta-blockers
   d. Calcium channel blockers
   e. Other antihypertensives
   f. Sedative medications
     The treatment of medication-associated hypovolemia is often fluid support, Trendelenberg position, and time.
5. Some medications have specific antidotes.
   a. Opiates can be reversed with **naloxone (Narcan) 0.2 to 2 mg IV, intramuscularly (IM), SC, or endotracheal tube (ET) with repetition of the dose every 5 minutes to a total dose of 10 mg.**
   b. Some benzodiazepines can be reversed with **flumazenil (Romazicon) 0.2 mg IV over 30 seconds. A dose of 0.3 mg may be given** if there is no response in 5 minutes, **followed by subsequent doses of 0.5 mg every 5 minutes to a total dose of 3 to 5 mg.** The effective dose may be repeated every 20 minutes, delivered at a rate of **0.2 mg/minute to a total of 3 mg/hour.**

SEPTIC SHOCK

Hypotension and Fever

Note that the onset of septic shock may be increased tissue warmth associated with tachycardia, as the peripheral beds initially dilate. During the early stages of sepsis, respiratory alkalosis is the rule. As hypoperfusion worsens, acidosis becomes apparent. In addition to supportive measures, the treatment of septic shock is based on identification of the offending microorganism, correction of the source, and administration of appropriate IV antibiotics. This usually starts off as empirical wide-spectrum therapy, which is subsequently narrowed as the organism is identified. Fluid resuscitation is usually supported with vasopressor administration. Prolonged hypotension requires transfer to the ICU/CCU.

ANAPHYLACTIC SHOCK

Hypotension, Hives, and Wheezing

The onset of anaphylactic shock is usually associated with an identifiable source (e.g., penicillin and contrast dye). Treatment of anaphylactic shock is outlined in Chapter 8.

NEUROGENIC SHOCK

Hypotension and History of Recent Spinal Cord Injury

Neurogenic shock may follow spinal cord injury or transection. It results from a functional sympathectomy. Treatment consists of fluid resuscitation and alpha$_1$-adrenergic pressors (such as phenylephrine).

IRREVERSIBLE SHOCK AND MULTIPLE ORGAN FAILURE SYNDROME

Prolonged or refractory shock will lead to the complications of hypoperfusion. This affects most organ systems and is termed multiple organ failure syndrome (MOFS). The etiology of MOFS is unclear. There is no specific treatment other than ICU/CCU level support. Despite aggressive treatment of injuries and infections and adequate delivery of oxygen to the tissues, the mortality of patients with MOFS remains quite high.

SPECIAL SURGICAL CONSIDERATIONS

Preoperative Considerations

1. Shock may be the reason to operate.
   If a septic source cannot be found in a patient with abdominal pain, consider necrotic bowel as a source.
2. Shock is an indication to cancel an elective case.
   Contact your resident or attending physician.

Postoperative Considerations

1. Sequestration (third-spacing) of fluids may result in hypovolemic shock.

    This is common after major abdominal procedures. Adequate preoperative and intraoperative hydration may not be sufficient to maintain hydration in a postoperative patient.

2. In a recent postoperative patient who develops hypotension, always consider postoperative bleeding as a possible source.

    Remember that the initial hemoglobin may be normal despite significant blood loss. A change may not be noted until after rehydration has occurred.

REMEMBER

1. Prolonged hypotension with decreased tissue perfusion may have late complications such as MI, acute tubular necrosis, and stroke. These usually happen 2 to 3 days after a significant hypotensive event.

2. Though toxic shock syndrome is most common in pre-menopausal women, it can occur in any patient, regardless of sex or age.

3. Nearly all forms of shock will require ICU/CCU care and monitoring. Do not hesitate to discuss transfer of the patient with your resident.

Insomnia

The hospital is unfamiliar to many patients. Routine sleeping hours in hospitals often are interrupted with disruptions from other patients, nursing checks, and noisy monitoring equipment. Many patients become very fatigued, yet are unable to sleep. Calls requesting "sleepers" for patients will be common. For this type of call, it is generally not necessary to examine the patient at the bedside. Ordering a safe, effective sleep-inducing medication is appropriate.

PHONE CALL

Questions

What is the patient's reason for hospitalization, and is the patient preoperative or postoperative?

Learn why the patient is in the hospital. If the patient is postoperative, is he or she in pain? If so, order an appropriate analgesic. If the patient is preoperative, is he or she anxious?

A preoperative patient may benefit from a sleeping medication.

Does the patient have any medical problems?

Ask the RN about the patient's pertinent medical history. Benzodiazepines are among the most commonly prescribed sedative/hypnotics. These drugs are oxidized in the liver. Care must be used when administering these drugs in patients with liver disease. Also be careful when using benzodiazepines in patients who have recently consumed alcohol, because alcohol increases the toxicity of benzodiazepines.

What is the patient's age?

Beware of using benzodiazepines for elderly or frail patients. The half-life of these drugs may be increased up to fourfold in elderly patients. Think about using a sleeping medication with a short half-life. Some elderly patients do best with a nonbenzodiazepine drug.

Does the patient have any drug allergies or a history of adverse reactions to drugs?

Obviously, avoid using a drug to which a patient has had an allergic or adverse reaction. Common adverse reactions to sedative/hypnotic drugs include excessive sedation, prolonged drowsiness, and nightmares.

Has the patient been provided a sleeping medication recently that was effective?

There is no reason to change a medication that has been effective previously.

Orders

The key to selecting an appropriate sleeper is to choose a drug that causes the least long-term sedation and the fewest side effects. The following are important suggestions:

1. **Diphenhydramine hydrochloride** *(Benadryl)* is a safe drug to use in elderly or frail patients.

   It has both an antihistamine and a sedative effect. It is metabolized in the liver, so the drug will have a prolonged half-life in patients with cirrhosis. In frail or elderly patients, consider a dose of **25 mg orally (PO) just before sleep.** If this is not effective, the dose can be repeated.

2. **Chloral hydrate** is especially safe and effective in children.

   This drug is metabolized in the liver and has an active metabolite that determines the half-life of action. The usual dose is **500 to 1000 mg PO at the hour of sleep.** In children, the dose is **25 to 50 mg/kg.**

3. **Zolpidem** *(Ambien)* acts at the gamma-aminobutyric acid receptor. It has relatively few side effects and a short half-life and is a safe drug. The usual dose is **5 to 10 mg PO at the hour of sleep.**

   The benzodiazepines are the most commonly prescribed sleeping medications and are useful in many adult patients with normal liver function.

   The benzodiazepines combine sedation with an anxiolytic effect. Beware that the benzodiazepines may be habit forming with long-term use and have the potential for abuse. In addition, some benzodiazepines are more useful for anxiolytic purposes than for insomnia (e.g., **diazepam** *[Valium]* **and lorazepam** *[Ativan]*.

   Table 18–1 gives common drugs useful for insomnia.

TABLE 18-1 **Drugs Useful for Insomnia: Sedative/Hypnotics**

Drug	Dose	Half-life
Common Benzodiazepines		
Triazolam (Halcion)*	0.125–0.5 mg PO just before sleep	2–3 hr
Flurazepam HCl (Dalmane)	15–30 mg PO just before sleep	50–100 hr
Temazepam (Restoril)*	15–30 mg PO just before sleep	9–12 hr
Nonbenzodiazepine Agents		
Diphenhydramine HCl (Benadryl)	25–50 mg PO just before sleep	2.4–9 hr
Zolpidem tartrate (Ambien)	5–10 mg PO just before sleep	2.5 hr
Chloral hydrate	25–50 mg/kg, to 1000 mg maximum, PO or PR just before sleep	8–11 hr

*Benzodiazepine drugs with inactive metabolites. Benzodiazepines with inactive metabolites are useful in patients with liver disease.
PO, orally; PR, rectally.

Intravascular Access

Intravascular access is a means to administer fluids and medications, and it is a valuable tool for gathering hemodynamic information. The loss of "access" is a common reason for a phone call. This chapter provides orientation to various types of intravascular access, procedures to attain them, and common complications and problems. Some hospitals require informed consent before some of these procedures are performed; find out what the specific regulations are at your institution. Proprietary kits for intravascular line placement have specific instructions to follow for safe placement. The suggestions below do not attempt to supersede the written instructions supplied with each kit. Read the kit instructions, and follow the steps carefully. Perform procedures only if you are comfortable with them; enlist the help of more experienced personnel if you are unsure. Many hospitals have protocols for placing lines. Follow the protocols at your institution.

LOSS OF LINE FUNCTION

PHONE CALL

Questions

Why does a patient need intravascular access?
    Reasons may range from hemodynamic monitoring by arterial or central venous lines, nutrition or medication delivery through central access, need for hemodialysis, or administration of medication or fluids through peripheral lines.

Is the access still necessary?
    Often lines remain in place long after their usefulness is gone. There may be enteral routes or other options available for use. Even if you determine continued need for intravascular access, the patient may be stable enough to wait for intravenous (IV) line placement in the morning by the regular care team.

Are there immediate problems with the access?
    These are discussed in the sections for the individual lines, but the question should be asked, because some problems such as severe bleeding or shortness of breath (SOB) may be life threatening.

225

How long has the existing line been in place?

Long-term access lines such as long-arm or PICC (peripherally inserted central venous catheter) lines or Hickman-type catheters are designed to remain in for weeks to months but may have thrombotic or infectious complications. Other "medium-term" lines such as multilumen central venous access catheters or arterial lines may require removal and reinsertion with a clean line at intervals to minimize infectious risk.

Are there any other symptoms?

Are there any changes in vital signs?

Orders

1. Have the means available to restart the access, if necessary, which may include peripheral IV trays or specific kits for arterial line or central venous access.
2. Respond to any immediate problem such as bleeding or SOB as necessary.

Degree of Urgency

Loss of peripheral access is not an emergency unless a specific, important medication such as heparin is interrupted. If there is a significant change in vital signs or symptoms, the patient must be evaluated immediately.

ELEVATOR THOUGHTS

What causes loss of IV access?

1. Reevaluate the need for intravascular access.
2. Think about the various options for vascular access.
   There may be more than one approach that is appropriate in an individual patient.
3. Causes of loss of function of a line are as follows:
   - Kinking of the line
   - Loose or disconnected line
   - IV pump failure
   - Intraluminal blockage
   - Thrombosis of the vessel
   - Thrombophlebitis
   - Misplacement of the line by initial insertion or migration
   - IV site infection

MAJOR THREAT TO LIFE

Loss of vital hemodynamic information
Interruption of important medication

Life-threatening complication following line placement, such as pneumothorax after central venous line placement, or arterial thrombosis of a peripheral limb associated with an arterial line

BEDSIDE

Quick Look Test

If there is a specific complaint related to the line, such as SOB or pain, the patient may look distressed. A malfunctioning line usually produces no symptoms. The patient may be distressed by the IV infusion pump alarms or by a leak in the IV tubing.

Airway and Vital Signs

There is generally no derangement in vital signs due to the nonfunction of the line, unless the medications delivered are responsible for altering cardiopulmonary physiology (such as inotropic agents). If thrombophlebitis is present, fever may be apparent.

Selective Physical Examination

VS:	Repeat as necessary.
Line site:	Inspect the line: look for kinks and loose connections. Inspect the IV pump: is it on and functioning correctly? Inspect the fluid: is there fluid remaining in the IV bottle?
Skin:	Is there redness, swelling, purulence, or clear fluid collection under the dressing?
Extrem:	If the IV is in a peripheral site, look for swelling or discoloration of the limb; feel for distal pulses.
Additional tests:	

1. CXR: This is for evaluation of internal jugular (IJ) and subclavian central line tip placement. The tip should be at the superior vena cava (SVC). Occasionally, after placement of a subclavian line, the tip can be found in the IJ vein. If out of place, the line must be repositioned. The CXR is also diagnostic when evaluating for pneumothorax following central line placement.
2. Aspiration: Aspiration should be done in a sterile fashion. Wipe the connection with a small amount of iodine. Disconnect the IV tubing from the hub of the line, and immediately attach a 5- to 10-mL syringe to the hub. For a central line, wait for exhalation before detaching the IV tubing. Gently aspirate. Removal of a

small-tip thrombus is usually sufficient to clear the line. Continue to aspirate until 3 to 5 mL of blood have been collected. Discard the blood and reconnect the line to the IV tubing. Replace a sterile dressing. Never flush the line, because this might dislodge a larger clot propagating from the tip of the catheter into the vena cava and result in a pulmonary embolus.

MANAGEMENT

1. If repositioning or aspiration of the line is unsuccessful in restoring function, another way of delivering medication is required. Ask a few basic questions:
   a. Does the patient still need intravascular access?
   b. Is the patient taking food or medication orally (PO)?
   c. Can current medication be switched to PO or intramuscular (IM) administration?
   d. Must the access be central access?
   e. Is the patient on medication that requires central access, such as total parenteral nutrition (TPN), chemotherapy, inotropic drugs, or irritating medication such as amphotericin?
   f. Are there other ports on an existing central catheter that are usable? If the site is clean, the line may be changed to a new one over a wire (Seldinger technique). If there is a problem with the site, such as erythema, the existing line must be removed regardless of the patency of the other lumens.
2. A new site is required if the current skin site is red or purulent and the patient is febrile, or the line is clogged through the distal port (this also may dislodge a clot propagating from the tip of the catheter).
3. Restart IV access, if required.
4. If removal of the existing central line is required, remember to send the catheter tip for culture, if required; also hold pressure at the skin site after removal for 10 minutes (by the clock) to ensure adequate hemostasis.

SPECIAL SURGICAL CONSIDERATIONS

Occasionally, a surgical house staff member is called to remove a longer term line such as a Hickman catheter. These differ from temporary central venous access in that a Dacron fiber cuff is present under the skin a short distance from the insertion site. The toughness of the adherence of the subcutaneous tissue to this cuff depends on the length of time during which the catheter has been in and on the healing properties of the patient. The removal of these lines is discussed below.

BLEEDING FROM THE SITE

PHONE CALL

Questions

Is this the only site of bleeding?
Blood oozing from more than one site may be evidence of coagulopathy.

Is the line functional?

Did the patient undergo a surgical procedure, and if so, how long ago?

Are there any other symptoms?

Are there any changes in vital signs?

Orders

1. Have the means available to restart the access, if necessary; this may include peripheral IV trays or specific kits for arterial line or central venous access.
2. Respond to any immediate problems.
3. Have the nurses hold pressure on actively bleeding sites until you arrive.

Degree of Urgency

If there is a significant change in vital signs or symptoms, the patient must be evaluated immediately.

ELEVATOR THOUGHTS

What causes bleeding from an IV site?
1. A new site will ooze slightly, which should stop within several hours.
2. Coagulopathy, causing bleeding, may result from the following:
Medications including heparin, warfarin, streptokinase, and tissue plasminogen activator (t-PA). Platelet dysfunction from thrombocytopenia or nonsteroidal anti-inflammatory drugs (NSAIDs). Clotting factor deficiency, dilutional coagulopathy, disseminated intravascular coagulation (DIC).

MAJOR THREAT TO LIFE

Soft-tissue swelling; subcutaneous blood can exert pressure on surrounding structures; depending on the site of the line, the hematoma can displace lung (with a subclavian line) or trachea (with an IJ line)

Loss of vital hemodynamic information

Interruption of important medication

Life-threatening complication, such as pneumothorax after central venous line placement, or arterial thrombosis of a peripheral limb associated with an arterial line.

BEDSIDE

Quick Look Test

Minor bleeding is not associated with discomfort. If the bleeding is due to impending sepsis, the patient may appear ill.

Airway and Vital Signs

If the line is in the IJ site, pay special attention to the patient's airway. Is the patient breathing well? If a significant amount of blood is lost, pulse rate may be elevated and blood pressure (BP) may drop.

MANAGEMENT

1. Inspect the wound.
   Remove the dressing and clean around the site. Try to identify a specific site of oozing, which is often not possible.
2. If no specific site can be identified, apply pressure (with a gloved hand) at the site for 20 minutes (by the clock).
3. Recheck the site, being careful not to dislodge any clot that may have formed; if bleeding continues, hold pressure for another 20 minutes.
4. If bleeding continues, consider evaluation of the patient for coagulopathy.
   See Chapter 26 for evaluation and treatment of bleeding disorders.
5. Bleeding may compromise the function of the line, and if this is the case, consider replacement of the line but at another site.

PURULENCE AT THE SITE

PHONE CALL

Questions

Is the patient febrile?

Are there other signs of infection?

Is the line functional?

Did the patient undergo a surgical procedure, and if so, how long ago?

Are there any other symptoms?

Are there any changes in vital signs?

Orders

1. Have the means available to restart the access, if necessary. This may include peripheral IV trays or specific kits for arterial line or central venous access.
2. Respond to any immediate problems.

Degree of Urgency

If there is a significant change in vital signs or symptoms, the patient must be evaluated immediately.

ELEVATOR THOUGHTS

What causes purulence at an IV site?
1. Local site infection
2. Suppurative thrombophlebitis
3. Line sepsis

MAJOR THREAT TO LIFE

- Sepsis
- Suppurative thrombophlebitis

BEDSIDE

Quick Look Test

A local wound infection may cause only minor discomfort at the site. If the patient has suppurative thrombophlebitis or impending sepsis, he or she will appear ill.

Airway and Vital Signs

Evaluate the patient as if sepsis is impending. Look at fluid status, pulse rate, and BP, including orthostatics. Fever is the hallmark of severe infection and usually indicates that the line must be removed.

MANAGEMENT

1. Evaluate the site.
    If there is redness of the skin or any purulence from the wound site, the line must be removed. Clean the site carefully before removal. Do this sterilely so that the tip of the line may be sent for culture.
2. Express pus from the skin site, if possible; this may also be sent for Gram stain and culture.
3. If the patient is febrile, blood cultures should be sent.
    It is possible to draw one sample through the existing line, but be sure to draw one elsewhere from a new skin puncture.
4. Appropriate antibiotics must be started.
    Most site infections are staphylococcal; these respond best to synthetic penicillins, first-generation cephalosporins, or vancomycin. Focus the antibiotic therapy based on culture and Gram stain results.
5. If IV access is still required, the line must be replaced.
    Try not to do this while the patient is febrile and is at risk for exhibiting bacteremia. Avoid skin sites that are red, macerated, or breaking down.
6. Suppurative thrombophlebitis must be suspected if the white blood cell (WBC) count is elevated or if the patient is septic.
    Do not be fooled by the absence of skin findings. The hallmarks include tenderness at an existing or previous IV insertion site in the setting of fever and elevated WBC count. Vein sites must be explored surgically in the patient who has no other source of fever. Recovery of normal vein is a negative result. Vein occluded with clot or pus is evidence of thrombophlebitis, and the entire infected vein must be excised. The skin is left open to drain. Send a portion of the excised vein to pathology for histology and a portion to microbiology for culture and sensitivities. Antibiotics must be initiated.
7. If the patient is hemodynamically unstable, resuscitate aggressively and treat shock as outlined in Chapter 17.

SHORTNESS OF BREATH AFTER INSERTION OF A CENTRAL LINE

Pneumothorax is a common complication of central line placement in IJ and subclavian sites. It should be suspected in a patient who has a central line in place that is recent. There are other, less common causes of SOB that must also be considered. See also Chapter 28 for a complete discussion on diagnosis and management of SOB.

PHONE CALL

Questions

How long has the patient been short of breath?

How long has the line been in place?
Complications of central line placement may happen immediately after insertion or may be delayed by days.

Did the patient undergo a surgical procedure, and if so, how long ago?

Are there any other symptoms?

Is the patient complaining of chest pain? Is the patient cyanotic or hypoxic?

Are there any changes in vital signs?
Hypotension and increased respiratory rate are indicative of pneumothorax.

Orders

1. If the line is new, order posterior-to-anterior (PA) and lateral chest x-rays (CXRs) immediately.
   This may be done at the bedside, if necessary. Order inspiratory and expiratory films, as pneumothorax is often best noted on the expiratory film.
2. Check oxygenation with a pulse oximeter, and treat hypoxia as necessary.
3. Treat hypotension with fluid resuscitation and pressors, as necessary.
4. Have sterile gloves, dressing supplies, and 16-gauge needle at the bedside for diagnosis and treatment of tension pneumothorax (as in Chapter 28).

Degree of Urgency

The patient must be evaluated immediately.

ELEVATOR THOUGHTS

What causes SOB after central line placement?

   1. Local hematoma at a neck site causing pressure on the trachea
   2. Pneumothorax (including tension pneumothorax)
   3. Hemothorax
   4. Tamponade
   5. Air embolus
   6. Pleural effusion

MAJOR THREAT TO LIFE

- Obstruction of the upper airway due to tracheal pressure
- Tamponade
- Tension pneumothorax
- Air embolus

BEDSIDE

Quick Look Test

Patients will tend to look sick. If tension pneumothorax, tamponade, or air embolus is present, the patient may look moribund.

Airway and Vital Signs

Tachypnea is generally apparent regardless of the cause. Tachycardia is present in tamponade and in tension pneumothorax or may be present simply because the patient is in distress. Hypotension is ominous and indicates tension pneumothorax or tamponade.

Selective Physical Examination

VS:	Check again now
HEENT	Tracheal deviation and swelling at the insertion site in the neck (local hematoma)
CVS:	Pulsus paradoxus and elevated jugular venous distention (tamponade and tension pneumothorax). Muffled heart tones (tamponade or pericardial effusion)
Resp:	Unilateral decrease in breath sounds, and hyperresonance (pneumothorax)
	Dull to percussion (pleural effusion)
Line site:	Are connections tight? (Air embolus)

MANAGEMENT

1. Each of these situations is life threatening; contact your resident immediately.
2. See Chapter 28 for evaluation and emergency treatment of tension pneumothorax and tamponade.
3. If there is upper airway obstruction, be prepared to intubate.

    Contact your resident and the intensive care unit (ICU) or the cardiac care unit team for airway protection and transfer of the patient.
4. Air embolism is treated by placement of the patient on the right side in Trendelenburg position to sequester the air bubbles in the right ventricle.

    These will generally resorb, although some authors recommend aspiration of the air from the ventricle.

PLACEMENT OF INTRAVASCULAR LINES

Sterile Technique

In many procedures, it is imperative that sterile technique be observed. This is especially true about the placement of long-term intravenous access lines. Although most sterile techniques are performed in a controlled fashion in the operating room (OR), the procedures described here may be done at the bedside and require special care and preparation to maintain sterility. The preparation and maintenance of a sterile field represent a skill that, once acquired, will become second-nature. For those new to surgery or the infrequent user of sterile techniques, here are a few tips:

1. Prepare your environment.

    Make sure that your workspace is well lit and comfortable. Place the bed at a comfortable height, have the bedrails down, and get a chair, if appropriate. Sterility is often broken by having to reposition lighting or draping. Clear the area of objects that might catch your sleeves or your feet. Have room to move.
2. Make sure that all the instruments are available.

    Anticipate what supplies and instruments you will need. Have them opened and within easy reach. This requires planning, but it will soon become routine.
3. Have help standing by, if needed.

    You will need an extra pair of hands in many cases; make sure it is someone who is familiar with sterile technique. If you need more senior supervision, give that individual plenty of notice.
4. Know the steps of the procedure.

Do a mental walk-through of the procedure before you put on your gloves. Check to ensure that the equipment needed for each step is available. It often is possible to line up the instruments in the order in which they are needed.

5. Inform the patient that a sterile field is going to be used.

Instruct the patient not to touch areas of sterility. It also is important to reassure the patient if the drapes are going to temporarily cover the eyes or airway. Always explain if there are uncomfortable or painful steps in the procedure, and warn the patient before the pain. Sterility often is broken when a patient jumps after a painful stimulus such as a needlestick.

6. Position the patient.

Place the patient in the position in which you want him or her, ensuring that any positioning aids (such as towel rolls) are in place before beginning. The nurses will appreciate if you place a pad or diaper under the region of the body that is to be prepped to protect the bed from drips of blood or soap.

7. Prepare the insertion site.

Use chlorhexidine, or an iodine-based disinfectant soap and clean (or "prep") the area well. Solution on a gauze or prepackaged swab sticks may be used. Start from the center of the desired field and work your way outward, cleaning an area wider than you think necessary. Repeat with a fresh gauze or swab for a total of three cleanings. If desired, more than one area may be initially prepared. The second site may be kept sterile with a drape while the first site is being used.

8. Don protective gear.

Put on a mask and cap, especially if the patient is immunocompromised or if an invasive line will be needed for a long time. Many hospitals have protocols as to how much sterile clothing is required. Don't forget eye protection. Use Universal Precautions at any time that there is potential for contamination with blood or other bodily fluid.

9. Scrub your hands with a disinfectant soap.

Remove rings and jewelry first. Scrub your hands with disinfective soap for 5 minutes.

10. Put on sterile gloves and gown.

Get help if you do not know how to do this in a sterile fashion.

11. Drape the area with sterile towels.

Ensure that the only thing visible through the "window" made with the towels is "prepared" skin. The towel may come fenestrated, or a window may be made using two or more towels. The drapes may be held in place with towel clamps, if desired.

12. Try not to move from the sterile field unless absolutely necessary.

 Once the sterile field is in place and you are working, be mindful of the nonsterile areas of your body (elbows, hair, waist). If you have forgotten an instrument or some supplies, ask for help.

13. Work quickly but carefully.

14. Admit easily if there has been a break in sterility.

 The constraints of time and pride may tempt you to overlook a minor break in sterility, but any time saved here will be more than taken up by the time required to care for a sicker patient if a complication arises.

 Do not hesitate to "break scrub," rewash, redrape, and begin again if you think that you compromised sterility.

 Do not put the patient at risk.

15. The procedure is not done until the line is secured.

 Secure the line or tube by taping, suturing, or tying down. Do this before removing the drapes. Make sure the line is secure even if a chest x-ray (CXR) is required to assess placement of the line before its use. You do not want your well-placed line to be dislodged during the confirmatory x-ray or while repositioning the patient.

16. Protect the sterility of the line.

 Place a dressing over the site, including an antimicrobial ointment as needed. Confirm that all connections and joints are secure before careful removal of the drapes.

17. "Reprep" and drape the area if repositioning of the line is necessary.

 Start with step one. The preparation of the area is no less vigorous if the line must be repositioned.

18. When the procedure is completed, clean the area of soap.

 The soaps used often are very irritating, so protect the skin by cleaning away the irritant.

19. Be responsible for your own "sharps" disposal.

 Do not leave this job to a nurse or a student. Only you know where all of the sharps are on the tray.

20. Many hospitals have protocols for placing lines. Follow the protocols at your institution.

Seldinger Technique

Some intravascular access is achieved by using a preplaced guide wire. This technique is also useful for replacing existing lines with clean catheters. It is based on cannulating the vessel with a needle and passing a wire through the needle into the vessel. Once the wire is placed in the vessel, the passageway through the tissues may be suitably widened by means of a rigid dilator. A large-bore catheter then may be placed over the wire.

Contraindications and Precautions

1. Infection or lesion at the proposed insertion site
2. Occlusion or thrombosis of the desired vessel
3. Coagulopathy
   Abnormalities in platelet count or function, or in clotting factor concentrations should be corrected before insertion of the line.
4. Ongoing systemic infection
   A peripheral site may be advisable until the source of infection is identified and suitable treatment has begun. This may not always be possible.
5. Vessel perforation
   This is a risk any time a guide wire is used.
6. Dislodgment or loose connections to the line
   This can result in rapid exsanguination.

Equipment Needed

There are specific kits available for many approaches. Refer to the instructions supplied with these kits for complete information.

1. Skin preparation supplies (iodine, chlorhexidine, or alcohol)
2. Local anesthetic (1% or 2% lidocaine, 25-gauge needle, 3-mL syringe)
3. Sterile gloves, eye protection
4. Sterile towels or drapes
5. Supplies for Seldinger technique (or specific intravascular access kit)
   a. Needle (16- to 18-gauge)
   b. 10-mL syringe
   c. Guide wire
   d. Scalpel
   e. Dilator
   f. Catheter
6. If the Seldinger technique is not used, a catheter-over-needle system may be used.
7. Heparinized saline for flushing the catheter
8. Suture for securing the catheter
9. Equipment for continuous monitoring of arterial or venous pressure, if desired
10. Sterile dressing supplies

Procedure

1. Prepare the patient.
   a. Explain the procedure.
   b. Explain the risks and alternatives. Obtain consent, if necessary.
   c. Answer any questions.
2. Position the patient.

   a. Confirm that all the equipment is available.
   b. Prepare the equipment for use. Remove any unnecessary tags or covers, crack the seals of syringes, and remove the cap from the distal port of the line to be placed.
   c. Position the patient as per each individual technique.
3. Identify the desired vessel
   a. Choose the most appropriate site.
      Many lines have a hierarchy of desirable placement sites.
      These are based on the ease of placement and safety of the lines. Know the preferences for the line you wish to start.
         The most favorable sites for placement of a Swan-Ganz catheter are (in order of preference):
      i. The right internal jugular vein
      ii. The left subclavian vein
   b. Consider the use of ultrasound.
      Knowledge of anatomic relationships is important and is stressed in this book. However, in recent years, many operators are beginning to rely on ultrasound to locate and confirm the patency of a desired vessel.
      A hand-held 7.5 MHz linear phase probe is used. In experienced hands, ultrasound can increase the speed and accuracy of a line placement.
4. Prepare the skin.
   a. Use sterile technique.
   b. Prepare and drape the skin.
   c. Infiltrate the entry site with 1% to 2% lidocaine.
   d. Confirm that adequate anesthesia has been achieved.
      Test the skin over where the local anesthetic has been injected for a pain response.
5. Place the 10-mL syringe on the needle.
      Identify appropriate anatomic landmarks with the index finger of your non-dominant hand.
6. Insert the needle into the vessel.
   a. Many operators will use a 22- to 25-gauge "finder needle" to confirm the location of the vessel before switching to the larger needle through which the wire will pass. In the event of an inadvertent arterial penetration, a smaller defect is made in the artery.
   b. Aspirate during insertion and during withdrawal, as often the vessel is encountered on the way out.
   c. When blood is encountered, note the depth and angle of the finder needle penetration.
   d. Pull out the finder needle and switch to the larger needle.
   e. Reinsert the larger needle at the same angle and to the same depth.
7. When blood flows freely into the syringe, remove the syringe from the needle.
      Immediately place your finger over the hub to stop the outflow of blood and to avoid the inflow of air.

8. Gently place the guide wire through the needle (Fig.19–1A)

A Passage of guide wire through the needle

B Removal of the needle

C Passage of the catheter over the guide wire

Figure 19–1 Seldinger Technique for placing intravascular lines. *A*, Passage of guide wire through the needle; *B*, removal of the needle; *C*, passage of the catheter over the guide wire.

Keep a good hold on the wire throughout this procedure.

Ensure that the wire passes without resistance. It should feel like passing through warm butter. If you examine the guide wire before starting the procedure, you will note that as the wire bumps against a wall it will bend toward the curve of the "J" (Fig. 19–2). This may be exploited when a difficult placement is anticipated. Insert the wire in the orientation such that it will tend to bend toward the direction that you desire.

If the wire does not pass easily, do not force it. Remove the needle and the guide wire together, and reposition the needle before reinsertion of the wire.

If the patient is monitored, watch for ventricular dysrhythmias. This is an indication that the wire is too deep (i.e., in the heart) and should be pulled back until the dysrhythmias stop.

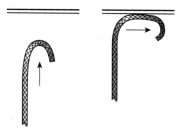

Figure 19–2 Typical 2 pattern of J-wires.

9. Remove the needle over the wire (see Fig. 19–1B)

Always keep one hand on the wire to maintain its position in the vessel and to avoid the calamity of losing the wire completely in the vessel. (Do not let your patient's x-ray be the subject at the next interventional radiology grand rounds.)

10. If the needle must be removed because of inability to pass the wire, **DO NOT REMOVE THE WIRE FROM THE NEEDLE.**

The bevel of the needle is sharp enough to shear off the end of the guide wire, which will remain in the vessel or in the tissues. Remove the needle and the guide wire simultaneously. Once out of the body, the guide wire may be removed by passing it completely through the needle from hub to tip.

11. Nick the skin at the entry site with a scalpel.

Make the skin defect just large enough to allow passage of the catheter.

12. Place the dilator over the wire, dilate the entry path, and then remove.

Often, a twisting motion is required. Apply pressure to the dilator close to the skin insertion site.

Anticipate increased bleeding at the skin site on removal of the dilator. This is easily controlled with gentle pressure. **Be careful to maintain the wire position.**

13. Place the catheter over the wire into the vessel (see Fig. 19–1C)

a. Maintain control of the wire.

b. Remember to have removed the appropriate (distal) cap on multilumen catheters so that the wire passes through easily.

c. It is advisable to have flushed the lumens of the catheter with heparinized saline before placement.

d. Introducer sheaths for Swan-Ganz catheters should be introduced slowly because they become warm and more compliant as they enter the body. The introducers are very large, and rapid movements can damage a wider area.

e. Real time fluoroscopy can be used while passing large dilators or introducers into the chest to ensure their safe passage into a vessel.

    f. If the catheter slides easily into the lumen of the vessel, remove the wire. Hold your finger over the hub of the catheter until it is flushed and tightly capped.

    g. Confirm that each cap is in place and is tightly fastened.

14. Confirm placement by aspirating blood from each port. Flush each port with heparinized saline. Some lines require placement confirmation by x-ray before use.

15. Secure the catheter at the skin level with suture.

16. Sterilely dress the site.

17. Confirm the position of the line with CXR, if necessary.

18. Document the procedure.

FORMS OF INTRAVASCULAR ACCESS

Arterial Lines

Indications: Hemodynamic monitoring, arterial blood sampling, and frequent blood draw requirements. This is generally done in an ICU setting where the patient is under close observation, and is non-ambulatory.

Peripheral Arterial Line with Angiocatheter

The most straightforward approach involves use of a simple angio-catheter in the wrist. There are arterial line kits available that use the Seldinger (guide wire) technique that are also acceptable. The dorsalis pedis artery may also be used with this technique.

Indications

Indications are hemodynamic monitoring, arterial blood sampling, and frequent blood draw requirements in the nonambulatory patient. Placement of arterial lines is generally done in an ICU setting, where the patient is under close observation.

Contraindications and Precautions

1. Infection or lesion at the proposed insertion site
   Consider choosing another site.
2. Occlusion or thrombosis of the desired vessel
   Consider choosing another site.
3. Coagulopathy
   Abnormalities in platelet count or function, or in clotting factor concentrations should be corrected before insertion of the line.
4. Ongoing systemic infection
   A peripheral site may be advisable until the source of infection is identified and suitable treatment has begun. This may not always be possible.
5. Vessel perforation
   This is a risk any time a guide wire is used.

6. Dislodgment or loose connections to the line
   This can result in rapid exsanguination.

Equipment Needed

1. Skin preparation supplies (iodine, chlorhexidine, or alcohol)
2. Local anesthetic (1% or 2% lidocaine, 25-gauge needle, 3-mL syringe)
3. Sterile gloves, eye protection
4. Sterile towel or drapes
5. Angiocatheter (20- or 22-gauge, 2 inches in length) or specific arterial line kit
6. Heparinized saline in a pressurized delivery system
7. Blood gas syringe, if needed for arterial blood sampling
8. Additional 5-mL syringe with heparinized saline
9. Suture for securing the catheter
10. Arm board with a small terry cloth roll to help secure line and prevent kinking
11. Equipment for continuous monitoring of arterial pressure
12. Sterile dressing supplies

Procedure

1. Prepare the patient.
   a. Explain the procedure.
   b. Explain the risks and alternatives. Obtain consent, if necessary.
   c. Answer any questions.
2. Position the patient.
   a. The patient may be seated or supine. The selected wrist should be immobilized on an arm board with a roll under the wrist in slight dorsiflexion.
   b. Get a chair for yourself.
   c. Raise the bed to a comfortable height.
   d. Confirm that all the equipment is available.
   e. The pulse of the radial artery is easily palpable on the volar surface of the wrist at the radial head.
      Perform an Allen test to confirm the collateral circulation in the hand. The Allen test is performed by compression of both the radial and ulnar arteries until the palm blanches; then, release the ulnar artery and confirm reperfusion of the palm. A delay of more than 5 seconds is considered abnormal, and another site should be chosen.
   f. Whenever possible, choose the nondominant hand.
3. Prepare the skin.
   a. Use sterile technique.
   b. Prepare and drape the skin.
   c. Infiltrate the entry site with 1% to 2% lidocaine. Also infiltrate over the sites of anchoring sutures.

    d. Confirm that adequate anesthesia has been achieved.
4. Insert the catheter.
    a. Locate the pulse with the index finger of your nondominant hand.
    b. Some operators like to nick the skin over the entry site with a scalpel in order not to damage the catheter as it enters the skin.
    c. Insert the angiocatheter at a 30-degree to 45-degree angle to the artery.
    d. When bright red blood pumps freely into the catheter, continue to advance the catheter slowly until the flow just stops.
    e. Back off slightly until the blood pumps again, and advance the catheter over the needle into the vessel.
5. If blood does not immediately flow into the needle
    a. Pull out, reconfirm the landmarks, reposition, and try again.
    b. Occasionally, the needle needs to be flushed of clogging tissue before reinsertion. Use a syringe of heparinized saline.
    c. If the catheter cannot be placed in three attempts, try another site.
6. When the catheter is successfully placed
    a. Secure the catheter to the skin with suture.
      Some angiocatheters have wings for this purpose.
    b. Obtain arterial blood samples as needed.
    c. Attach to manometer for continuous monitoring.
    d. Apply a sterile dressing.
7. Document the procedure.
8. General considerations
    a. Reassess daily the need for the arterial line.
    b. Confirm daily adequate blood flow to the hand and fingers.
    c. If fever occurs, remember to draw blood for cultures from this site as well as from other indwelling sites.
    d. If the site remains clean, the catheter may be changed over a wire as needed.

FEMORAL ARTERIAL LINE BY SELDINGER TECHNIQUE

Arterial lines and especially femoral lines are for nonambulatory patients. The femoral technique is used in supine patients in whom the radial or dorsal pedal approach has failed or is not possible.

Indications

Indications are hemodynamic monitoring, arterial blood sampling, and frequent blood draw requirements in the nonambulatory patient. Placement of arterial lines is generally done in an ICU setting, where the patient is under close observation.

Contraindications and Precautions

1. Infection or lesion at the proposed insertion site
   Consider choosing another site.
2. Occlusion or thrombosis of the desired vessel
   Consider choosing another site.
3. Coagulopathy
   Abnormalities in platelet count or function, or in clotting factor concentrations should be corrected before insertion of the line.
4. Ongoing systemic infection
   A peripheral site may be advisable until the source of infection is identified and suitable treatment has begun. This may not always be possible.
5. Vessel perforation
   This is a risk any time a guide wire is used.
6. Dislodgment or loose connections to the line
   This can result in rapid exsanguination.

Equipment Needed

1. Skin preparation supplies (iodine, chlorhexidine, or alcohol)
2. Local anesthetic (1% or 2% lidocaine, 25-gauge needle, 3-mL syringe)
3. Sterile gloves, eye protection
4. Sterile towels or drapes
5. Supplies for Seldinger technique (or specific arterial line kit)
   a. Needle (16- to 18-gauge)
   b. 10-mL syringe
   c. Guide wire
   d. Scalpel
   e. Dilator
   f. Catheter
6. If the Seldinger technique is not used, a catheter-over-needle system may be used
7. Heparinized saline in a pressurized delivery system
8. Blood gas syringe, if needed for arterial blood sampling
9. Additional 5-mL syringe with heparinized saline
10. Suture for securing the catheter
11. Equipment for continuous monitoring of arterial pressure
12. Sterile dressing supplies

Procedure

1. Prepare the patient.
   a. Explain the procedure.
   b. Explain the risks and alternatives. Obtain consent, if necessary.
   c. Answer any questions.

2. Position the patient.
   a. The patient must be supine.
   b. Raise the bed to a comfortable height.
   c. Confirm that all the equipment is available.
3. Prepare the skin.
   a. Use sterile technique.
   b. Prepare and drape the skin. Hair removal may be necessary.
   c. Infiltrate the entry site with 1% to 2% lidocaine. Also infiltrate the sites of anchoring sutures.
   d. Confirm that adequate anesthesia has been achieved.
4. Insert the catheter.
   a. Locate the pulse with the index finger of your nondominant hand.
      The vein is found halfway between the anterior iliac spine and the symphysis pubis.
      Recall the orientation of the artery to the vein (NAVELS):
      Nerve → Artery → Vein → Empty space → Lymphatics → Symphysis pubis.
      The artery is found halfway between the anterior iliac spine and the symphysis pubis (Fig. 19–3).
   b. Nick the skin over the entry site with a sterile scalpel so as to not damage the catheter as it enters the skin.
   c. Place the 10-mL syringe on the needle.
   d. Insert the needle at a 45-degree angle to the artery (about 3 to 4 cm). Aspirate during insertion and withdrawal. Often the vessel is encountered on the way out.
   e. When bright red blood pumps freely into the syringe, remove the syringe and immediately place your finger over the hub of the needle.
   f. Place the guide wire through the needle.

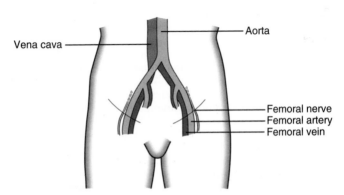

Figure 19–3 Anatomy of groin vasculature.

Make sure that the wire passes without resistance. Remove the needle over the wire.

Be sure to control the wire.

g. Extend the nick in the skin to allow for the size of the dilator.

h. Place the dilator over the wire and then remove. Watch for increased bleeding at the skin site. This is easily controlled with gentle pressure.

i. Place the catheter over the wire into the wound.

j. Remove the wire, confirm appropriate placement by brief observation of bright red pulsatile blood emitting from the catheter hub, and cap the catheter.

5. If blood does not immediately flow into the needle
   a. Pull out, reconfirm the landmarks, reposition, and try again.
   b. Occasionally, the needle needs to be flushed of clogging tissue before reinsertion. Use a syringe of heparinized saline.
   c. If the catheter cannot be placed in three attempts, try another site.

6. When the catheter is successfully placed
   a. Secure the catheter to the skin with suture.
   b. Obtain arterial blood samples, as needed.
   c. Attach to manometer for continuous monitoring.
   d. Apply a sterile dressing.

7. Document the procedure.

8. General considerations
   a. Reassess daily the need for the arterial line.
   b. Confirm daily adequate blood flow to the lower extremity.
   c. If fever occurs, remember to draw blood for cultures from this site as well as from other indwelling sites.
   d. If the site remains clean, the catheter should be changed over a wire as needed.

Removal of Arterial Lines

1. Have a scissors or blade, gauze, and tape ready.

2. Always wear gloves and eye protection when there is a potential for exposure to blood or other body fluids.

3. Remove sutures.

4. Remove the catheter.

   Confirm that the catheter has been removed intact.

5. Apply firm pressure at the entry site for 10 minutes (by the clock).

   Hold pressure longer if the lumen was large or if the patient was anticoagulated.

6. After 10 minutes, confirm that bleeding has stopped.

7. Place a pressure dressing.

8. Check the site and confirm adequate blood flow to the extremity the next day.

Complications and Problems of Arterial Lines

Procedures

1. Nonplacement of the line
2. Air embolus
   Arterial air may cause distal ischemia.
3. Entry site infection
   The line must be removed and a new site used, if necessary.
4. Suppurative thrombophlebitis
   This may require surgical drainage and IV antibiotics.
5. Catheter-related sepsis
   This requires removal of the line and treatment with IV antibiotics
6. Vessel thrombosis
   Transient occlusion is common, occurring in about 10% of arterial line placements. It is treated with removal of the line.
7. Distal ischemia
   Remove the line.
   Confirm distal pulses.
8. Hemorrhage
   a. Dislodged line or loose connections
      Be sure to check the connections. Under arterial pressures, a poor coupling of lines can result in rapid exsanguination.
   b. Bleeding or hematoma at the vessel entry site
      Hold pressure for 10 minutes (by the clock).
      Occasionally, a stitch at the entry site will suffice.
9. Nonfunction of the line

CENTRAL VENOUS LINES

These include hemodynamic lines such as central venous pressure (CVP) lines and Swan-Ganz catheters, dialysis ports, and lines with multiple lumens for TPN or prolonged medication delivery. Venous blood sampling may also be possible through these sites.

Subclavian Approach

This is a common approach to central venous access. It is the most comfortable site for a conscious patient, an easy and relatively safe placement technique, and a very easy site to keep clean and protected. There is a higher risk of pneumothorax during placement of this line than during internal jugular or femoral lines.

Indications

1. Delivery of high concentrations of nutrition or medication
2. Delivery of inotropic medications
3. Prolonged delivery of medication

4. Hemodialysis
5. Hemodynamic monitoring of CVP

Contraindications and Precautions

1. Infection or lesion at the proposed insertion site
   Consider choosing another site.
2. Occlusion or thrombosis of the desired vessel
   Consider choosing another site.
3. Coagulopathy
   Abnormalities in platelet count or function, or in clotting factor concentrations should be corrected before insertion of the line.
4. Ongoing systemic infection
   A peripheral site may be advisable until the source of infection is identified and suitable treatment has begun. This may not always be possible.
5. Vessel perforation
   This is a risk any time a guide wire is used.
6. Dislodgment or loose connections to the line
   This can result in rapid exsanguination.

Equipment Needed

There are specific kits available for many approaches. Refer to the instructions supplied with these kits for complete information.
1. Skin preparation supplies (iodine, chlorhexidine, or alcohol)
2. Local anesthetic (1% or 2% lidocaine, 25-gauge needle, 3-mL syringe)
3. Sterile gloves, eye protection
4. Sterile towels or drapes
5. Supplies for Seldinger technique (or specific intravascular access kit)
   a. Needle (16- to 18-gauge)
   b. 10-mL syringe
   c. Guide wire
   d. Scalpel
   e. Dilator
   f. Catheter
6. If the Seldinger technique is not used, a catheter-over-needle system may be used
7. Heparinized saline for flushing the catheter
8. Suture for securing the catheter
9. Equipment for continuous monitoring of central venous pressure, if desired
10. Sterile dressing supplies

Anatomic Landmarks (Figs. 19–4 and 19–5)

1. The subclavian vein is found anterior to the first rib and the anterior scalene muscle.

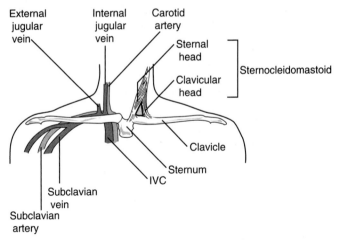

Figure 19–4 Anatomy of neck vasculature.

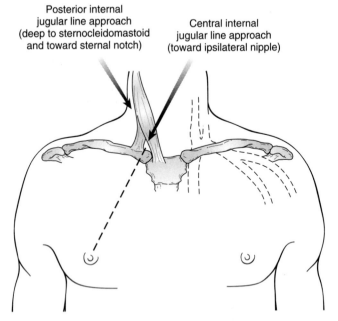

Figure 19–5 Needle entry site and directions.

2. The vein lies posterior to the clavicle and crosses under it medially and superiorly at the distal third of the clavicle and joins the internal jugular vein at the base of the neck.
3. If right-sided heart cannulation is desired, the left subclavian is more desirable than the right side, because this allows a more smooth arc of the catheter once in place.
4. The most common approach is from an infraclavicular site, although it is possible to approach from a supraclavicular site.
5. The insertion site is generally from a point 1 cm inferior to the distal third of the clavicle (see Fig. 19–5).
6. Figure 19–6 shows the cross-sectional anatomy of the subclavian approach.
7. The use of ultrasound can increase the speed and accuracy of line placement.

Procedure

Kits have specific instructions.
1. Prepare the patient.
   a. Explain the procedure.
   b. Explain the risks and alternatives. Obtain consent, if necessary.
   c. Answer any questions.

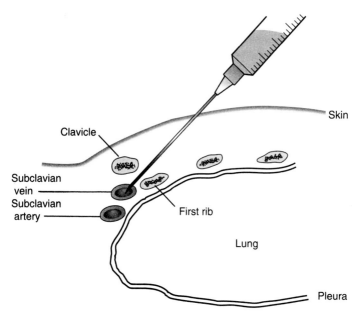

Figure 19–6 Intraclavicular approach to subclavian vein cannulation.

2. Position the patient.
   a. Supine and 15-degree Trendelenburg positioning will increase the venous filling of the subclavian vein.
   b. Elevate the bed to a comfortable height.
   c. Turn the patient's head away from the chosen site.
   d. Confirm that all the equipment is available.
   e. Place a roll under the spine between the shoulder blades (optional).
3. Prepare the skin.
   a. Use sterile technique.
   b. Prepare and drape the skin.
   c. Infiltrate the entry site with 1% to 2% lidocaine; then, infiltrate toward the clavicle. Once the clavicle is reached, march stepwise down the bone, infiltrating the periosteum.
   d. Estimate the length of catheter required to reach the superior vena cava (SVC) by placing the catheter on the sterile field and approximating its anatomic position after placement. It is often not necessary to insert the catheter to its hub.
   e. Confirm that adequate anesthesia has been achieved.
4. Insert the catheter.
   a. Place the 10-mL syringe on the needle.
   b. Insert the needle at a 20-degree to 30-degree angle to the skin. Direct the needle superiorly and medially toward the suprasternal notch (Fig. 19–7.) Place a finger in the notch over the drapes to define this landmark (see Fig. 19–7A). Insert the needle just below the clavicle such that it is necessary to step down the bone to find the space beneath it. Advance along the dorsal surface of the bone and aspirate during insertion (about 5 cm).
   c. If the vessel is not encountered during insertion, slowly withdraw while aspirating because often the vessel is found on the way out.
   d. When dark venous blood flows freely into the syringe, remove the syringe from the needle. Immediately place your finger over the hub of the needle to avoid air embolus.
   e. Place the guide wire through the needle (see Fig. 19–7B). Ensure that the wire passes without resistance. Remove the needle over the wire. Be sure to control the wire.
   f. Nick the skin at the entry site with a scalpel (see Fig. 19–7C).
   g. Place the dilator over the wire and then remove. Watch for increased bleeding at the skin site. This is easily controlled with gentle pressure.
   h. Place the catheter over the wire into the wound (see Fig. 19–7D).
   i. Remove the wire, and confirm appropriate placement by aspiration of blood through each lumen, followed by flushing each lumen with heparinized saline, and cap the catheter.

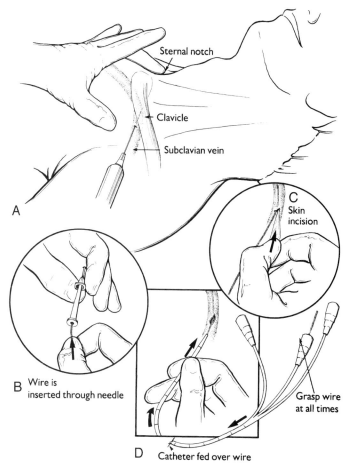

Figure 19–7 Subclavian vein cannulation (Seldinger technique). (From Dunmire SM, Paris PM: Atlas of Emergency Procedures. WB Saunders, Philadelphia, 1995, p. 199.)

5. If blood does not immediately flow into the needle
   a. Pull out, reconfirm landmarks, reposition, and try again.
   b. Occasionally, the needle needs to be flushed of clogging tissue before reinsertion. Use a syringe of sterile normal saline.
   c. If the catheter cannot be placed in three attempts, try the other side. Obtain a CXR first, to rule out pneumothorax.
   d. Confirm the position of the vessel with ultrasound.

6. If arterial blood is encountered
   a. Remove the needle immediately. Discontinue the procedure.
   b. Because of the anatomy of this site, pressure applied to the site may be inadequate to prevent bleeding (see Fig. 19–7). It may be wise to consider the internal jugular or femoral approaches in settings of platelet dysfunction or coagulopathy.
   c. Monitor the patient carefully for the next 24 hours for signs of respiratory distress, swelling at the entry site or evidence of severe blood loss.
7. If air is encountered
   a. Remove the needle immediately. Discontinue the procedure.
   b. Obtain a stat upright CXR, PA, and lateral. Repeat in 12 to 24 hours.
   c. Monitor the patient carefully for the next 24 hours for signs of pneumothorax.
   d. After the CXR has been checked and pneumothorax ruled out, an attempt may be made to place the line on the contralateral side.
8. When the catheter is successfully placed
   a. Secure the catheter to the skin with suture.
   b. Obtain blood samples as needed.
   c. Apply a sterile dressing.
   d. Obtain an upright CXR to confirm placement before infusion of fluids.
   e. Reposition as needed based on the CXR results.
   f. Attach to a manometer for continuous CVP monitoring, if desired.
9. Document the procedure.
10. General considerations
   a. Reassess daily the need for the central venous line.
   b. Check daily the site for infection.
   c. If fever occurs, remember to draw blood for cultures from this site as well as from other indwelling sites.

Internal Jugular Vein Approach

This is a common approach to central venous access. The line is not as comfortable as the subclavian line, but many operators believe that it is a simpler approach and that it may involve a lower incidence of pneumothorax during placement. As the vessels at this site are easy to compress, this approach may be preferable to the subclavian approach in settings of platelet dysfunction or coagulopathy.

Indications

1. Delivery of high concentrations of nutrition or medication
2. Delivery of inotropic medications
3. Prolonged delivery of medication

4. Hemodialysis
5. Hemodynamic monitoring of CVP

Contraindications and Precautions

1. Infection or lesion at the proposed insertion site
   Consider choosing another site.
2. Occlusion or thrombosis of the desired vessel
   Consider choosing another site.
3. Coagulopathy
   Abnormalities in platelet count or function, or in clotting factor concentrations should be corrected before insertion of the line.
4. Ongoing systemic infection
   A peripheral site may be advisable until the source of infection is identified and suitable treatment has begun. This may not always be possible.
5. Vessel perforation
   This is a risk any time a guide wire is used.
6. Dislodgment or loose connections to the line
   This can result in rapid exsanguination.

Equipment Needed

There are specific kits available for many approaches. Refer to the instructions supplied with these kits for complete information.
1. Skin preparation supplies (iodine, chlorhexidine, or alcohol)
2. Local anesthetic (1% or 2% lidocaine, 25-gauge needle, 3-mL syringe)
3. Sterile gloves, eye protection
4. Sterile towels or drapes
5. Supplies for Seldinger technique (or specific intravascular access kit)
   a. Needle (16- to 18-gauge)
   b. Syringe (10-mL)
   c. Guide wire
   d. Scalpel
   e. Dilator
   f. Catheter
6. If the Seldinger technique is not used, a catheter-over-needle system may be used
7. Heparinized saline for flushing the catheter
8. Suture for securing the catheter
9. Equipment for continuous monitoring of central venous pressure, if desired

Anatomic Landmarks (see Figs. 19–4 and 19–5)

1. The IJ vein exits the skull and runs posteriorly and laterally to the carotid artery. Both lie in the carotid sheath in the midcervical region.

2. The vein runs medial to the sternocleidomastoid muscle at the top of the neck, and then passes under the muscle to join the subclavian vein behind the medial clavicle.
3. The path that defines the internal jugular vein may be traced between a point just anterior to the mastoid process and a point just lateral to the sternoclavicular joint.
4. At the inferomedial portion of the neck a triangle is defined by the two heads of the sternocleidomastoid muscle—medially by the sternal head and laterally by the clavicular head. The base of the triangle is defined by the medial clavicle. The internal jugular vein enters this triangle at the apex and runs lateral to the sternal head of the muscle.
5. The insertion site for the middle or central approach is at the apex of the triangle, aimed toward the ipsilateral nipple (see Fig. 19–5).
6. The insertion site for the posterior approach is lateral to the sternocleidomastoid muscle starting 4 to 5 cm above the clavicle; the needle is inserted under the sternocleidomastoid muscle, aimed toward the suprasternal notch (see Fig. 19–5).
7. The approach from the right side has several advantages:
   a. It provides the straightest approach to the right atrium.
   b. There is less of a chance of pneumothorax because the right pleural dome is somewhat lower than the left.
   c. The right jugular vein is often larger than the left.
   d. The position of the right jugular vein relative to the carotid artery is somewhat less variable than on the left.
   e. There is no risk to the thoracic duct.
8. The use of ultrasound can increase the speed and accuracy of line placement.

Procedure

The general steps are similar to the subclavian approach. Refer also to the placement of that line. Where steps differ, they are outlined here.

1. Prepare the patient.
   a. Explain the procedure.
   b. Explain the risks and alternatives. Obtain consent, if necessary.
   c. Answer any questions.
2. Position the patient.
   a. The patient must be supine.
   b. Confirm that all the equipment is available.
   c. Pull the bed away from the wall. Ensure that it is at a comfortable height.
   d. Remove the patient's pillow.
   e. Remove the headboard of the bed if there is one.
   f. Turn the patient's head 30 degree away from the side of choice. Further rotation will defeat the purpose.

g. From 10 degrees to 15 degrees of Trendelenberg will facilitate engorgement of the veins.

3. Prepare the skin.
   a. Use sterile technique.
   b. Prepare and drape the skin. The drape may cover the face of the patient; ensure that the patient is comfortable and able to breathe.
   c. Infiltrate the entry site with 1% to 2% lidocaine. Also infiltrate over the sites of anchoring sutures.
   d. Estimate the length of catheter required to reach the superior vena cava by placing the catheter on the sterile field and approximating its anatomic position after placement.
   e. Confirm that adequate anesthesia has been achieved.

4. Insert the catheter.
   a. Place the 10-mL syringe on the needle.
      Often, a 22-gauge "finder" needle is used to sound for the jugular vein. The theory is that if the carotid artery is penetrated, the hole made is smaller than if a larger-gauge needle is used. The subsequent bleeding is less, and the risk of air embolism is less. Once the direction and depth of the jugular vein are determined, switch to the larger needle and proceed with the line placement.
   b. With your nondominant hand, palpate the carotid pulse. You may feel comfortable putting gentle pressure medially on the carotid to retract it from the insertion site.
   c. Use ultrasound, if desired, to confirm the position and patency of the vessel. Patency is confirmed by compressibility.
   d. Insert the needle at a 20-degree to 30-degree angle to the skin.
      i. Central or middle approach (thought to be the most reliable approach)
      Direct the needle inferiorly and laterally toward the nipple on the ipsilateral side (Fig. 19–8A). Aspirate during insertion (approximately 1 to 4 cm).
      ii. Posterior approach
      If the posterior approach is used, direct the needle inferiorly and anteriorly toward the suprasternal notch (approximately 5 cm) (see Fig. 19–8B).
   e. If the vessel is not encountered during insertion, slowly withdraw while aspirating because often the vessel is found on the way out.
   f. When dark venous blood flows freely into the syringe, remove the syringe from the needle. Immediately place your finger over the hub of the needle to avoid air embolus.
   g. Place the guide wire through the needle and complete the procedure according to the Seldinger technique.

5. If blood does not immediately flow into the needle
   a. Pull out, reconfirm landmarks, reposition, and try again.

Figure 19–8 Technique of internal jugular vein cannulation. Direct the needle inferiorly and laterally toward the nipple on the ipsilateral side. *A*, Central approach; *B*, posterior approach.
(Redrawn from Dunmire SM, Paris PM: Atlas of Emergency Procedures. WB Saunders, Philadelphia, 1995, p. 201.)

    b. Occasionally, the needle needs to be flushed of clogging tissue before reinsertion. Use a syringe of sterile heparinized saline.

    c. If the catheter cannot be placed in three attempts, try the other side.

       Obtain a CXR first, to rule out pneumothorax.

    d. Reconfirm the position of the vessel with ultrasound.

6. If arterial blood is encountered

    a. Remove the needle immediately. Discontinue the procedure.

    b. Hold pressure at the site for 10 minutes (by the clock).

    c. Once bleeding has been controlled locally, the procedure may be resumed.

    d. Monitor the patient carefully for the next 24 hours to watch for signs of respiratory distress, swelling at the entry site or evidence of severe blood loss.

7. If air is encountered

    a. Remove the needle immediately. Discontinue the procedure.

    b. Obtain stat upright CXR, PA, and lateral. Repeat in 12 to 24 hours.

    c. Monitor the patient carefully for the next 24 hours for signs of pneumothorax.

    d. After the CXR has been checked and pneumothorax ruled out, an attempt may be made to place the line on the contralateral side.

8. When the catheter is successfully placed

    a. Secure the catheter to the skin with suture.

    b. Obtain blood samples, as needed.

    c. Apply a sterile dressing.

    d. Obtain an upright CXR to confirm placement before infusion of fluids.

    e. Reposition, as needed based on the CXR results.

    f. Attach to a manometer for continuous central venous pressure monitoring, if desired.

9. Document the procedure.

10. General considerations

    a. Reassess daily the need for the central venous line.

    b. Check daily the site for infection.

    c. If fever occurs, remember to draw blood for cultures from this site as well as from other indwelling sites.

Femoral Vein Approach

This femoral vein approach is the easiest and safest site for line placement. The tip of the line will reside in the inferior vena cava (IVC); this is not a good site for an ambulatory patient or one in whom pulmonary wedge pressures might need to be monitored. This line also has a higher site infection rate because of its placement in skin folds. Also, it is often hidden under bedding, and concerted effort is required to check the site for bleeding or infection.

Indications

1. Delivery of high concentrations of nutrition or medication
2. Delivery of inotropic medications
3. Prolonged delivery of medication
4. Hemodialysis
5. Hemodynamic monitoring of CVP (the femoral site is not the best for this)

Contraindications and Precautions

1. Infection or lesion at the proposed insertion site
   Consider choosing another site.
2. Occlusion or thrombosis of the desired vessel
   Consider choosing another site.
3. Coagulopathy
   Abnormalities in platelet count or function, or in clotting factor concentrations should be corrected before insertion of the line.
4. Ongoing systemic infection
   A peripheral site may be advisable until the source of infection is identified and suitable treatment has begun. This may not always be possible.
5. Vessel perforation
   This is a risk any time a guide wire is used.
6. Dislodgment or loose connections to the line
   This can result in rapid exsanguination.

Equipment Needed

There are specific kits available for many approaches. Refer to the instructions supplied with these kits for complete information.

1. Skin preparation supplies (iodine, chlorhexidine, or alcohol)
2. Local anesthetic (1% or 2% lidocaine, 25-gauge needle, 3-mL syringe)
3. Sterile gloves, eye protection
4. Sterile towels or drapes
5. Supplies for Seldinger technique (or specific intravascular access kit)
   a. Needle (16- to 18-gauge)
   b. 10-mL syringe
   c. Guide wire
   d. Scalpel
   e. Dilator
   f. Catheter
6. If the Seldinger technique is not used, a catheter-over-needle system may be used.
7. Heparinized saline for flushing the catheter
8. Suture for securing the catheter

9. Equipment for continuous monitoring of central venous pressure, if desired
10. Sterile dressing supplies

Anatomic Landmarks (see Fig. 19–3)

1. The vein is found halfway between the anterior iliac spine and the symphysis pubis.
2. Remember the orientation of the artery to the vein (NAVELS):

Nerve → Artery → Vein → Empty space → Lymphatics → Symphysis pubis

(The vein resides between the pulse and the pubis.)

Procedure

The general steps are similar to the subclavian approach.
1. Prepare the patient.
   a. Explain the procedure.
   b. Explain the risks and alternatives. Obtain consent, if necessary.
   c. Answer any questions.
2. Position the patient.
   a. The patient must be supine.
   b. Confirm that all the equipment is available.
   c. Ensure that it is at a comfortable height.
3. Prepare the skin.
   a. Use sterile technique.
   b. Prepare and drape the skin. Hair removal may be necessary.
   c. Infiltrate the entry site with 1% to 2% lidocaine. Also infiltrate over the sites of anchoring sutures.
   d. Confirm that adequate anesthesia has been achieved.
4. Insert the catheter.
   a. Place the 10-mL syringe on the needle.
   b. With your nondominant hand, palpate the femoral pulse.
   c. Insert the needle at a 30-degree to 40-degree angle to the skin, medially to the pulse. Direct the needle superiorly. Aspirate during insertion (about 4 cm).
   d. If the vessel is not encountered during insertion, slowly withdraw while aspirating because often the vessel is found on the way out.
   e. When dark venous blood flows freely into the syringe, remove the syringe from the needle. Immediately place your finger over the hub of the needle to avoid air embolus.
   f. Place the guide wire through the needle and complete the procedure according to the Seldinger technique.
5. If blood does not immediately flow into the needle.
   a. Pull out, reconfirm landmarks, reposition, and try again.

b. Occasionally, the needle needs to be flushed of clogging tissue before reinsertion. Use a syringe of heparinized saline.

c. If the catheter cannot be placed in three attempts, try the other side.

6. If arterial blood is encountered.

a. Remove the needle immediately. Discontinue the procedure.

b. Hold pressure at the site for 10 minutes (by the clock).
   Hold pressure longer if the lumen was large or the patient is anticoagulated.

c. Once bleeding has been controlled locally, the procedure may be resumed.

7. When the catheter is successfully placed.

a. Flush all lumens with heparinized saline.

b. Secure the catheter to the skin with suture.

c. Obtain blood samples as needed.

d. Apply a sterile dressing.

e. Chest x-ray (CXR) is not necessary before the use of this line.

8. Document the procedure.

9. General considerations.

a. Reassess daily the need for the central venous line.

b. Check daily the site for infection.

c. If fever occurs, remember to draw blood for cultures from this site as well as from other indwelling sites.

Removal of Central Venous Lines

1. Ensure that the patient has no need for continued central venous access.

2. If a peripheral line is necessary, ensure that it is in place and patent.

3. Have a scissors or blade, gauze, and tape ready.

4. Always wear gloves and eye protection when there is a potential for exposure to blood or other body fluids.

5. Place the patient in the supine position.

6. Clean around the catheter entry site with sterile soap if blood for culture is to be drawn.

7. Remove the sutures.

8. Remove the catheter.

a. Remove all IV lines from the catheter.

b. Clamp off or occlude all of the catheter ports.

c. For subclavian and internal jugular lines, have the patient hold his or her breath.
   This increases the intrathoracic pressure and decreases the risk of air embolism.

d. Some long-term catheters have subcutaneous cuffs, which adhere to surrounding tissue (e.g., Hickman, Broviac). It will be necessary to break the adhesions between the subcutaneous tissues and the cuff. If the distance is short between the cuff and the skin insertion site, the adhesions may be broken using a hemostat inserted through the skin entry site. Be sure to use local anesthetic and clean the skin well. Occasionally a separate skin incision will be needed over the palpable portion of the cuff, and the adhesions should be broken through that incision. Occasionally the cuff will detach from the catheter with gentle pressure and may be safely left behind in the subcutaneous tissues.

  e. Remove the catheter with smooth, constant pressure.
  f. Confirm that the entire catheter has been removed. If a portion of the catheter breaks off during removal it may migrate and cause dysrhythmias or respiratory difficulties. It must be removed by vascular surgery or interventional radiology personnel.
 9. Apply firm pressure at the vein entry site for 10 minutes (by the clock).
    Hold pressure longer if the lumen was large or the patient is anticoagulated.
10. Also apply light pressure to the skin entry site.
11. After 10 minutes, confirm that the bleeding has stopped.
12. Place an occlusive dressing for 24 to 48 hours.
13. Culture the catheter tip if clinically indicated.
14. Document the line removal.
15. Check the skin site the next day for evidence of infection or continued bleeding.

Complications and Problems of Central Venous Line Procedures

 1. Venous air embolism
 2. Pneumothorax
    a. Obtain a stat upright CXR to confirm the diagnosis.
    b. Place the patient on 100% O_2.
    c. If respiratory compromise is present, place a tube thoracostomy (see Chapter 30).
    d. This complication may occur up to 24 hours following placement of a line.
 3. Guide wire embolism
    Embolus must be removed by vascular surgery or interventional radiology personnel.
 4. Carotid arterial puncture
    Apply pressure at the puncture site.
 5. Nonplacement of the line
    Obtain a CXR to rule out pneumothorax prior to considering attempting a line on the other side.
 6. Misplacement of the line

     Occasionally lines will end up in the wrong vessel (i.e., in the subclavian vein rather than the SVC). Be sure to orient the point of the J-wire in the desired direction during placement (see Fig. 19–2).

7. Cardiac tamponade

     Remember Beck's triad: systemic hypotension, distended neck veins, muffled heart tones.

     This may require emergency pericardiocentesis (see Chapter 28).

8. Entry site infection

     This requires removal of the line.

9. Suppurative thrombophlebitis

     This may require surgical drainage and IV antibiotics.

10. Catheter-related sepsis

     This requires removal of the line and treatment with IV antibiotics

11. Vessel thrombosis

     Remove the line.

12. Hemorrhage

   a. Dislodged line or loose connections

     Be sure to check the connections. Poor coupling of lines can result in rapid exsanguination.

   b. Bleeding or hematoma at the vessel entry site

     Hold pressure for 10 minutes (by the clock).

     Occasionally, a stitch at the entry site will suffice.

13. Non-function of the line

PERIPHERAL VENOUS LINES

This is the most common access and is used for routine fluid replacement and medication delivery.

Indications

1. Requirement of IV fluid replacement for maintenance or rehydration purposes
2. Delivery of medication or nutrition

Contraindications and Precautions

1. Infection or lesion at the proposed insertion site
     Consider choosing another site.
2. Occlusion or thrombosis of the desired vessel
     Consider choosing another site.

Equipment Needed

1. Skin preparation supplies (iodine, chlorhexidine, or alcohol)
2. Local anesthetic (1% or 2% lidocaine, 25-gauge needle, 3-mL syringe), optional

3. Nonsterile gloves, eye protection
4. Angiocatheter (18- to 22-gauge needles commonly used)
5. Heparinized saline for flushing the catheter
6. 10-mL syringe for flushing the catheter
7. Tape for securing the catheter
8. Sterile dressing supplies

Anatomy

1. Most frequently, distal upper extremity sites are chosen. It is best to start more distally and then move proximally.
2. Palpable veins often are easier to cannulate than visible ones.
3. If no veins are apparent, try to warm the extremity, or place it in a dependent position to increase venous dilation.
4. In supine, nonambulatory patients, the lower extremity may be used.
5. Whenever possible, try to avoid sites that would be inconvenient to the patient. These might include the dorsum of the patient's dominant hand, antecubital veins, or painful sites such as the volar surface of the forearm.

Procedure

1. Prepare the patient.
   a. Explain the procedure. All needle sticks are painful.
   b. Explain the risks and alternatives.
   c. Answer any questions.
2. Select the site.
3. Position the patient.
   a. The patient should be comfortable, sitting or supine.
   b. Get a chair for yourself.
   c. Occasionally, armboards are required to immobilize sites such as the dorsum of the hand or the antecubital site.
   d. Confirm that all the equipment is available.
4. Prepare the skin.
   a. Use clean technique.
   b. Prepare the skin.
   c. If the patient desires, or if a large needle is to be used, consider infiltration of the entry site with 1% to 2% lidocaine.
5. Apply the tourniquet.
   a. Apply the tourniquet on the upper arm because this gives better dilation of the distal superficial venous system.
   b. Do not apply so tightly as to impair arterial flow into the extremity.
6. Insert the catheter.
   a. Confirm that adequate anesthesia has been achieved (if used).
   b. Palpate the vein with the index finger of your nondominant hand. Apply gentle pressure to stretch the vein away from yourself.

    c. An optional step is to nick the skin over the entry site with a sterile scalpel in order not to damage the catheter as it enters the skin.

    d. Insert the angiocatheter at a 30-degree to 45-degree angle to the vein.

    e. When dark venous blood pours freely into the catheter, continue to advance the catheter slowly until the flow just stops.

    f. Back off slightly until the blood flows again, and advance the catheter over the needle into the vessel.

7. If blood does not immediately flow into the needle
    a. Pull back but not completely out of the skin, reconfirm the landmarks, reposition, and try again.
    b. Occasionally, the needle needs to be flushed of clogging tissue before reinsertion. Use a syringe of heparinized saline.
    c. If the catheter cannot be placed in three attempts, try another site. To avoid venous bleeding from the unsuccessful site, leave the catheter in the skin wound, and retry with a fresh angiocatheter. The unsuccessful angiocatheters may be removed later after the tourniquet is removed.

8. When the catheter is successfully placed
    a. Remember to remove the tourniquet.
    b. Secure the catheter to the skin with tape.
    c. Attach tubing for delivery of appropriate IV fluid.

9. Document the procedure.

Removal of Peripheral Lines

1. Make sure the patient no longer needs the IV site.
2. Always wear gloves and eye protection when there is a potential for exposure to blood or other body fluids.
3. Remove securing tapes.
4. Remove the catheter.
5. Apply firm pressure at the entry site for 5 to 10 minutes.
    Hold pressure longer if the lumen was large or the patient is anticoagulated.
6. Confirm that bleeding has stopped.
7. Place a clean dressing.
8. Check the site the next day.

Complications and Problems of Peripheral Lines

1. Nonplacement of the line
2. Entry site infection
    This requires removal of the line.
3. Vessel thrombosis
    This requires removal of the line.
4. Suppurative thrombophlebitis
    This requires removal of the line and may require surgery.
5. Hemorrhage (usually minor)
6. Nonfunction

Leg Pain

Leg pain is common with lower extremity surgery, trauma, vascular problems, inflammatory or degenerative conditions, infection, or referred pain. Some of these conditions can be managed by telephone, whereas others require that you examine the patient. A careful discussion with the RN will help to show which patients should be examined.

PHONE CALL

Questions

1. **What area of the leg is painful?**
   Pain in the region of a joint may be indicative of an inflammatory or an infectious process, but pain in the calf may suggest a vascular cause of the pain.

2. **What are the vital signs? Is there any shortness of breath (SOB)?**
   Deep venous thrombosis (DVT) and subsequent pulmonary embolus may first present with leg pain. SOB with a history of recent leg pain may suggest pulmonary embolus.

3. **Did the patient have surgery or a traumatic accident? If the patient had surgery, what type of operation was performed, and when was it performed?**
   Surgery on the lower extremities, the pelvis, and the abdominal wall predisposes a patient to development of DVTs. Investigate a traumatic cause of leg pain with a clinical examination and appropriate radiographs.

4. **Why was the patient admitted? Is there any history of recent trauma?**
   Pelvic and lower extremity trauma may be associated with leg pain and increased risk of DVTs. Posttraumatic leg pain in the presence of a loss of pulses may suggest an arterial injury.

5. **Is there a pulse in the leg? Is there swelling or discoloration of the skin?**
   An acute loss of pulses in a lower extremity represents an emergency. It often suggests acute embolism or thrombosis. Leg pain and pallor of the skin may suggest insufficiency of arterial inflow. This may accompany arterial injury, thrombosis, or

compartment syndrome. Bluish discoloration of the skin with or without leg pain suggests venous insufficiency.

6. Has the patient lost any sensation in the leg acutely?

An acute loss of sensation suggests arterial insufficiency or compartment syndrome.

7. Is there a dressing or a cast in place on the leg?

Increasing pain in the presence of a cast or a dressing usually requires investigation. A dressing may be covering an infected wound; a cast may be too tight. Fractures under the cast may also hurt.

8. Does the patient have known medical problems?

A patient who has known atherosclerosis, degenerative changes of the lower extremity, or history of DVT may be more likely to present with leg pain.

Inform RN

Will arrive at the bedside in . . . minutes.

Sudden-onset, severe leg pain may be a sign of arterial or venous compromise and should be assessed immediately. Leg pain associated with fever, loss of pulses, new-onset swelling, or SOB may represent a limb-threatening or life-threatening process and requires immediate evaluation.

ELEVATOR THOUGHTS

What causes leg pain?
1. Vascular diseases
   - DVT
   - Acute arterial insufficiency (thrombus and embolus)
   - Arterial vasospasm
   - Chronic arterial insufficiency (arteriosclerosis obliterans)
   - Buerger disease
   - Popliteal artery entrapment
   - Ischemia due to constrictive dressing or cast
   - Superficial thrombophlebitis
   - Venous stasis disease
2. Inflammatory and degenerative diseases
   - Degenerative arthritis (hips, knees, and ankles)
   - Lumbar disk disease (sciatica)
   - Acute gout and pseudogout
   - Rheumatoid arthritis
   - Systemic lupus erythematosus
   - Periostitis
3. Infectious processes
   - Cellulitis
   - Septic arthritis
   - Septic thrombophlebitis
   - Necrotizing fasciitis
   - Osteomyelitis

4. Soft-tissue and bone processes
   - Compartment syndrome
   - Neuropathy (diabetic)
   - Erythema nodosum
   - Neuroma or other soft-tissue mass
   - Skeletal tumors
   - Benign leg cramps
   - Postsurgical pain
   - Traumatic causes of pain (fracture, sprain)

MAJOR THREAT TO LIFE

The following are either limb-threatening or life-threatening processes:

1. Arterial occlusion
2. Pulmonary embolus resulting from DVT
3. Infectious processes
   - Septic arthritis
   - Septic thrombophlebitis
   - Necrotizing infection
4. Compartment syndrome

Acute Arterial Insufficiency

Acute arterial insufficiency often presents with an acute increase in pain, pallor, and loss of pulses in the affected extremity. In the lower extremity, it most frequently affects the foot. If circulation is not re-established rapidly (within 6 hours), irreversible tissue damage and loss of limb may result.

Deep Venous Thrombosis

DVT is very common in postsurgical and bedridden patients. Although DVTs originate in the leg or pelvis, they may become blood borne and travel to the pulmonary artery. This may lead to a life-threatening pulmonary embolus.

Infectious Processes

Infectious processes of the lower extremity may involve joints, blood vessels, and other soft tissues. Many of these processes are rapidly progressive due to the poor blood supply to the lower extremities in patients with vascular disease. Diabetic patients are particularly susceptible to infectious processes of the lower extremities. Diabetics generally have a component of small-vessel and large-vessel disease, with decreased blood flow to the legs. These patients often have neuropathies, making trauma and late detection of skin breakdown commonplace. The decreased immune function of diabetic patients makes infections especially troublesome and may lead to blood-borne infection and sepsis.

Compartment Syndrome

Compartment syndrome may follow leg trauma or reperfusion of an ischemic extremity. Failure to recognize elevated lower extremity compartmental pressures may result in soft-tissue necrosis and ultimate limb loss.

BEDSIDE

Although the list of causes of leg pain is long, careful discussion of the on-call problem with the RN will help determine if examination and treatment of the patient is necessary. Loss of lower extremity pulses and foot pain (acute ischemia) is an emergency. New-onset lower extremity swelling must also be evaluated immediately and may represent DVT or compartment syndrome. Fever and leg pain may indicate infection or DVT; this presentation requires your evaluation.

Quick Look Test

Most patients with leg pain will give a history that helps to provide a narrowed differential diagnosis. Patients with infectious processes often look sick, and patients with ischemia or DVT appear uncomfortable.

Airway and Vital Signs

By itself, leg pain should not lead to instability of the vital signs. However, when SOB, severe pain, or infection is associated with leg pain, changes in vital signs may be seen.

Heart Rate, Blood Pressure, and Respiratory Rate

Severe leg pain is stressful to patients, and it may lead to tachycardia, tachypnea, and hypertension. A DVT that migrates from the lower extremity to the pulmonary vessels may cause acute SOB and tachypnea.

Temperature

Leg pain associated with an infectious process often presents with fever. DVT may present with leg pain, fever, and swelling.

Selective History and Chart Review

Does the patient have a history of leg pain? Is the current pain similar to or worse than prior pain episodes?
     Many patients with advanced atherosclerosis of the lower extremity vessels will have a history of intermittent claudication and foot pain. Patients with inflammatory or degenerative conditions will often give a history of chronic pain. It is important to establish a baseline to allow comparison with the patient's current leg pain.

Pain that is different or more severe than prior pain episodes requires you to perform a careful examination of the leg.

Is there a history of prior vascular surgery?

Patients who have undergone revascularization of the leg generally have significant peripheral vascular occlusive disease. These patients may have re-occlusion of their bypass grafts or occlusion of arteries acutely in the other lower extremity.

Does the patient have a history of atrial fibrillation? Does the patient have prosthetic heart valves?

Atrial fibrillation is a leading cause of embolization and acute arterial occlusion in the lower extremities. Other causes of embolization include embolism from prosthetic heart valves or peripheral emboli (aortic and other vessels).

Is there a history of deep venous thrombosis or venous disease of the lower extremities?

Patients who have had prior DVTs are at an increased risk for having another one. Patients with a hypercoagulable state (e.g., cancer, pregnancy, and congenital conditions) are more likely to develop DVTs. Any history of venous insufficiency or venous stasis disease should be ascertained. Prolonged surgical procedures, surgery in lithotrophy position, pelvic fractures, and pelvic surgery predispose a patient to DVT formation.

Selective Physical Examination

The physical examination is directed toward finding a cause for the leg pain. Examination will be directed at looking for signs of inflammation, infection, arterial insufficiency, or venous disease.

VS: Obtain a set of vital signs; look for signs of fever (infection and DVT).

Resp: If the patient has SOB, listen for friction rub or evidence of pulmonary effusion (pulmonary embolus).

CVS: Look for pulse regularity; irregularity of the rhythm and rate suggests atrial fibrillation. Listen for evidence of a prosthetic heart valve (metallic click).

Extrem: Perform a complete vascular examination of the lower extremities, including an evaluation of femoral, popliteal, dorsalis pedis, and posterior tibial arteries. Recall that the posterior tibial vessels and the great saphenous vein are on the medial aspect of the ankle, with the posterior tibial vessels posterior to the medial malleolus and the saphenous vein about 1 cm anterior to the medial malleolus (Fig. 20–1). Evaluate for tenderness, sensory function, and motor strength, and compare results with those of the opposite leg.

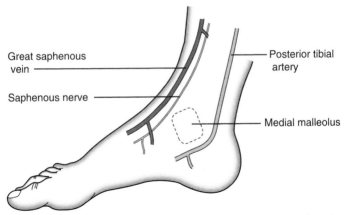

Figure 20–1 Medial view of ankle region and structures of major importance.

> Remember that patients with prior vascular surgery may have altered pulses. Look for historical documentation of pulses in the chart.

Skin: Look for erythema, cyanotic changes, mottling, pallor, and edema.

ABI: The ankle brachial index (ABI) is a straightforward measurement of lower extremity perfusion. It is performed by taking a blood pressure on an arm, and on each leg. The ABI is calculated by dividing the leg systolic pressure by the arm systolic pressure. Normal is 0.9 to 1.1. Rest pain is apparent below 0.5.

MANAGEMENT

Management is directed at treating the cause of the leg pain, as follows:

VASCULAR DISEASES

Acute Arterial Insufficiency

Selective History

Is there a history of peripheral vascular disease or intermittent claudication?

Is there a history of cardiac or vascular disease (e.g., atrial fibrillation, prior embolus, prosthetic heart valve, left ventricular aneurysm, or aortic disease)?

Was pain, temperature change, or color change in the leg of sudden onset?

How does the symptomatic leg compare with the other leg?

Selective Physical Examination

Look for the "six P's" for evidence of acute arterial insufficiency, as follows:

Pain:	An early sign of ischemia
Pallor:	An early sign of ischemia
Poikilothermia:	Cool to the touch
Pulselessness:	An early sign of gross arterial occlusion
Paresthesia:	Sensory loss in ischemic region
Paralysis:	Usually a late finding and indicative of tissue damage

In addition, look for the following:

VS:	Signs of shock, hypovolemia, or orthostasis
Skin:	Pallor, mottling, gangrenous changes, and chronic changes including hair loss, thin skin, and shiny skin
CVS:	Heart sounds: listen for regularity; pulse examination: radial, femoral, popliteal, dorsalis pedis, and posterior tibial; comparison of symmetry with other leg; use of Doppler probe if pulses are not palpable
Neuro:	Evaluation of light touch sensation (first neurologic deficit seen in ischemia); evaluation of muscle strengths

The diagnosis of acute arterial insufficiency or occlusion is best made by history and careful physical examination. Always compare the symptomatic leg with the nonsymptomatic leg.

Patients who are sensate will often complain of leg pain in the presence of an acute arterial occlusion. Temperature changes and skin changes are also seen shortly after acute arterial occlusion. The leg will often show a distinct line of demarcation, below which the skin temperature is cooler and more mottled or pale than the region proximal to the suspected occlusion. Mark the line of demarcation, and evaluate the lower extremity pulses to see if pulse changes correspond to other changes.

Take care when treating patients undergoing cardiac catheterization or other invasive arterial procedures. These patients are at risk for embolization and may shower emboli to the lower extremity. Common locations for emboli include the foot and the toes. When circulation to the foot is compromised by an embolus, a cold foot or "trash foot" results. A cold foot represents an emergency that requires rapid action. Recent arterial catheterization may also lead to pseudoaneurysm formation at the insertion site and result in occlusion.

Management

Acute arterial occlusion is an emergency. In the event of acute occlusion, observe the following protocol:

1. Notify the chief resident or attending physician immediately.
2. If there are no contraindications, start heparinization immediately. The patient may be given **5000 to 10,000 U heparin intravenous (IV) bolus, followed by a continuous infusion of 1000 U/hour (18 mg/kg/hour).** Adjust the infusion rate to keep the partial thromboplastin time (PTT) at 70 to 80 seconds.
3. Arrange for an arteriogram immediately. Many institutions follow heparin using anti-X_a levels. The range varies depending on whether thrombocytics are used.
4. Review the case with the attending physician and a consulting vascular surgeon.
   The patient will likely require emergent angiography and either surgical embolectomy or angioplasty.
5. Fibrinolytic therapy is used only for surgically inaccessible peripheral arterial occlusions.

Do not confuse acute arterial insufficiency with chronic arterial insufficiency. Patients with long-standing arteriosclerosis and chronic intermittent claudication may present with pain at rest. The key finding is a change in the exam. If there is no concern with limb viability, the patient may be treated with analgesics and by having the leg placed in a more dependent position. Consultation with a vascular surgeon may be made on a nonemergent basis. Platelet-inhibiting medications such as **aspirin,** or rheostatic agents such as **clopidogrel** *(Plavix)* are often prescribed.

Deep Venous Thrombosis

Selective History

Is there a history of prior DVT or coagulopathy?

Is there a history of trauma or surgery to the lower extremity or pelvis?

Is there a history of cancer?

Is there a history of prolonged immobilization?

Remember that the incidence of DVT is increased in the following patients:

1. Postoperative patients
2. Patients undergoing major orthopedic procedures
3. Patients more than 40 years of age
4. Obese or immobilized patients
5. Patients undergoing pelvic surgery or abdominal cancer surgery
6. Patients with pelvic or lower extremity fractures
7. Pregnant patients or those taking estrogen-based medications
8. Patients undergoing surgery in lithotomy position.

Selective Physical Examination

VS:	Rule out tachypnea and blood pressure changes suggestive of a pulmonary embolus.
Extrem:	Evaluate lower leg and foot for new-onset edema; use a measuring tape if available to document a difference in size of the two extremities; look for erythema and warmth of the skin; palpate calf posteriorly and medially to feel for venous cords; gently compress the calf muscles against the tibia to evaluate for tenderness; also palpate the popliteal space, the adductor canal, and the groin to evaluate for tenderness; tenderness over a thrombosed vein is usually present if palpated.
Test for *Homans' sign:*	With patient supine, straighten the leg and dorsiflex the foot; passive stretching of gastrocnemius and soleus muscles occurs with this maneuver, which may elicit pain in the presence of a deep calf venous thrombosis.

DVT is a difficult diagnostic and therapeutic problem that can lead to pulmonary embolus. The most common veins affected are veins associated with the deep system of the lower extremity or veins within the pelvis (Fig. 20–2). It is generally difficult to palpate these structures directly. Diagnosis is made by clinical signs (e.g., noting new-onset edema in one extremity) and a high level of suspicion.

Diagnostic Testing

Ultrasound studies (duplex) are the most accurate noninvasive test for diagnosing proximal DVT. However, duplex is less accurate at diagnosing isolated calf venous thrombosis. Another reliable noninvasive technique for diagnosing proximal thrombosis is **impedance plethysmography. Contrast venography** is the most reliable technique for diagnosing DVT. However, this technique is invasive and has fallen out of favor as a first-line diagnostic procedure.

Management

Patients with a significant venous thrombosis of the lower extremity require bed rest, elevation of the affected extremity, and anticoagulation. Although isolated venous thromboses of the calf can eventually extend proximally in up to 20% of cases, some physicians treat small, isolated DVTs with bed rest, elevation, and observation alone.

Patients with proximal DVT should receive anticoagulation with IV heparin. Therapy can be initiated with a bolus of 5000 U heparin IV (60 to 80 U/bolus/kg of body weight) followed by a continuous infusion starting at 1000 U/hour (18 U/hour/kg of body weight). Check PTT 6 hours after initiating therapy and every 6 to 8 hours thereafter until a steady state is reached. The goal of the therapy is to achieve a PTT value 1.5 to 2 times the control value. This is usually

Figure 20–2 Common patterns of venous thrombosis. *A*, Superficial thrombophelebitis; *B*, the most common form of deep thrombophlebitis; *C* and *D*, deep thrombophlebitis from the calf to the iliac veins. These patterns produce phlegmasia alba dolens, or if more complete, phlegmasia cerulea dolens. The usual locations of thrombosis in milk leg are shown in *C*. (From Haller JA Jr: Deep Thrombophlebitis: Pathophysiology and Treatment. Philadelphia, WB Saunders, 1967, p. 12.)

a PTT of 50 to 80 seconds. Adjust the hourly rate of infusion accordingly. Most patients require 800 to 1600 U/hour. Anti-X_a levels may also be followed.

By the second day of IV heparin therapy, consider starting patients on warfarin sodium (Coumadin) therapy. Patients may be given warfarin sodium 10 mg/day for the first several days. Recall that warfarin interferes with the vitamin K-dependent carboxylation of clotting factors. It generally takes several days to see the effects of warfarin. Remember that the prothrombin time (PT) reflects a warfarin dose given about 48 hours earlier. Follow anticoagulation by evaluating the PT on a daily basis. As the PT value begins to rise, consider decreasing the dose of warfarin. Many patients do well with about 5 mg/day. Elderly patients and patients with liver disease often require smaller daily doses. The international normalized ratio (INR) has been calculated to standardize warfarin anticoagulation. An INR of 2 to 3 is generally therapeutic. Once a patient is adequately anticoagulated on warfarin, IV heparin therapy may be stopped. Therapeutic doses of low-molecular-weight heparin may also be used in lieu of heparin or warfarin.

There are risks in using heparin or warfarin. Bleeding is a serious complication. Avoid these anticoagulants in acute trauma patients, neurosurgical patients, or patients with active peptic ulcer disease. In addition, avoid the use of warfarin in pregnant patients. Warfarin crosses the placenta and causes birth defects. Also beware of the numerous drugs that may interact with warfarin and alter PT. A list of some of the common drugs that alter PT are listed in Table 20–1.

Perioperative Prophylaxis for DVTS

Thigh-high TED hose and sequential compression devices should be used on the patient intraoperatively if the operation is expected to last more than 2 hours.

Subcutaneous heparin 5000 mg twice a day may also be used. Discuss the heparin dose with a resident or attending physician prior to administering it.

TABLE 20–1 **Common Drugs That Interact with Warfarin and Alter Prothrombin Time**

Increases Prothrombin Time	Decreases Prothrombin Time
Metronidazole	Cholestyramine
Trimethoprim and sulfamethoxazole	Barbiturates
Disulfiram	Rifampin
Amiodarone	Carbamazepine
Omeprazole	Griseofulvin
Cimetidine	Penicillins
Some cephalosporins	
Heparin	
Thyroxine	
Clofibrate	

Low-molecular-weight heparin (e.g., enoxaparin or dalteparin) may be used.

Avoid the use of heparin or low-molecular-weight heparin in the setting of recent trauma, head injury, or known coagulopathy.

INFLAMMATORY AND DEGENERATIVE DISEASES

Acute Gout and Pseudogout

Acute Gout

Acute gout is an extremely painful condition in which monosodium urate crystals are released into the joint space from the synovium. Definitive diagnosis is made by demonstrating negative birefringent monosodium urate crystals by using polarizing microscopy. Gout most commonly affects the foot and ankle. Patients may be managed with the nonsteroidal anti-inflammatory drug (NSAID) **indomethacin 100 mg orally (PO) followed by 50 mg PO every 6 hours. Ketorolac tromethamine (Toradol) 30 mg intramuscularly (IM), followed by 15 to 30 mg IM every 6 hours** may be used for pain control in more severe cases but should not be used for more than 3 days. An alternative is **colchicine 0.5 to 0.6 mg PO every 1 to 2 hours, which may be repeated until gastrointestinal side effects occur or when a maximum dose of 6 mg has been given in a 24-hour period.**

Pseudogout

Pseudogout is caused by the release of calcium pyrophosphate crystals from the joint surface into the joint space. Joint aspiration shows weakly positive birefringent rods in the joint fluid. Patients may also be managed with an NSAID such as indomethacin. Intra-articular steroids may be used in patients in which NSAIDs are contraindicated. As an alternative, **prednisone 40 to 60 mg PO every day** may be given for several days until a response is obtained and then rapidly tapered.

SOFT-TISSUE AND BONE PROCESSES

Compartment Syndrome

Compartment syndrome is a group of signs and symptoms resulting from increased pressures in the compartments of the lower extremity. The diagnosis is based on clinical examination and history. Patients usually present with pain, diminished sensation, and weakness or diminished muscle function. Clinical examination also shows tenseness and tenderness in compartment(s) of the lower extremity. Passively stretching the foot (dorsiflexion and plantarflexion) will often cause severe pain.

Close observation and repeated examinations spaced no more than 30 minutes apart is important for demonstrating progression. Symptoms that worsen progressively suggest increasing compartmental pressures and the need for compartment release. The most common causes of compartment syndrome are trauma and reperfusion injury. Table 20–2 lists injuries known to cause compartment syndrome of the lower extremity.

Selective Physical Examination

Clinical examination is the key to diagnosis. Rate the status and the function of the following:

1. Muscle function should be graded from 0 to 5 and followed serially.
2. Sensation should be evaluated as normal, slightly diminished, significantly diminished, or absent. Sensation should be tested by both pinprick and two-point discrimination.
3. Tenseness is palpated and recorded as normal, slightly increased, significantly increased, or rock-hard.

Clinical findings alone are generally used to diagnose compartment syndrome. However, in patients in whom the diagnosis cannot be made or ruled out by clinical examination (e.g., unconscious patient), evaluate the compartmental pressures. If you are rotating on a surgery service, ask the senior resident for help with measuring compartmental pressures. In some hospitals, orthopedic surgery performs these measurements, and a consultation can be obtained immediately.

TABLE 20–2 **Common Causes for Compartment Syndrome of the Leg**

Vascular
Bleeding into a compartment
Reperfusion edema
Venous obstruction
Intra-arterial drug injection
Traumatic
Fracture
Tissue crush
Contusion
Burns
Snakebite and spider bite
Other
Infection
Tight casts
Lying on limb

Two common techniques for measuring compartmental pressures include the infusion technique and the wick catheter technique. Both techniques involve inserting either a needle or a catheter into the leg compartment and measuring pressures with the aid of a transducer. A knowledge of the anatomy of the leg is also essential to interpreting the results of these tests. The lower leg is divided into three compartments by projections of fascia, tibia, fibula, and interosseous membrane. These compartments contain muscles, nerves, arteries, and deep veins. Figure 20–3 shows the cross-sectional anatomy and compartments of the lower leg.

Management

Fasciotomy is recommended when compartmental pressures approach 30 mm Hg, or when the pressure is within 20 mm Hg of the diastolic blood pressure. In most cases, however, the decision to perform decompressing fasciotomy will be based on the progression of symptoms and the clinical picture. If a patient requires surgical treatment, general surgery, orthopedic surgery, or plastic surgery services can perform fasciotomies of the lower extremity. It is critical to not postpone fasciotomy if indicated. Delayed surgical treatment may result in muscle necrosis, permanent nerve damage, and limb loss.

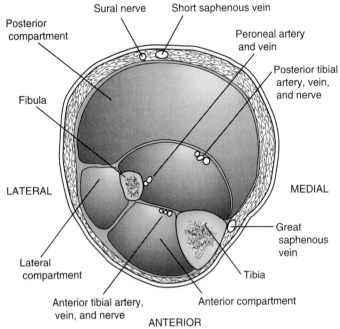

Figure 20–3 Cross-sectional anatomy and compartments of the lower leg.

INFECTIOUS PROCESSES

Cellulitis

Cellulitis in otherwise healthy patients commonly involves *Staphylococcus aureus* or *Streptococcus* species. The first-generation cephalosporins, such as **cefazolin 1 g IV every 8 hours,** are effective against staphylococcus. Adding **penicillin G potassium 2 to 3 million units IV every 4 hours** to a first-generation cephalosporin adds good *Streptococcus* coverage. **Nafcillin 1 to 2 g IV every 6 hours** covers both *Staphylococcus* and *Streptococcus.* Diabetic patients or patients with compromised lower extremity circulation have a higher incidence of gram-negative and anaerobic infections. For these patients, consider a broader spectrum antibiotic, such as **ticarcillin disodium (Timentin) 3.1 g IV every 6 hours, piperacillin and tazobactam (Zosyn) 3.375 g IV every 6 hours,** or **ampicillin sodium and sulbactam (Unasyn) 2.1 g IV every 6 hours.** Elevate the cellulitic extremity and treat with appropriate analgesics.

Septic Arthritis

Selective History

Septic arthritis may lead to systemic sepsis and permanent joint dysfunction. Patients usually present with a tender, erythematous, swollen joint. The affected joint is usually painful to both passive and active flexion. The patient will often have a fever. In a patient with a polyarticular rheumatologic disorder, a joint that is acutely inflamed significantly out of proportion to the other joints may be infected.

Septic arthritis is usually divided into nongonococcal or gonococcal disease. Nongonococcal septic arthritis is most often caused by *Staphylococcus aureus* and *Streptococcus* species and is most common in immunocompromised patients or in those with joint trauma. Gonococcal disease accounts for more than one-half of all septic arthritis in otherwise healthy, sexually active adults.

Look for predisposing factors.

Has there been recent joint pain, discomfort with movement of the extremities, or recent skin rash?

The cardinal signs of a gonococcal arthritis are migratory or additive polyarthralgias, tenosynovitis (inflammation of the tendons), and dermatitis.

Is there a history of penetrating trauma in the region of a joint?

Trauma to a joint may introduce organisms and lead to tissue injury. Open joint trauma greatly increases the incidence of *Staphylococcus* and *Streptococcus* infections.

Does the patient have a joint prosthesis?

Septic arthritis in the presence of a prosthetic joint is disastrous, and usually, removal of the prosthesis is required. Consult an orthopedic surgeon in these cases.

Management

1. Using sterile technique, aspirate the joint.

   If unsure of how to aspirate the joint, call the chief resident, or a consulting rheumatologist or an orthopedic surgeon. Collect fluid for an immediate Gram stain, culture (aerobic and anaerobic, gonococcal, and tuberculous), white blood cell (WBC) count and differential, and glucose levels. In septic arthritis, the joint fluid is usually cloudy or turbid. The WBC count is usually greater than 10,000 cells/mm^3.

2. Send for blood cultures and serum glucose; the synovial glucose will be less than 50% of the serum glucose in a true septic joint.

3. Start IV antibiotics immediately.

Remember that a negative Gram stain does not mean the patient does not have bacterial infection. Gram stain is frequently negative in culture-positive gonococcal arthritis.

Gram Stain-Positive for Organisms

Gram-positive cocci:	Consider nafcillin 1 to 2 g IV every 4 hours or vancomycin 1 g every 12 hours
Gram-negative bacilli:	Initial coverage, consider ceftriaxone 2 g IV every 24 hours. If *Pseudomonas* is suspected, consider piperacillin 2 to 3 g IV every 4 to 6 hours plus gentamicin 1 mg/kg IV every 8 hours.

Gram Stain-Negative for Organisms

Otherwise healthy adult:	Consider antistaphylococcal agent. If patient is at risk for gonococcal infection, add **ceftriaxone 1 g IV every 24 hours** or **penicillin G potassium 2 to 3 million units IV every 4 hours.**
Immunocompromised adult:	Consider *Staphylococcus* and Gram-negative coverage.

1. Elevate and splint the joint.
2. Consider surgical drainage in the following situations:
   * Septic hip joint
   * Loculated joint abscess
   * Prosthetic joint infection
   * Osteomyelitis or joint cartilage infection concomitant with septic arthritis.

Necrotizing Fasciitis

Selective History

This devastating, life-threatening infection involves extensive necrosis of the superficial fascia, with wide undermining of the skin and sepsis. Most of these cases are caused by mixed infections of beta-hemolytic streptococci and staphylococci; however, either of these groups of pathogens alone can cause necrotizing fasciitis. Gram-negative organisms are responsible for about 10% of cases.

Most cases of necrotizing fasciitis occur as secondary infections of abrasions, cuts, insect bites, and bruises. Susceptible patients include those with diabetes and peripheral vascular disease.

Look for predisposing factors.

Is there a history of a skin trauma?

Does the patient have diabetes, peripheral vascular disease, or an immunologically compromised state?

Selective Physical Examination

VS: Fever, tachycardia, and hypotension
Skin: Edema (mild to massive); cellulitis is usually present; color is often pale red without distinct borders (early); color becomes purple, and may turn black later in the rapid course; bullae and blisters frequently present; serosanguineous exudate or seropurulent exudate; rapidly advancing involvement of tissue

Management

The mortality rate in necrotizing fasciitis exceeds 30%. Treatment must be definitive and rapid.

1. Start IV antibiotic therapy.

    Consider triple antibiotic coverage (ampicillin, gentamicin, and metronidazole) until cultures demonstrate a specific flora to which to direct therapy. Clindamycin is often added due to bacteriocidal properties.

2. Contact your chief resident or attending physician immediately.

    Patients with necrotizing fasciitis require aggressive surgical debridement in the operating room. All undermined, necrotic fascia must be debrided and wounds must be opened. Frequent redebridements are generally required. Definitive culture and Gram stain can be taken in the operating room. Frequently, organisms will grow in culture despite the initiation of IV antibiotics several hours earlier.

Mental Status Changes

The cognitive functioning of a patient is the most complex of all physiologic processes, and it is therefore affected by derangements in many organ systems. Appropriate assessment of mental status changes requires a knowledge of a prior mental status examination. This information may be available from the chart or from the bedside caregiver. It is useful to organize your thinking according to that baseline and how the patient appears. The etiologies of confusion fall into two major categories: delirium and dementia.

Delirium: Delirium is an acute change and is characterized by clouded sensorium, agitation, confusion, and misinterpretations of the environment (hallucinations, illusions, and delusions). Delirium is potentially reversible and may be recurrent. For example, a common cause of a confusion in a postoperative patient is hypoperfusion. Remember that mental status is one of the three readily identifiable end-organ functions that are acutely affected by shock (the others being skin perfusion and urine output). Correction of the hypoperfusion will, in many cases, also reverse the confusion. Untreated, delirium increases morbidity and mortality.

Dementia: Dementia is an irreversible state of loss of memory, loss of cognitive function, and recognition. This is a baseline finding and should be well documented in the chart. A patient who has elements of dementia may still become delirious. It is necessary to compare the current state with how the patient was described at the time of his or her best recent cognitive functioning.

Most concerning acute are mental status changes in patients after head trauma or recent neurosurgical procedures or in patients at risk for sepsis.

PHONE CALL

Questions

1. **What symptoms is the patient exhibiting?**

   Clarify whether the patient is a risk to him- or herself or to others.

2. **Is this level of consciousness a change?**

   What was the baseline level of consciousness? Has the patient exhibited this sort of behavior before?

3. Are there other medical problems?

This may include metabolic derangements such as diabetes, hypocalcemia, hypomagnesemia, or thyroid malfunction; primary central nervous system (CNS) disease such as seizure disorder, stroke, or organic brain syndrome; or infectious disease such as meningitis or sepsis.

4. What medications is the patient currently taking?

Many will cause a change in mental status.

5. Has the patient undergone a surgical procedure, and if so, how long ago?

If this was a neurosurgical procedure, consider ordering a noncontrast computed tomographic (CT) head scan immediately. If the patient is taking narcotic medication, depressed cognitive functioning may result.

6. Did the patient fall?

See Chapter 10.

7. Are there any other symptoms?

8. Are there any changes in vital signs?

Orders

1. Make sure the patient and the bedside caregivers are safe. Often delirious patients exhibit combative behavior.
2. Order a bedside finger stick glucose level check immediately. Send for complete blood count and electrolyte level immediately.
3. Check oxygen saturation of arterial blood (SaO_2) with pulse oximetry.

    Supply O_2 if necessary. Be careful when delivering O_2 to patients with chronic obstructive pulmonary disease (COPD).
4. Hold all medications that could further alter the patient's sensorium.
5. If the patient is currently taking narcotic medication, have **naloxone hydrochloride (Narcan) 2 mg for intravenous (IV) administration** at the bedside.

Degree of Urgency

The patient must be evaluated immediately. A recurrent benign problem that is well documented in the chart, or that is expected, may wait if there is more urgent work to do. If there is any uncertainty in your mind, see the patient immediately.

ELEVATOR THOUGHTS

What causes a change in mental status?

1. Central nervous system
   - Infection (meningitis, abscess, infected appliance, human immunodeficiency virus [HIV], and encephalitis)
   - Cerebral vascular accident and transient ischemic attack

- Head trauma
- Tumor
- Primary dementia (Alzheimer, multi-infarct dementia, and Parkinson disease)
- Encephalopathies (Wernicke and alcoholic)
- Seizures (petit mal and postictal state)
- CNS vasculitis

2. Medications
- Narcotics
- Sedatives
- Hypnotics
- Anesthetic agents
- Antidepressants
- Anticonvulsants
- Nonsteroidal anti-inflammatory drugs (NSAIDs)
- Steroids
- Other medications; for example, histamine H2 receptor antagonists, other antihistamines, lidocaine, and digoxin

3. Medication withdrawal
- Alcohol
- Anxiolytics

4. Metabolic derangements
- Hypoglycemia and hyperglycemia
- Hyponatremia and hypernatremia
- Hypercalcemia
- Acid–base disorders
- Endocrinopathies (hypothyroidism, hyperthyroidism, and adrenal malfunction)

5. Organ failure
- Renal
- Liver (encephalopathy)
- Respiratory system (hypoxia and hypercapnia)
- Circulatory system (hypoperfusion)
- Multiorgan failure

6. Other global infection or serious illness
- Sepsis
- Polytrauma

MAJOR THREAT TO LIFE

- Alcohol withdrawal
- CNS mass lesion (herniation, tumor, and epidural or subdural fluid collections)
- Hypoxia
- Medication overdose
- CNS infection
- Sepsis
- Injury to self or staff

BEDSIDE

Quick Look Test

The degree of change in a patient's mental status is an indication of the severity of the underlying condition. A patient may be described as

Awake and alert
Agitated or uncontrollable
Lethargic
Stuporous
Comatose

Patients who need emergent treatment include those for whom lethargy, stupor, or coma is an acute change.

A Glasgow Coma Scale is often used (Table 21–1).

Airway and Vital Signs

Confirm adequate air movement and oxygenation. Check a pulse oximeter reading and supply supplemental O_2 as required. Remember that supplemental O_2 may cause respiratory depression in patients with COPD. Early sepsis may present with tachycardia and hypotension. The febrile patient may be delirious just by virtue of the fever. Hypoxic patients may hyperventilate; patients who are narcotized will hypoventilate.

Initial Management

1. Support ventilation and oxygenation, if necessary.
2. Support circulation and blood pressure, if necessary.

TABLE 21–1 **Glasgow Coma Scale**

Function	Response	Score
Eye opening (E)	Spontaneously	4
	To voice	3
	To pain	2
	None	1
	Eyes swollen closed	C
Best motor response (M)	Obeys commands	6
	Localizes pain	5
	Withdraws from pain	4
	Decorticate to pain	3
	Decerebrate to pain	2
	None	1
Best verbal response (V)	Oriented, appropriate	5
	Confused	4
	Inappropriate words	3
	Incomprehensible sounds	2
	None	1
	Intubated/trach	T

3. Check blood glucose result, and correct, if necessary.
4. Perform and document a complete neurologic examination including mental status (see Selective Physical Examination).

Selective History and Chart Review

Look for causes of mental status changes (see Elevator Thoughts).
Review the patient's current medications.
Look also at the list of medications normally taken at home. Was an important medication forgotten in the hospital orders?
Compare the most recent neurologic examination to previous ones in the chart.

Selective Physical Examination

VS:	Repeat now.
HEENT:	Is there papilledema (see Fig. 15–1) or nuchal rigidity (meningitis)? What are pupil size and reactivity? (Pinpoint pupils suggest narcosis. Dilated pupils suggest sympathomimetic medications. Unequal pupils suggest intracranial mass lesion.) Is there evidence of head injury secondary to a fall (bruises, abrasions, skull bony abnormalities, or blood behind the tympanic membrane)?
Skin:	Is it cool and clammy (poor perfusion)? Is there icterus? Are there spider angiomata (organ failure)?
MS:	A complete mental status examination is required for the assessment of a confused or lethargic patient. Document this well. This may not always be possible for patients who are stuporous or comatose.

1. Consciousness: Is the patient alert, lethargic, stuporous, or comatose?
2. General appearance: What is the behavior, and what is the physical condition?
3. Mood: Is the patient depressed, restless, agitated, or labile?
4. Form of thought: How does information flow? Are there loose associations, flights of ideas, or perseverations?
5. Content of thought: What is the information that flows? Is it composed of delusions or concrete ideations?
6. Perceptions: Is the environment being misinterpreted? Are there illusions or hallucinations (auditory or visual)?

7. Orientation: Does the patient know who and where he or she is and what the time and the date are?
8. Registration: Is the patient able to take in and repeat new information?
9. Recall: Is the patient able to repeat the new information in short- and long-term fashions?
10. Long-term memory: Is the patient able to recognize famous dates or famous people?
11. Language: How is language used? Is it understood (spoken and written)?
12. Judgment: What is the response to hypothetical situations?

Neuro: A complete physical and neurologic examination is also important to evaluate for lateralizing signs that might suggest a CNS lesion or disease. Compare this with other neurologic examinations documented in the chart.

Tubes: Does the patient have a CNS drain such as a ventricular shunt? Is it functioning? Has the disoriented patient removed other important lines or drains?

Wound: Is the dressing intact? Any evidence of wound infection?

Additional tests: Perform additional tests as indicated.

MANAGEMENT

Further management is dictated by the suspected diagnosis. The treatments of sepsis, hypoxemia, metabolic derangement, and seizures are covered elsewhere in this book.

Medications

If a specific medication can be identified as the cause of the confusion, stop the drug and replace it with another appropriate medication as necessary. Often in elderly patients, a simple dose adjustment is necessary. Many medications require individualization of dosages.

If there has been a change in renal or liver function, look at the medications that are excreted or detoxified by these organs and make adjustments as necessary. It is important to review all the medications that a patient is taking—not just those that affect mental status, but also those that are nephrotoxic or hepatotoxic and other medications that are affected by a change in organ function. In these cases, a consultation with a nephrologist or a hepatologist is often helpful.

If a patient requires a medication that was omitted from the admission record or the postoperative orders, re-administer it.

Some medications have antidotes that may be administered. Before treatment with further medication, be certain that the drug to be reversed is responsible for the change in mental status.

Narcotic Medication

Administer **naloxone hydrochloride *(Narcan)* 0.2 to 2 mg IV, intramuscularly (IM), subcutaneously (SC), or by endotracheal tube (ET) every 5 minutes until there is a response (to a total of 10 mg);** the effective dose may be repeated every 20 to 60 minutes.

Benzodiazepine Medication

Administer **flumazenil *(Romazicon)* 0.2 mg IV over 30 seconds.** If there is an initial response in 30 seconds after the first dose, **an additional 0.3 mg may be given over 30 seconds.** If there is still no response, further doses of **0.5 mg may be administered every 1 minute to a total dose of 3 to 5 mg.** The effective dose may **be repeated every 20 minutes at a rate of 0.2 mg/minute (to a total of 3 mg/hour).** Administration of flumazenil is associated with a risk of seizure, and it should be given carefully.

Specific Drug Overdose

Consult a pharmacology text, and contact the poison control department in your county to determine specific therapy. Treatment may include activated charcoal, ipecac, dialysis, and psychiatric consultation in addition to support of the patient's respiration and circulation.

HERNIATION OR MASS LESION

Patients who have lateralizing signs on neurologic examination (unequal pupils and unilateral loss of sensation or motor function) require a noncontrast head CT scan immediately. This is especially true of patients after recent neurosurgical procedures or of those who have had serious head trauma. If necessary, make sure that the patient's airway and circulatory system are supported. If the CT scan is abnormal or changed from baseline, contact the resident. Neurosurgical consultation may be required to drain fluid collections or to place a bolt for pressure manometry. These patients will require surgical therapy and transfer to the intensive care unit or the cardiac care unit.

ALCOHOL WITHDRAWAL

This is a potentially fatal complication of a hospitalized patient. It is important to establish a history of drinking, because withdrawal symptoms occur 24 to 48 hours after the last drink. Medical or psychiatric consultation is often required to help in the treatment of these patients.

Signs and Symptoms

Change in mental status (insomnia, hallucinations, restlessness, and anxiety)

Autonomic hyperactivity (sweating and tachycardia)

Nausea and vomiting

Hand tremors: coarse, fast frequency, and made worse with activity

Delirium tremens (DTs)

Seizures

Korsakoff's psychosis or Wernicke's encephalopathy

Management

1. Benzodiazepines

   Chlordiazepoxide hydrochloride *(Librium)* **at 25 to 100 mg IM or IV every 6 hours.**

   Do not exceed 300 mg in a 24-hour period.

   Or

   Diazepam *(Valium)* **at 5 to 10 mg orally (PO) every 6 hours.**

   Maintain the administration of these medications for 24 hours, and then begin to reduce, as possible, by 20% per day over 5 to 7 days. Additional doses may be used to control agitation as necessary.

2. Fluid and electrolyte support

3. Thiamine 100 mg IM or IV; repeat dose every day until a regular diet is resumed

4. Folate 1 mg PO every day for 4 days

5. Multivitamin 1 PO every day

6. Magnesium sulfate and antiepileptics (may be useful to help control postwithdrawal seizures)

7. **Haloperidol lactate** *(Haldol)* **2 to 5 mg PO/IM twice per day** (useful to control symptoms of withdrawal psychosis [DTs])

8. Enlist medical or psychiatric consultation as needed to help care for the patient.

Complications

- Seizures
- Aspiration

PRIMARY PSYCHIATRIC DISEASE

Symptoms of psychosis, schizophrenia, depression, mania, or other organic brain dysfunction will affect the treatment and the healing potential of the patient. These diagnoses require evaluation and treatment by a specialist. Do not hesitate to enlist the help of psychiatric colleagues.

SPECIAL SURGICAL CONSIDERATIONS

Preoperative Considerations

1. An acute change in mental status may affect a scheduled elective procedure.

   Check with the chief resident or the attending physician about canceling the procedure, if necessary.

2. A history of cyclic changes in mental status, such as "sundowning" in elderly patients, is common and will be exacerbated postoperatively.

   Anticipate this, and make sure the patient is safe and the staff is made aware.

3. Many preoperative sedatives and pain relievers will affect mental status.

Postoperative Considerations

1. Many postoperative medications, such as anesthetic agents, narcotics, and sedatives, affect mental status.

   Expect some drowsiness and disorientation in any patient for a day after a general anesthetic, and expect a longer recuperation and more severe symptoms in elderly patients.

2. Postoperative neurosurgical patients should have well-documented neurologic examinations in the chart, which should be used as standards of comparison.

   A significant change in mental status requires a noncontrast head CT scan immediately to rule out mass lesion.

3. Postoperative neurosurgical patients also may have appliances in place to drain fluid collections or to monitor intracranial pressures.

   These can be a source of CNS infection or they may malfunction, causing increased intracranial pressure.

   In addition, a normally functioning drain does not preclude the presence of problematic fluid collections elsewhere in the skull.

4. Mental status changes are often the first sign of impending sepsis.

Remember

1. High fever can be a source of delirium.
2. Sleep deprivation is a source of disorientation.

   (Many residents can vouch for this fact.)

Nausea and Vomiting

Nausea and vomiting are common on-call problems. There are many causes of nausea and vomiting. It is believed that the medulla contains two distinct centers that mediate vomiting, a chemoreceptor zone and a vomiting center. Toxic substances, drugs, and input from the cerebral cortex, the gastrointestinal (GI) tract, and other organs stimulate these centers to induce nausea and vomiting. Surgical patients are frequently exposed to medications that can stimulate the chemoreceptor zone. In addition, patients undergoing abdominal surgery frequently have a functional ileus and changes in GI function that predispose them to nausea. To be effective on call, you must know the common causes of and the treatments for nausea and vomiting.

PHONE CALL

Questions

1. **How severe is the nausea, and did the patient vomit?**

   Clarify the severity of the nausea and whether the patient has vomited. A patient who has mild nausea may benefit from orally (PO), rectally (PR), or intramuscularly (IM) administered antinausea medication. These methods of medication delivery are effective, yet they require time for the medication to be absorbed. A patient who has severe nausea and active vomiting may benefit more quickly from medication delivered intravenously (IV).

2. **Was anything associated with the nausea and the vomiting?**

   Did the patient recently eat a meal? Did the patient recently receive a medication or general anesthesia? Has the patient recently received chemotherapy?

3. **Has this patient had surgery? If so, what was the operation, and when was it performed?**

   It is critical to know what type of surgery and when the surgery was performed. Some types of surgery are associated with changes in GI function. For example, abdominal surgery frequently causes a postoperative ileus. Nausea and vomiting are common after major abdominal surgery unless decompression with a nasogastric (NG) tube is performed. Knowing exactly when surgery was performed is also important when dealing appropriately with nausea or vomiting problems. Patients are frequently nauseated in the first 12 hours postoperatively. This is often due to postanesthetic recovery. Many currently used anesthetic agents require several hours for metabolism. Patients are frequently nauseated during this early postoperative period. Although anesthesiologists frequently give patients an antiemetic agent at the end of an operation, the antiemetic agent dosing may need to be repeated.

4. Has the patient had abdominal surgery?

Always suspect that a patient who has had abdominal surgery may have a functional ileus. As discussed in Chapter 6, a functional ileus may last 4 to 5 days or longer. Patients having upper abdominal surgery are generally maintained with nothing by mouth (kept NPO) and are decompressed with an NG tube until they pass flatus. Patients having lower colonic surgery are usually kept NPO, but they generally do not need NG tube decompression.

5. Does the patient have an NG tube?

After abdominal surgery or certain GI problems (e.g., bowel obstruction), NG tubes are placed. Nonfunctioning NG tubes are a common cause of nausea and vomiting.

NG tubes are removed when it is believed that acceptable GI function has returned (patient is passing flatus). Frequently, NG tubes are removed prematurely, and patients become nauseated. If the patient vomits repeatedly, replacement of the NG tube may be warranted.

6. Is there hematemesis or coffee-ground emesis?

Hematemesis may indicate active GI bleeding. Hematemesis of bright-red or dark blood indicates that the source is proximal to the ligament of Treitz. This bleeding is frequently from the esophagus or the stomach (see Chapter 13). Coffee-ground emesis indicates that old blood has been metabolized in the stomach by gastric acid. Blood is a strong emetic agent.

7. Are there any changes in vital signs?

A patient who has been vomiting repeatedly may become dehydrated and suffer from acid–base imbalance. The patient may also have a severe electrolyte disturbance or suffer from diabetic ketoacidosis.

8. Does the patient have an IV? Does the patient have any drug allergies? What are the patient's weight and age?

Check to see if the patient has IV access. If the patient has been vomiting repeatedly and is dehydrated, he or she will need IV fluids. In addition, many effective antiemetic medications may be delivered by an IV route. Also, clarify if the patient has any drug allergies. Some patients may have adverse reactions to antiemetic medications. Finally, have the nurse give the patient's weight and age. These will help to determine the dosing of an appropriate antiemetic agent. Beware of using inappropriate doses of antiemetic agents in children or in elderly patients.

Inform RN

Will arrive at the bedside in . . . minutes.

Many of the calls for nausea and vomiting will be routine and do not require examination of the patient. However, if a patient has unstable vital signs, hematemesis, or significant distress, inform the RN that you will be coming to evaluate the patient.

ELEVATOR THOUGHTS

What causes nausea and vomiting?
1. Gastroenteritis
   - Viral illness
   - Food poisoning (e.g., *Staphylococcus* and *Salmonella*)
2. Drugs
   - Narcotics (e.g., morphine and meperidine hydrochloride)
   - Common therapeutic drugs (e.g., digoxin and theophylline)
   - Chemotherapeutic agents
   - Recovery from anesthesia (anesthetics)
3. Abdominal causes
   - Functional ileus
   - Bowel obstruction
   - Inflammation or irritation of GI tract structures
   - Hepatobiliary and pancreatic disorders
   - Nonfunctional NG tube
4. Electrolyte, endocrine, and metabolic disturbances
   - Acidosis
   - Hypernatremia
   - Hyponatremia
   - Hypercalcemia
   - Diabetic acidosis
   - Pregnancy
   - Uremia
5. Associations with shock
   - Hypotension
   - Sepsis
   - Acute myocardial infarction
6. Central nervous system (CNS) disorders
   - CNS infection, e.g., meningitis or encephalitis
   - Subarachnoid hemorrhage and stroke
   - Increased intracranial pressure secondary to trauma
   - Intracranial mass
   - Migraine
7. Conditions related to the inner ear
   - Infection

- Motion sickness
- Meniere syndrome
8. Psychiatric conditions
  - Anxiety disorder
  - Anorexia nervosa
  - Bulimia
  - Psychosis

MAJOR THREAT TO LIFE

- Aspiration pneumonia
- Intractable vomiting leading to GI bleeding (e.g., Mallory–Weiss tear)
- Unrecognized electrolyte or metabolic emergency (e.g., diabetic ketoacidosis)
- Postemetic rupture of the esophagus

A weakened patient or a patient with altered mental status is at high risk for aspiration. **Aspiration pneumonia** is a common cause of morbidity and death in debilitated patients. Severe and prolonged nausea and vomiting should be treated aggressively. Life-threatening complications of forceful vomiting include severe **GI bleeding** and **esophageal rupture.** In addition, it is important to identify and to treat **dehydration** and **electrolyte abnormalities** in vomiting patients. Frequently, nausea and vomiting signal serious electrolyte and metabolic disturbances.

BEDSIDE

It is necessary to examine and to evaluate patients with nausea and vomiting who also show signs of significant dehydration, hematemesis, or alterations in normal vital signs.

Quick Look Test

Does the patient look well (mildly nauseated), sick (very distressed), or critical (about to die)?

Patients with all types of medical problems will present with nausea and vomiting. A patient who is vomiting in response to a life-threatening problem (e.g., severe ketoacidosis, CNS bleeding, and hypotension) will often have an altered mental status and will look sick. If the patient is mildly nauseated with a normal mental status, the patient is probably stable.

Airway and Vital Signs

The airway is of concern in weakened patients or in patients with altered mental status. If these patients vomit, they are likely to aspirate. Aspiration may cause airway obstruction, tachypnea, hypoxemia, chemical pneumonitis, or pneumonia. You should make sure that the airway is clear after a compromised patient has vomited. With a gloved hand, sweep any vomitus from the mouth and the throat. Use bedside suction and a large suction tip to clear the airway. Once the airway is clear, the patient should be positioned in a lateral decubitus position. Any additional emesis will tend to drain from the mouth and not be aspirated. A patient in respiratory failure, or who is unable to protect their airway (no gag reflex), may need to be intubated.

Patients who have had severe and repeated bouts of vomiting may demonstrate changes in vital signs. They may show signs of dehydration and acidosis. On examination, look for tachycardia, tachypnea, and hypotension.

Selective History

Are there changes in neurologic status?

A patient who starts vomiting and who demonstrates a change in neurologic status may have a life-threatening problem. Consider stroke, meningitis, and increased intracranial pressure. Also, examine the abdomen quickly to look for abdominal distention and tenderness.

Selective Physical Examination

HEENT: Nuchal rigidity may indicate meningitis or subarachnoid hemorrhage. Papilledema indicates increased intracranial pressure (see Fig. 15–1).

Neuro: Assess mental status. Look for pupil symmetry and equal muscle strength on both sides of the body. A change in mental status, the finding of pupil asymmetry, or focal weakness may represent a neurosurgical emergency. Call a neurosurgeon for these problems.

GI: Assess if the abdomen is distended or tender. Abdominal distention may indicate a functional ileus. Abdominal tenderness may indicate peritoneal irritation, bowel obstruction, or peritonitis. Evaluate the groins for hernias.

Management

The Unstable Patient with Severe Vomiting

1. Management should begin by stabilization of the vital signs.

    An unstable, vomiting patient who shows signs of hypovolemia or acidosis should be resuscitated with IV fluids (lactated Ringer's or normal saline). However, be careful not to over-resuscitate patients who show evidence of increased intracranial pressure. Resuscitate to the point of hemodynamic stability.

2. Make sure the airway is secure.

    Do what is possible to minimize the chance that the patient will aspirate. Consider intubating a patient who has both respiratory distress and intractable, severe vomiting. Use a cuffed endotracheal tube, which will protect the airway from vomitus.

3. Look for electrolyte or metabolic causes of vomiting.

Once resuscitation with IV fluids has begun, draw an electrolyte panel, a complete blood count, and a glucose level. Be sure to draw the blood from a site distal to or away from the IV. Correct any electrolyte or glucose abnormalities.

4. Look for mechanical causes of the vomiting.

Has the patient had recent abdominal surgery? Should the patient have an NG tube? If a patient is vomiting repeatedly and has evidence of obstruction or ileus, place an NG tube to decompress the stomach and to remove residual gastric contents. **Do not place an NG tube if the patient has had recent oropharyngeal, esophageal, or stomach surgery (to avoid the risk of perforation through the suture line).** In these patients, NG tubes must be placed with fluoroscopic guidance.

The Stable Patient with Nausea and Vomiting

1. Many patients with a self-limited illness such as viral gastroenteritis will need no therapy. These patients benefit from a clear liquid diet.

2. Look for mechanical causes of vomiting.

If the patient appears to have a functional ileus or a bowel obstruction, an NG tube will decompress the upper GI tract and the patient will feel better. If possible, discuss the need to place an NG tube with the patient before attempting to place it.

3. Look for any adverse drug reactions.

Frequently, morphine, meperidine hydrochloride, and other drugs induce nausea. Simply discontinuing the offending drug will often stop or slow the nausea and vomiting. If the patient requires a narcotic for adequate analgesia, combining an antiemetic agent with the narcotic may be effective; for example, meperidine is frequently combined with promethazine hydrochloride *(Phenergan)* for IM administration.

4. Look for electrolyte or metabolic disturbances that can explain the nausea and vomiting.

Draw an electrolyte panel and a glucose level. Correct any significant abnormalities.

5. Consider providing an antiemetic drug. These agents may be given IV, IM, PO, or PR. They fall into four distinct classes. See Table 22–1 for a list of common antiemetic agents.

Special Surgical Considerations

Vomiting can put strain on recent upper GI tract anastomoses. Always evaluate a patient who has had recent abdominal surgery before administering antiemetics. Rule out nonfunctioning nasogastric tubes, hernias, or wound problems first.

TABLE 22–1 **Common Antiemetic Agents**

Drug Name	Drug Type	Dose
Promethazine hydrochloride (Phenergan)	Phenothiazine	25–50 mg PO, PR every 4–6 hr 25 mg IM every 4–6 hr 12.5 mg IV every 4–6 hr Peds: 0.5–1 mg/kg/dose PO, PR, or IM
Prochlorperazine maleate (Compazine)	Phenothiazine	5–10 mg PO, PR 3 or 4 times per day 5 mg IV over 2–3 min Peds: 0.13 mg/kg/dose
Trimethobenzamide HCl (Tigan)	Related central agent	250 mg PO 3 times per day 200 mg PR, IM every 6–8 hr Peds: 100 mg/dose if patient is >30 lb
Metoclopramide Monohydrochloride monohydrate (Reglan)	Dopamine antagonist	10 mg PO, IM, IV 1 hr before meals and at bedtime
Cisapride (Propulsid)	Prokinetic agent	10–20 mg PO before meals and at bedtime
Ondansetron hydrochloride (Zofran)	Serotonin 5-HT$_3$ blocker	8 mg PO, IV 3 times per day (IV form may be given in a single 32-mg dose every day, if desired)

PO, orally; PR, rectally; IM, intramuscularly; IV, intravenously; Peds, pediatric.

Pain Management

Surgical patients have pain. Pain may be caused by a disease state or the therapies used to treat that disease state. Historically, pain has been under-recognized and under-treated, but recent emphasis by regulatory and government groups have brought into focus the need to adequately assess and treat pain. As an on-call physician, you will receive many calls requesting pain medication for patients. Many of these calls are for reordering or adjusting doses of medications. However, some of the calls will be for new-onset or poorly controlled pain. It is important to know how to control pain. Having an understanding of the various analgesic agents and delivery systems will allow you to order appropriate pain medication for patients.

Specific pain in the abdominal, chest, head, and leg are discussed in separate chapters.

PHONE CALL

Questions

1. **Where is the patient's pain, and how severe is the pain?**

   It is important to know what hurts the patient. Frequently, a patient will have pain in a location unrelated to the main medical problem or surgical site; for example, patients may develop back pain from prolonged bed rest. In addition, you should ask about the severity of a patient's pain. Severe pain is treated differently than mild pain. Visual analog scales work well.

2. **Has the patient had surgery? If so, what operation did the patient have, and when was it performed?**

   A patient who has had recent surgery or a traumatic injury will have pain. It is important that you know what type of operation the patient had and when it was done. This will help you decide what treatment to offer.

3. **Does the patient have any drug allergies?**

   You should know about any allergies or adverse drug reactions in a patient's history. You do not want to order a pain medication that will cause complications or allergic reactions. Also avoid ordering analgesic medications that have given a patient significant side effects or unpleasant experiences.

4. What pain medication, if any, is the patient taking now?

It is important to know whether a patient is currently taking pain medication and whether the patient has pain while taking the medication. This will help you decide what changes to make in dosing or in analgesic selection.

5. What is the patient's weight and age?

Elderly patients and pediatric patients are especially sensitive to narcotics. It is important to know the age and the weight of a patient when prescribing pain medication. For pediatric patients of less than 75 lb (35 kg), dose medications by kilograms of body weight. For elderly debilitated patients, consider reducing the normal adult dose. Use your best judgment; you can always supplement with additional pain medication, if necessary.

6. Does the patient have a history of chronic pain?

Patients with chronic pain present significant challenges to the on-call physician. These patients are frequently demanding and will ask specifically for a particular medication (usually a narcotic). Try to assess what pain medications have been used recently in their care. Remember that non-narcotic preparations should be used to treat chronic pain whenever possible. Try to limit use of the narcotic pain medications to the treatment of acute pain or acute pain episodes within the baseline chronic pain.

7. Does the patient have a history of renal or liver disease or any history of peptic ulcer disease?

Avoid the use of acetaminophen in patients with liver disease. Acetaminophen can cause serious liver damage in these patients. Aspirin may cause gastrointestinal (GI) bleeding in patients with peptic ulcer disease. Although nonsteroidal anti-inflammatory drugs (NSAIDs) are generally safe and effective analgesics, they may cause adverse GI and renal effects; dyspepsia, gastritis, and peptic ulceration may occur with the use of NSAIDs. Impairment of renal filtration, nephritis, papillary necrosis, and acute renal failure can occur with use of NSAIDs; avoid use of NSAIDs in patients with impaired renal function.

8. Does the patient have a history of narcotic drug abuse?

Those with a history of drug abuse will pose particular problems. It is important to differentiate between drug-seeking behavior and true acute pain. In addition, when treating acute pain, it will frequently take higher doses of narcotic medication to achieve the desired results, due to acquired tolerance.

Orders

1. If pain is severe and not controlled by oral (PO) or intramuscular (IM) analgesics, ask the RN to place an intravenous (IV) line.
2. After ordering an appropriate pain medication, ask the RN to phone back in an hour if the pain has not been relieved by the medication.

3. If ordering high-dose or IV narcotic agents, ask the RN to monitor the patient's respiratory rate (RR), blood pressure (BP), and heart rate (HR).

Inform RN

Will arrive at the bedside in . . . minutes.

If a patient has new-onset pain, previously undiagnosed pain, or pain significantly greater than you might expect otherwise, you need to examine the patient. For example, a stable ward patient complaining of sudden-onset, severe abdominal pain radiating to the back may have an expanding abdominal aortic aneurysm. Only by examining the patient will you find a pulsatile mass characteristic of an abdominal aortic aneurysm. Thus, make a habit of examining patients who have pain uncharacteristic of a particular medical problem or operation.

ELEVATOR THOUGHTS

What causes pain?
1. Postoperative conditions
   - Incisional wound
   - Expanding hematoma
2. Infections
   - Cellulitis
   - Abscess
   - Osteomyelitis
3. Inflammatory conditions
   - Arthritis
   - Neuritis and neuropathies
   - Erythema nodosum
   - Reflex sympathetic dystrophy
4. Traumatic injuries
   - Fractures
   - Contusions
   - Open wounds
   - Posttraumatic inflammation
   - Compartment syndrome
5. Skeletal system
   - Lumbar disk disease (sciatica)
   - Metastatic tumors to bone
   - Primary skeletal tumors
   - Expansile bone lesions
6. Vascular disease
   - Angina or myocardial infarction
   - Arterial occlusion
   - Venous thrombosis or thrombophlebitis
   - Thromboangiitis (Buerger disease)

7. Psychological factors
  • Chronic pain disorder
  • Narcotic dependence

MAJOR THREAT TO LIFE

Pain that is classic for a life-threatening medical problem (e.g., myocardial infarction, aortic aneurysm, and stroke).

Untreated, severe, stressful pain leading to arrhythmia or myocardial infarction.

BEDSIDE

The purpose of evaluating a patient at the bedside is to rule out the major threats to life. Pain is a classic presentation for a variety of severe medical problems. Start your evaluation of the patient at the bedside by obtaining a pertinent history and performing a quick chart review.

Quick Look Test

Does the patient look well (mild pain), sick (moderate pain and distressed), or critical (severe pain and about to die)?

If a patient's pain is far greater than you would expect based on the operation or medical problem, rule out a major threat to life. Severe pain associated with pale appearance, altered mental status, and overall distress may signal a severe problem such as dissecting or expanding aneurysm, contained ruptured vessel, expanding hematoma, stroke, myocardial infarction, or other emergency.

You do not need to have made a diagnosis before administering pain medications. If the patient is in significant distress, and is clinically stable, consider treating this pain while you are searching for a cause. Parenteral narcotics will not erase significant peritoneal signs.

Airway and Vital Signs

Poorly treated pain may make a patient tachycardic and hypertensive. This occurs because pain may lead to sympathetic nervous system activation. In addition, abdominal pain (epigastric or subcostal) or musculoskeletal chest wall pain may contribute to shallow breathing and splinting. However, pain should not compromise the vital signs. Hypotension, bradycardia, or hypoxia generally indicate an underlying, significant medical problem or process. When evaluating the airway and vital signs, ask the following:

What is the HR, and is it regular or irregular?

Sinus tachycardia is common in patients with poorly treated pain. However, tachycardia associated with hypotension or irregular rhythm may signal a severe medical problem. For example, leg pain or chest pain associated with tachycardia and shortness of breath could be the presentation of pulmonary embolus.

What is the patient's temperature?

Pain alone does not cause fever. When pain is associated with fever, there are several types of processes to think about. For example, in postoperative surgical patients, incisional pain frequently leads to immobilization. Atelectasis is common in these patients and is a likely cause of fever. Other common causes of fever and pain include infectious or inflammatory processes and pulmonary embolism.

Selective History and Chart Review

Where is the pain?

It is important to have the patient pinpoint the location of the pain. This will give you insight as to the likely cause.

When did the pain start, and has the patient experienced similar pain before?

Quickly review the chart noting the patient's medical history, date of surgery (if any), and postoperative course. Review the analgesics that the patient has been taking.

Selective Physical Examination

The goal of this examination is to rule out a serious medical problem that could be responsible for the pain. The examination should include a careful evaluation of both the site of the pain and the major organ systems.

VS:	HR, BP, RR, and temperature
HEENT:	Site of pain or surgical site
CVS:	Pulse volume
	Skin temperature and color
	Capillary refill (should be less than 1.5 seconds)
Resp:	Equal breath sounds
	Rales or rhonchi
Abd:	Softness
	Tenderness
	Rebound
Neuro:	Mental status
	Movement of all extremities
	Symmetric muscle strengths
Surgical site:	Examine for evidence of erythema, swelling, infection, dehiscence

MANAGEMENT

Once you have ruled out a major threat to life and have diagnosed the cause of the pain, you may treat the patient with an appropriate analgesic. The most common analgesics used in hospitals fall into the following three categories:

1. Non-narcotic agents

   These are best for mild to moderate pain, and they include acetaminophen and NSAIDs. NSAIDs may be nonselective (such as **ibuprofen** or **naproxen**).

2. Combination agents

   These agents are best for moderate pain, and they include oral agents that contain both a non-narcotic (**acetaminophen, ibuprofen,** or **aspirin**) and a narcotic.

3. Narcotic agents

   These drugs are for moderate to severe pain, and they include **morphine, meperidine hydrochloride,** and **fentanyl.**

Non-Narcotic Agents

These drugs are very useful for managing mild to moderate pain. Most are available for PO use. Acetaminophen is useful for mild pain and headache. It has analgesic and antipyretic properties but no anti-inflammatory properties. The NSAIDs are very useful for both analgesia and anti-inflammatory purposes. They are commonly used for musculoskeletal and arthritic pain. Most of these agents are in PO form, and one of these agents (ketorolac) is available in both IM and PO forms. Table 23–1 provides a list of some of the more popular non-narcotic agents.

Combination Agents

These drugs combine oral narcotics with non-narcotic analgesics. The combination of these two types of agents gives a synergistic effect. These are effective and potent drugs for moderate pain. The non-narcotic component is either acetaminophen, ibuprofen, or aspirin. Choose the agent based on both the non-narcotic and the narcotic ingredients. Remember to avoid ordering aspirin-containing combination agents in preoperative patients (aspirin interferes with platelet aggregation). In addition, do not use aspirin-containing drugs in the immediate postoperative period because of the increased risk of postoperative bleeding. Table 23–2 provides common combination agents. Note that some of these agents are available in different strengths. The strengths vary based on the narcotic component. Combination agents, especially the hydromorphone- and the oxymorphone-containing agents, have the potential for abuse.

Narcotic Agents

The narcotics are best reserved for moderate to severe pain. Some of these drugs are available in PO form, others are limited to parenteral use. Table 23–3 provides a list of commonly used narcotics.

The narcotic agents are generally class II or III substances, and they require controlled substance prescription forms for outpatient use. All of the narcotics generally have side effects, which include sedation, respiratory depression, and nausea. In overdose, severe respiratory depression, altered mental status, and hypotension can result. Care must be taken when administering parenteral narcotics.

TABLE 23–1 **Common Non-Narcotic Analgesics**

Drug	Dose and Route (Adult)	Comments
Acetaminophen (Tylenol)	650 mg PO or PR every 4 hr Pediatric dose: 10 mg/kg/dose	Avoid in patients with liver disease
Aspirin (Bayer varieties and Ecotrin)	650 mg PO every 4–6 hr	Avoid in patients with peptic ulcer disease Antiplatelet aggregation action
Ibuprofen (Motrin and Advil)	300–800 mg PO 4 times per day	NSAID (nonselective) Avoid in patients with liver or renal disease Avoid in patients with peptic ulcer disease Some antiplatelet aggregation action
Indomethacin (Indocin)	25–50 mg PO 3 times per day	NSAID (nonselective)
Sulindac (Clinoril)	150–200 mg PO twice per day	NSAID (nonselective)
Diflunisal (Dolobid)	1000 mg PO initially, then 500 mg PO twice per day	NSAID (nonselective)
Naproxen (Naprosyn)	200–500 mg PO 2–3 times per day	NSAID (nonselective)
Ketorolac (Toradol)	30 mg IM loading, followed by 15–30 mg IM	Potent parenteral NSAID, approved for short-term use (5 days) every 6 hr or 10 mg PO every 6 hr
Celecoxib (Celebrex)	100–200 mg PO twice per day	Selective COX-2 inhibitor Avoid in patients allergic to sulfa Cardiac risks

PO, orally; PR, rectally; NSAID, nonsteroidal anti-inflammatory drug; IM, intramuscularly.

Frequent nursing checks of the patient's level of sedation and vital signs should be performed.

Narcotic drugs are usually given parenterally (IM or IV) to hospitalized patients. Table 23–4 compares IM and IV routes for administration of a narcotic drug.

Patients have differing thresholds of pain, and likewise have variable responses to narcotic pain medicine. Table 23–5 shows equipotent dosing for a variety of narcotic medications. If one agent is ineffective, try another agent, or increase the dosage.

Patients who abuse narcotics will have low pain thresholds *and* high narcotic tolerances. They may need higher doses than patients who are narcotic naive.

One of the best ways to administer a narcotic IV is to use a patient-controlled analgesia (PCA) pump. A PCA pump is a device

TABLE 23–2 **Common Combination Analgesics**

Drug	Dose and Route (Adult)	Comments
Tylenol with Codeine	No. 2: 300 mg aceta + 15 mg codeine No. 3: 300 mg aceta + 30 mg codeine 1–2 tablets PO every 4 hr	2 strengths
Darvocet-N	50: 325 aceta + 50 mg propoxyphene napsylate 100: 325 aceta + 100 mg propoxyphene napsylate 1–2 tablets PO every 4 hr	2 strengths
Darvon Compound-65	325 mg ASA + 65 mg propoxyphene napsylate 1–2 tablets PO every 4 hr	
Fiorinal	325 mg ASA + butalbital 50 mg + 40 g caffeine 1–2 tablets PO every 4 hr	
Vicodin or Vicodin ES	500 mg aceta + 5 mg hydrocodone bitartrate ES: 500 g aceta + 7.5 hydrocodone bitartrate 1–2 tablets PO every 4–6 hr	2 strengths
Lortab	500 aceta + 2.5 or 5 or 7.5 mg hydrocodone bitartrate 1–2 tablets PO every 4–6 hr	3 strengths
Tylox	500 mg aceta + 5 mg oxycodone HCl 1 capsule PO every 6 hr	
Percocet	325 mg aceta + 5 oxycodone HCl 1 tablet PO every 6 hr	
Percodan	325 mg ASA + 5 mg oxycodone HCl 1 tablet PO every 6 hr	

Aceta, acetaminophen; PO, orally; ASA, acetylsalicylic acid.

that allows a patient to self-administer a narcotic based on need. The patient presses a button that is attached to the pump. When the button is pressed, a measured dose of narcotic is delivered to the patient. The pump allows regulation of the narcotic with respect to frequency (maximum doses per hour), dose (milligrams per dose), maximum narcotic delivered per hour (milligram maximum per hour), and basal rate (base rate of narcotic in milligrams per hour).

If properly used, the PCA pump is a safe narcotic delivery system. If the dosing or frequency settings are deliberately set a little too high, the patient will become sedate and less likely to continue self-administering dosing. However, only the patient should be allowed to give him- or herself narcotic doses; a patient can be overdosed on narcotics with a PCA if family members or friends press the dose button and give an already sedate patient additional drug. Frequent nursing checks of the patient's level of sedation and vital signs should be performed. In addition, you must make sure that a narcotic antagonist (**naloxone hydrochloride [*Narcan*]**) is available on

TABLE 23–3 **Common Narcotics for Treating Pain**

Drug	Dose and Route (Adult)	Comments
Fentanyl citrate (Sublimaze)	2–3 mcg/kg IV, to 50 mcg Transdermal patches: 2.5-mg patch every 3 days	Short-duration IV, but very effective; 1–2 hr duration
Hydromorphone hydrochloride (Dilaudid)	1–6 mg PO, IM, PR every 4–6 hr	4–5 hr duration
Meperidine hydrochloride (Demerol HCl)	1–1.5 mg/kg in 25-mg increments IV, up to 150 mg maximum IM, PO every 3 hours	More idiosyncratic rxns when given IV; 2–4 hr duration
Oxycodone (OxyContin)	10–40 mg PO every 12 hr	Do not break or chew
Methadone hydrochloride (Dolophine HCl)	1.5–20 mg PO, IM every 3–6 hr	Good for chronic pain and narcotic withdrawal; 4–6 hr duration
Morphine sulfate	0.1–0.2 mg/kg IV, in 2–4 mg IV increments	The "gold standard"; 2–4 hr duration
Sustained release morphine sulfate (MS Contin)	10–30 mg PO every 8–12 hr	Good for chronic pain 8–12 hr duration
Nalbuphine hydrochloride (Nubain)	5–10 mg IV, IM every 3–6 hr	3–6-hr duration
Pentazocine	30-60 mg IV, IM every 3–4 hr	2–3-hr duration
Propoxyphene hydrochloride	65 mg PO every 4 hr	Mild pain; 4–6-hr duration

IV, intravenous; PO, oral; IM, intramuscularly; PR, rectal.

the ward. Table 23–6 gives typical settings for a PCA pump using three different narcotics.

Dose

Select a dose that gives the patient measurable relief of pain without excessive sedation. If the patient does not obtain pain relief from your initial PCA set dose, try increasing the dose of narcotic without changing the lockout interval. If the patient's pain is relieved without excessive sedation or change in vital signs, the pain is being managed appropriately. Record the amount used during the shift.

Lockout Interval

If the patient achieves pain relief with activation of a dose, but the pain returns before the end of the lockout period, shorten the lockout period. Many patients will need a PCA lockout in the 10-minute range. Some patients may do best with a lockout interval of less than

TABLE 23–4 **Comparison of Intramuscular and Intravenous Routes of Narcotic Administration**

IM administration	Onset of action of narcotic is 15 to 20 minutes after injection
	Lower peak effect than IV administration
	Longer duration of action compared with IV route due to slower absorption
	Slower onset of narcotic side effects (e.g., respiratory depression)
IV administration	Immediate onset of action
	Greater peak effect than IM administration
	Shorter duration of action compared with IM route
	More rapid onset of potential side effects

IM, intramuscular; IV, intravenous.

10 minutes. You can always start the lockout interval in the 10- to 15-minute range and shorten the interval if needed.

Basal Rate

This feature of a PCA allows you to run a narcotic drip to supplement the patient-controlled dosing. A basal rate offers the advantage of allowing the patient a level of continuous analgesia. However, a basal rate also introduces some risks. If the basal rate of narcotic is excessive, a patient may develop respiratory depression and excessive sedation. If you are going to run a basal rate, it is suggested that it be at a relatively low and safe dose. Higher doses can be used safely only in continuously monitored units or the intensive care unit. Many practitioners do not use a basal rate or use them for only a defined period of time (e.g., 24 hours). Check with your chief resident to see if a basal rate is appropriate.

Narcotic Antagonists

If you are going to use parenteral narcotics, narcotic antagonists must be available. These agents are usually competitive inhibitors

TABLE 23–5 **Equianalgesia Table**

Drug	IV/SC/IM Dose	PO/PR Dose
Morphine	10 mg	30 mg
Oxycodone	NA	20 mg
Hydromorphone	1.5 mg	7.5 mg
Codeine	120 mg	200 mg
Fentanyl	0.1 mg	NA
Meperidine	75 mg	300 mg
Methadone	10 mg	20 mg

IV, intravenous; SC, subcutaneous; IM, intramuscular; PO, oral; PR, rectal; NA, not available.

TABLE 23–6 **Typical PCA Settings**

Narcotic	Dose	Lockout Interval	Basal Rate (Low Dose)
Morphine	1–3 mg	Every 10–15 min	None to 2 mg/hr
Meperidine HCl (Demerol)	5–15 mg	Every 10–15 min	None to 15 mg/hr
Fentanyl	15–25 mcg	Every 10–15 min	None to 25 mcg/hr

PCA, patient-controlled analgesia.

that act on the opiate receptors. If a patient receiving parenteral narcotics becomes oversedated, hypotensive, or hypoxic or has significant respiratory depression, you should consider reversing the narcotic agent with an antagonist. Use **naloxone hydrochloride (Narcan) 0.4 to 2 mg IV, IM, subcutaneously, or by endotracheal tube.** IV naloxone is most likely to give the most rapid reversal.

Other Pain Management Options

Pain is not merely a lack of an agonist binding to the mu narcotic receptor. Pain has components of physical discomfort, affected also by the patient's fears, anxiety, experience with pain, social situation, and culture. There are many other strategies for managing pain while on call. Simply sitting down and talking with the patient may give you other clues as to what might be effective. If there is a significant anxiety component to the pain, consider adding an anxiolytic. This often will decrease the dose of narcotic necessary to alleviate the pain. Simply explaining what to expect from a disease process or postoperative recovery is also very helpful.

Many hospitals have a pain service run by anesthesiologists, and consulting with them can be very useful. They can help manage pain with a variety of therapies including epidural catheters, IV lidocaine, and long-acting nerve blocks.

Patients having thoracic or abdominal surgery can frequently benefit from epidural anesthesia. An epidural catheter is usually placed at the time of surgery by an anesthesiologist. An epidural can also be placed postoperatively. Either a narcotic infusion or a local anesthetic infusion can be run through the epidural catheter to provide profound analgesia. The epidural catheter is usually placed and managed by the anesthesiology service. There are risks associated with epidural catheters, including infection, bleeding, and hypotension. Discuss the case with your chief resident or attending physician before consulting anesthesiology for placement of an epidural catheter. PCA pumps may also be used to control epidural infusions.

Preoperative Preparation

Ideally, a patient is prepared preoperatively for a procedure by the primary care team. Occasionally, an on-call physician will be asked to complete a workup or to check a laboratory result. Preoperative preparation encompasses those precautions that are aimed at decreasing the inherent risks of a procedure. A patient must be readied both physically and psychologically.

NUTRITION

Extensive surgical procedures are followed by an obligate catabolic period, the length of which is influenced by the extent of the operation, the natural history of the disease state, and the general health of the patient. Urgent and emergent conditions do not allow for the shoring up of metabolic stores. But in elective cases, enteral supplementation, especially with protein-rich foods, or even total parenteral nutrition may be beneficial. The diets of patients with documented malnutrition (albumin of <3 g/dL or a recent 15% weight loss) should be supplemented. There is value in supplementation in elderly patients or in patients with other degenerative diseases such as cardiac cachexia or pulmonary insufficiency. Benefit is measurable in 5 to 7 days.

HYDRATION

Surgery is associated with intravascular volume depletion. This may include fluid losses such as bleeding and insensible losses due to exposure of surgical fields to the air, and hemodynamic changes due to anesthetic agents. Patients should be well hydrated preoperatively to account for potential losses. In addition, patients may present with preexisting fluid deficits. Intra-abdominal infections and generalized sepsis are associated with sequestration of fluids or "third spacing." Intravascular volume may be further depleted by vomiting, diarrhea, or anorexia before presentation. Correction of preexisting fluid deficits should be done before a surgical procedure. Fluid replacement therapy is covered more fully in Chapters 12 and 17. Follow moderate fluid replacement therapy closely with adequate hemodynamic, urine output, and electrolyte monitoring. Care should be used when hydrating a patient with suspected congestive heart disease.

PROPHYLACTIC ANTIBIOTICS

Prophylactic antibiotic treatment has documented efficacy in many, but not all, surgical procedures. Table 24–1 lists those instances in which the inherent costs and risks of antibiotic therapy are outweighed by the potential costs and risks of infectious complications. A good reference is "Bratzler et al.: Antibiotic prophylaxis for surgery: an advisory statement from the National Surgical Infection Prevention Project. Am J Surg 189:395–404, 2005."

The following guidelines pertain to the use of prophylactic antibiotics:

1. Antibiotic infusion should be started within one hour before the skin incision to ensure adequate tissue levels of the agent.
2. Prophylactic antibiotics should not be given for more than 24 hours following a surgical procedure. Any antibiotic use thereafter is defined as therapeutic, and should be directed toward a particular agent or disease process.
3. Determine before the administration if a patient has a specific allergy to the recommended agent.

TABLE 24–1 **Operations for which Prophylactic Antibiotics Are Found to be Beneficial**

Procedure	Antibiotic
Oropharyngeal	Penicillin
Esophageal (includes hiatal hernia)	1st-generation cephalosporin
Gastroduodenal	1st-generation cephalosporin
Biliary tract (high risk)	Mechanical bowel preparation and 2nd-generation cephalosporin
Age >70 yr	
Cholecystitis	
Required choledochostomy	
Bowel resection (small or large)	Mechanical bowel preparation and 2nd-generation cephalosporin
Laparotomy for penetrating abdominal trauma	1st-generation cephalosporin
Colorectal	Mechanical bowel preparation and 1st-generation cephalosporin
Appendicitis with suspected perforation	2nd-generation cephalosporin
Hysterectomy	1st-generation cephalosporin
Abdominal or lower extremity revascularization	1st-generation cephalosporin
Foreign body implantation Cardiac valve Prosthetic joint	1st-generation cephalosporin

4. Antibiotics should be readministered intraoperatively if the case exceeds two half lives of the antibiotic used.

Attending surgeons often have their own preferences as to when antibiotics should be used and which agent is appropriate; for example, many physicians prefer the use of second-generation cephalosporins before bowel surgery. Always ask. Hair removal, if necessary, should be done immediately before the incision, and clippers are recommended over razors.

Additional measures which decrease the development of postoperative wound infection include maintenance of perioperative glucose control, maintenance of perioperative normothermia and administration of oxygen in the perioperative period.

MECHANICAL BOWEL PREPARATION

Alimentary tract cases, as described above, are contaminated with enteric bacteria. Mechanical bowel preps are used to decrease the bacterial burden in the GI tract preoperatively. This is performed the day before surgery. The patient is instructed to remain on a clear liquid diet. Four liters of electrolyte solution (e.g., GoLYTELY or Colyte) is administered by mouth and should be completely taken within the space of 1 hour. A nasogastric tube may be required for administration. If the efflux does not clear, supplemental saline enemas may be useful. Enemas may be the sole agent required for rectal surgery. In addition, oral antibiotics are administered as follows:

Neomycin 1 g and erythromycin base 1 g by mouth at 1 PM, 3 PM, and 11 PM on the day before surgery.

Always administer the oral antibiotics well in advance of or after the electrolyte solution, as any pills in the gastrointestinal tract will get washed out. The goal of mechanical bowel preparation is not to completely sterilize the bowel contents, but to decrease the bacterial count. The patient should be maintained with nothing by mouth for 6 to 8 hours before surgery to ensure adequate stomach emptying and to decrease aspiration risk. Be sure to maintain adequate intravenous hydration during this time. Routine medications may be given the morning of surgery with a small sip of water.

CARDIAC RISK ASSESSMENT

Myocardial ischemia is a significant risk factor for perioperative morbidity. As many as 50,000 patients have perioperative MIs each year, and up to 40% may die. Those at greatest risk include patients with a history of CAD, recent MI (within 3 months), heart failure, aortic stenosis, renal insufficiency, cerebrovascular disease, and age over 70 years. Other factors include poorly controlled diabetes or hypertension, and poor functional capacity.

History and physical examination alone can help stratify patients with respect to cardiac risk, reserving more invasive testing for those at significant risk for myocardial ischemia, or who are scheduled to undergo high-risk surgeries. As the risks of cardiac surgery often outweigh the risks of noncardiac surgery, it rarely is necessary to consider revascularization as a modality to make noncardiac surgery more safe. However, it is often possible to maximize a patient's cardiac status before surgery in order to minimize cardiac risks perioperatively.

The original preoperative risk index developed by Goldman in 1977 has been modified by Detsky and others in 1986 in this index (summarized in Table 24–2).

In general, patients should be adequately stratified to define their risks for prognostic discussion. In addition, specific steps need to be taken in some patients to decrease risk.

Hypertension: Wherever possible, severe hypertension (diastolic >100 mm Hg) should be controlled before surgery. Be sure to maintain existing antihypertensives perioperatively, especially beta-blockers or clonidine, which may be associated with a significant rebound phenomenon.

Valve disease: Severe stenotic lesions pose a great risk to a surgical patient, and consideration should be given in this subset of patients to repair of the valvular lesion before noncardiac surgery if possible. Patients with even moderate regurgitant valvular lesions may safely undergo noncardiac operation with appropriate monitor-

TABLE 24–2 **Detsky's Modified Cardiac Risk Index**

Predictor	Risk
Age older than 70 years	5
Myocardial infarction within 6 months	10
Myocardial infarction after 6 months	5
Angina with 1–2 blocks or one flight of stairs	10
Angina with minimal activity or at rest	20
Unstable angina within 6 months	10
Alveolar pulmonary edema within one week	10
Alveolar pulmonary edema at any time	5
Suspected critical aortic stenosis	20
Rhythm other than sinus (or sinus with occ. PATs)	5
More than 5 PVCs	5
Emergency operation	10
Poor general medical condition	5

Class	Points	Cardiac Risk
I	0–15	Low
II	20–30	Intermediate
III	>30	High

(Modified from Detsky et al.: Predicting cardiac complications in patients undergoing non-cardiac surgery. J Gen Intern Med 1:211–219, 1986).

ing and attention to fluid status. Care must be taken to decrease afterload with diuretics and antihypertensive agents such as ACE inhibitors or long-acting calcium channel blockers.

Myocardial disease: Those patients with myocardial dysfunction are at increased risk for perioperative CHF. Intensive perioperative monitoring and fluid management is necessary.

Beta blockade: Those patient with a history of CAD will benefit from perioperative beta-blockade. Multiple studies have now documented decreased cardiac morbidity and mortality with the use of these agents. Patients who qualify include any patients with at least two of the following risk factors:

Age >65 years
History of myocardial infarction
History of coronary artery disease or angina pectoris
History of congestive heart failure
History of diabetes mellitus
History of chronic renal insufficiency (serum Cr >2 mg/dL)
History of cerebrovascular accident (CVA)
Poor functional capacity (attributable to chest pain of shortness of breath)

Recent myocardial infarction (MI): A general surgical procedure within 6 weeks of an MI carries a 50% risk of a second MI. The risk of death approaches 25%. Therefore, elective procedures should be postponed for at least 6 months after MI, if possible, to decrease the risk of subsequent cardiac events. If this is not possible because of urgency, appropriate care should be taken, including afterload reduction, cardiovascular and hemodynamic monitoring, and arrhythmia precautions.

When in doubt about a patient's cardiac status, preoperative cardiology consultation will help define risks and offer suggestions for perioperative care. This is a very common call for the cardiologist.

PREOPERATIVE LABORATORY STUDIES

Blood is generally drawn preoperatively to evaluate potential risks of the procedure to the patient, for example, for measurement of hemoglobin and hematocrit when anemia is suspected. Another purpose is to establish a baseline for comparison, if the same study will be used to follow the patient postoperatively, for such things as tumor markers, or Ca^{2+} before parathyroid resection. Clotting studies (prothrombin time, partial thromboplastin time, Ivy bleeding time, and platelet count) are important for patients with liver failure, renal failure, or bleeding diathesis, and also for those patients treated with anticoagulants (including aspirin) or those who may require blood product replacement. Other studies (e.g., chest x-ray and electrocardiogram) may be considered as the patient's clinical condition indicates.

There is no "routine preoperative laboratory panel". Each test much have a specific purpose. History alone is often the only tool necessary to identify these risks.

BLOOD PRODUCT REPLACEMENT

The need for blood postoperatively is determined by the patient's cardiovascular reserve, the amount of blood lost anticipated during the procedure, and the ongoing postoperative losses due to leaks or hypocoagulability states. The need to have blood or products available is dependent on the type of surgery planned and the preferences of the surgeon. The blood bank requires a clot tube to be drawn well in advance of need so that the patient's serum can be matched with the product. There are several options for ensuring the availability of blood (Table 24–3). Check with the hospital blood bank for more information regarding specific times of preparation and the time interval for which each option is valid.

Patients may also have blood available from other sources. Autologous blood is that which has been donated by the patient in the weeks before in preparation for elective surgery. Directed donor blood has been donated by a friend or a relative of the patient and is crossmatched to the patient. It is important to confirm the readiness of these types of blood with the blood bank. Also, individual blood banks may have protocols for specific surgical procedures. If you know of a greater blood need before a procedure, let the blood bank know well in advance.

Blood products carry significant risk of viral contamination with HIV, hepatitis, or CMV. Most hospitals require a consent form to be signed by the patient before elective administration of blood. Some states also have specific laws requiring documentation of the discus-

TABLE 24–3 **Options for Ensuring the Availability of Preoperative Blood**

Type only	This gives only the ABO blood type and the Rh status of the patient.
Type and hold (no. of units)	This types the patient's blood and reserves the blood for use in the future. The blood may be released for use in another patient if it is not used
Type and crossmatch (no. of units)	This types the patient's blood and prepares the units of blood for subsequent administration. The blood cannot be released for use in any other patient.

sion held between the physician and the patient regarding the risks of blood transfusions before one may be given.

OTHER CONSIDERATIONS

Patients with other concurrent illnesses may have special requirements for pre- and postoperative care. Specific diseases require selective preparation. For example, a patient to be operated on for removal of pheochromocytoma must first be adequately hydrated, treated with nitroprusside, and then treated with alpha- and beta-blockade to protect against catecholamine storm. In a similar manner, patients with thyroid storm require beta-blockade and antithyroid measures.

Patients treated with recent or chronic steroid replacement therapy may require stress doses of hydrocortisone to bolster the physiologic postoperative adrenal response (Table 24–4). Not all attending surgeons feel that steroid "stress doses" are appropriate. Ask first. Do not hesitate to enlist specialists to help handle a complex series of problems, as your primary care team allows.

PSYCHOLOGICAL PREPARATION

Along with physiologic changes, the patient will also undergo psychological changes before and after a surgical procedure. Anticipation of these changes and proper preparation of the patient will make the postoperative period smoother for both patient and physician. Patients may already be depressed and frightened at the new onset

TABLE 24–4 **Perioperative Steroid Replacement Regimen**

Preoperative
100 mg hydrocortisone IV at midnight and 2 hr before surgery
Postoperative
100 mg hydrocortisone IV immediately postoperative, again in 8 hr, and again in 12 hr
POD 1
100 mg hydrocortisone IV every 12 hr
POD 2
50 mg hydrocortisone IV or PO every 12 hr
POD 3
Continue to taper rapidly over 4–5 days unless replacement steroids are necessary

IV, intravenously; POD, postoperative day; PO, by mouth.

of illness or the prospect of surgery. Listen to patients carefully; they often communicate their fears. Answer questions fully and honestly. Make enough time to talk. Be optimistic but not unrealistic. Explain to each patient and to significant others the full procedure, the risks, the alternatives, and the goals. Include descriptions of the scar and any disfiguring aspects of the procedure (including drains or tubes). Be sure to describe what the postoperative recovery period will be like and what will be expected of the patient. Include descriptions of what to expect with regard to pain and its management, incentive spirometry, bowel function, ambulation, and diet. Don't minimize any aspect of this discussion. The more details that are conveyed, the more honest you are, the better prepared the patient will be. It is far better to have a patient say, "Boy, you told me this would be hard," than to hear "I never knew that THIS could happen!"

Expect the patient to be depressed for 2 or 3 days after the procedure (the post-op blues). Encourage support from family and significant others during this time. Anticipate a psychological regression, which is common with anyone who enters the hospital. Hospitals, by their nature, remove part of a patient's individuality and reduce even strong-willed people to the common denominators of nursing schedules and bodily functions. Encourage questions; remind the patient to write questions down, because they may be difficult to remember later when the care team is making rounds. Most important is maintaining openness and approachability. Each patient will have different needs.

The night before surgery, patients often require a sedative for sleep. More important may be a reassuring visit from the attending surgeon to answer any last-minute questions.

Some patients have psychiatric or psychological comorbidities. Be mindful of these, allow for them in the postoperative care, and make sure to continue any medications that are necessary to treat them.

PREOPERATIVE NOTE

The above information should be summarized in a brief preoperative note. The following is an example:

Preop Note
Procedure anticipated:
Attending surgeon:
List of routine medications/therapies:
List of significant preoperative exam findings:
List of preoperative lab and study results:
Bowel preparation (if needed):
Diet orders:
Blood products available:

"On call to OR" instructions (e.g. antibiotics or beta-blockers):
Void:
Preoperative medications:
Consent signed and witnessed:
'PAR' (a brief statement that the procedure has been discussed with the patient, for example: "Procedure, alternatives, risks, complications and benefits described in detail to the patient [and family], questions were answered to his/her satisfaction. He/she elects to proceed. Consent signed. Surgical site was confirmed. [Translator needed]").

Pronouncing Death

One of the most unpleasant requirements of on-call responsibilities is pronouncing death. This important task represents a significant medicolegal responsibility. You may not have had much experience evaluating recently deceased persons, and there is some controversy as to what exactly constitutes the legal definition of death. This chapter provides a guide of the steps to follow when declaring a patient dead.

Different states in the United States may have differing criteria for declaring death. However, most states and neighboring countries, including Canada and Mexico, have adopted the concepts of both physiologic death and brain death. Physiologic death refers to absence of any spontaneous cardiac activity, no blood pressure, and no evidence of respiration. Pronouncing brain death is more complicated and is usually managed by neurology or neurosurgery services. There is more variability regionally as to what constitutes brain death. Remember that declaring death is a serious medicolegal responsibility. Be careful and studious in your evaluation of the person presumed deceased.

When you are paged by the RN to pronounce a patient dead, it is advisable that you come equipped with a stethoscope and a penlight. The most important thing to ascertain is that the patient has no spontaneous circulation or respiratory function. It is also important to perform a brief assessment of the neurologic system. Table 25–1 indicates the key criteria for declaring death. Using these criteria to declare death requires that the person presumed deceased has a body temperature of at least 34°C to 35°C. If the body is very cold (e.g., after ice water immersion or cold weather exposure), you may have to warm it before legally pronouncing death. Recall that hypothermia slows metabolic rate, heart rate, and respiratory rate. Hypothermic critically ill patients have been mistaken for dead. Also make sure that there is no history of use of paralytic drugs or seda-

TABLE 25–1 **Key Criteria for Pronouncing Death**

No cardiac activity (asystole)
No blood pressure
No respiratory activity

tives within a reasonable time period. If paralytic drugs were used within the last 6 to 8 hours before the presumed death, a paralytic reversing agent such as neostigmine methylsulfate *(Prostigmin)* should be administered.

STEPS FOR PRONOUNCING PHYSIOLOGIC DEATH

The Nonventilated Patient

1. Overview the chart briefly.

   Make sure that in examining the presumed deceased you will incur no infectious risk (e.g., human immunodeficiency virus or hepatitis). Wear gloves.

2. Check the identity of the patient by looking at the identification bracelet worn on the wrist.

   Make sure you know who you are pronouncing dead.

3. Make sure that the patient does not respond to verbal or tactile stimuli.

   You may want to perform a sternal rub to satisfy yourself that the presumed deceased does not respond to painful stimuli.

4. Check for radial and carotid pulses.

   The deceased patient will have no pulses anywhere.

5. Check the blood pressure.

   The deceased patient will have no blood pressure.

6. Listen for heart sounds; listen carefully over the entire precordium.

   You will hear no heart sounds in a deceased patient. You may also want to listen over the carotid artery in the neck. If the patient is in the intensive care unit and is attached to monitoring leads, you may wish to evaluate the rhythm strip.

7. Listen for spontaneous respirations over both lung fields

   A deceased patient will have no air movement whatsoever.

8. Examine the pupils.

   The pupils of a deceased patient will be fixed, and they may also often be dilated, but not always. The pupils will not respond to light.

The Ventilated Patient

If a mechanically ventilated patient has lost cardiac activity and has no blood pressure, you must alter the procedure by which you declare death. First, contact the attending physician for consent to turn off the ventilator. Once there is agreement to terminate mechanical ventilation, proceed to disconnect the ventilator. First, however, make sure that all the electrocardiographic (ECG) leads are properly connected and that the monitoring equipment is functioning. You do not want to disconnect from the ventilator a patient who actually does have cardiac activity. In addition, make sure that the patient has not been given any paralytic drugs within 6 to 8 hours of the examination.

1. After you have verified that the ECG monitoring equipment is functioning and all the connections are intact, proceed to disconnect the ventilator from the patient; leave the endotracheal tube in place.
2. Follow the procedure outlined in steps 1 to 8 in the preceding section for declaring death.
3. Observe the patient for a full 3 minutes for evidence of spontaneous respiration.
4. Record in the medical record that mechanical ventilation was terminated after consultation with the attending physician and after all evidence of circulatory function had ceased. Document the rest of your examination. Give a time and a date when you declared death.

AFTER YOUR EXAMINATION

Always remember to document your examination in the chart. Carefully list what your examination found. The time of death is the time you complete your examination. Record the time of death and the date. Sign the note. You may also be required to fill out and sign the death certificate. Some hospitals will also ask that you call the medical examiner's office to notify them of the death. Some states require contact with the local donor network or tissue bank.

It is appropriate to contact your supervising resident or the attending physician as soon as you pronounce the patient dead. Ask your superiors if they want you to contact the next of kin. It is appropriate to notify the family as soon as practically possible. Also ascertain from the attending physician whether an autopsy is necessary or appropriate. The attending physician may want to consult the family about this option.

If you are going to notify the family of the deceased and you did not know the patient, take some time to review the medical history and the recent events. Talk to the nursing staff about the family members who have visited the patient. Become aware of any difficult family situations that may be important.

First, contact the family member closest to the patient. Sometimes the RN will know which family member is the spokesperson for the family. You may also see a notation in the chart as to who is the next of kin. Once you have made telephone contact with the family member, identify yourself and the hospital where you work. In an apologetic and conciliatory tone, inform the family member that their loved one has passed away. Frequently, the family member will want to know the time of death and the circumstances. If appropriate, you may wish to offer the reassurance that death was painless and peaceful. Do not be shocked if a family member is not surprised or too upset. Many families have watched a loved one deal with chronic illness, pain, and suffering for many years. They are often relieved when they hear that the loved one's suffering has ended. Other families may show obvious grief and despair at the notification of the death of their loved one. Try to be supportive, and understand that distinct cultures deal with death in different ways.

BRAIN DEATH AND ORGAN DONATION

As the on-call physician, it is not your responsibility to pronounce brain death. This is a more complicated task than declaring physiologic death. Consult neurology or neurosurgery for help with this task. The declaration of brain death is important for obtaining legal clearance for organ donation. If you believe that a brain-dead patient may be a good candidate for organ donation and the family is supportive, contact the organ transplant program at your hospital or in your city. There is usually a transplant coordinator on call 24 hours a day to help make arrangements. You should maintain the brain-dead patient on supportive hydration and ventilation until the transplant service takes over the management of the organ donor. Some states require that the local transplant coordinator be contacted with every death.

The concept of brain death has been accepted throughout the United States, Canada, Mexico, and much of the world. The diagnostic criteria followed by most hospitals are shown in Table 25–2.

TABLE 25–2 **Criteria for Pronouncing Brain Death**

No cerebral or brain stem function
Fixed pupils
No response (including reflexes) to noxious stimuli
Apneic during oxygenation (for 10 min)
No oculovestibular responses (50-mL ice-water calorics)
Spinal reflexes may be intact
Circulatory function may be intact

Coma of known cause and duration
Known structural damage or disease
Known irreversible metabolic disease
No hypothermia, sedation, paralytic drugs, or drug intoxication
Minimum 6 hr observation of no brain function; if drugs or alcohol were involved, a minimum of 24 hr of observation of no brain function and a negative toxicology screen is required

Optional criteria
No cerebral circulation on angiogram
Electroencephalogram isoelectric for 30 min at maximal gain
Auditory evoked responses show no brain stem function

26

Postoperative Bleeding

Bleeding in the postoperative period is a concern for the on-call physician. You must decide whether the bleeding has a surgical cause (major vessel bleeding) or a medical cause (abnormal coagulation status). Some patients will require a return to the operating room for control of bleeding. Other patients may require bedside care or transfusion of blood products. Guidelines for evaluation of bleeding patients and for management of postoperative bleeding problems are discussed in this chapter.

PHONE CALL

1. **What are the patient's vital signs?**
   Rapid postoperative bleeding is occasionally associated with hypotension and tachycardia.
2. **How severe is the bleeding?**
   Ask the RN to describe the bleeding site. Is the dressing or the wound slowly oozing blood, or is there a large amount of blood on the dressing or in the patient's bed? Also ask the RN if the surgical site appears markedly swollen or bruised (hematoma).
3. **What operation did the patient have, and when was the operation performed?**
   Knowing the surgical site is critical when managing bleeding patients. For example, a bleeding patient who has undergone abdominal, chest, or pelvic surgery can easily bleed into the potential spaces of these anatomic areas.
4. **Does the patient have known bleeding problems, and is the patient taking anticoagulant medication?**
   Ask the RN if the patient has a history of bleeding diathesis (e.g., alcoholic liver disease). Also find out if the patient is taking, or has recently taken, aspirin, warfarin, or other medication that interferes with normal blood clotting.
5. **Does the patient have recent blood count and coagulation studies? Is there blood available for this patient in the blood bank?**
   If a postoperative patient is already anemic from a surgical procedure, significant postoperative bleeding is likely to lead to decompensation. Recent coagulation studies are important to

help you rule out coagulopathy as a cause of bleeding. Make sure that blood is available for any patient with significant postoperative bleeding.

Orders

1. Order intravenous (IV) line access.
   - For patients with significant bleeding, ask the RN to establish an IV if a functional IV is not present.
   - For patients with significant bleeding, one or two large-bore (14- to 16-gauge) antecubital IVs are necessary.
   - Large antecubital IVs are generally better than central lines for fluid resuscitation.
2. Give IV fluids.
   - Order a 500-mL fluid bolus (normal saline [NS] or lactated Ringer's [LR]) if a patient has hemodynamic compromise associated with active bleeding.
3. Order hematocrit immediately.
   - Ask the RN to draw a hematocrit immediately if possible. The RN should be sure to draw blood from a site distal to the IV or from the opposite upper extremity. If a patient has bleeding associated with hemodynamic compromise, blood should be drawn only after IV access and fluid resuscitation have been initiated.
4. Order platelet count and coagulation studies (prothrombin time [PT] and partial thromboplastin time [PTT]) immediately. Some hospitals monitor heparin with anti-X_a levels.

Inform RN

Will be at the bedside in . . . minutes.

Postoperative bleeding requires immediate bedside evaluation. The amount of bleeding may be underestimated by the RN.

ELEVATOR THOUGHTS

What are the causes of postoperative bleeding?

Surgical Causes

Technical Surgical Errors

1. Ties coming off vessels
2. Inadequate coagulation of vessels
3. Unrecognized vessel injury (traumatic or iatrogenic)
4. Transected vessels not bleeding at the time of surgery (vasospasm)

Bleeding from Surgical Sites

1. Bleeding associated with coughing or hypertension
2. Bleeding from vessel anastamoses (vascular surgery)

Medical Causes

Platelets

1. Thrombocytopenia
2. Platelet dysfunction
   - von Willebrand's disease
   - Uremia
   - Nonsteroidal anti-inflammatory drugs (NSAIDs) and other drugs

Soluble Blood Clotting Factors

1. Coagulopathy of liver disease
2. Other coagulation factor deficiencies
   - Hemophilia A and B (factors VIII and IX, respectively)
3. Vitamin K deficiency
4. Disseminated intravascular coagulation (DIC)
5. Dilutional coagulopathy
6. Coagulopathy associated with drugs
   - Heparin
   - Warfarin sodium (Coumadin)
   - Antibiotics (hypoprothrombinemia)

MAJOR THREAT TO LIFE

Major surgical bleeding (large vessel)
Bleeding in the neck leading to airway compromise
Intracranial bleeding leading to increased intracranial pressure or herniation
Severe coagulopathy or DIC

BEDSIDE

Quick Look Test

Does the patient look well (comfortable), sick (uncomfortable or distressed), or critical (about to die)?

Patients who have significant postoperative bleeding usually look distressed or critical. Rapid blood loss leads to activation of the sympathetic nervous system with resulting tachycardia and peripheral vasoconstriction.

These patients may appear pale and may be hypotensive. If a patient appears to have rapid, surgical-type bleeding, attend to the patient personally. Have the RN call for backup help from a senior or chief resident.

Airway and Vital Signs

Check that the patient has a patent, nonobstructed airway. Patients with significant bleeding in the upper aerodigestive tract are at high risk for aspiration of blood; they may need to be intubated.

What is the respiratory rate?

Tachypnea may suggest airway compromise or impending shock.

What is the heart rate (HR)?

Tachycardia in the presence of significant bleeding suggests intravascular volume depletion and impending hypotension.

What is the blood pressure (BP)?

Sympathetic activation in the presence of postoperative bleeding causes tachycardia and peripheral vasoconstriction in an attempt to maintain a normotensive blood pressure. Rapid or extensive blood loss overcomes the sympathetic drive and leads to hypotension.

What is the temperature?

Measuring the temperature is important, as abnormally low body temperature (hypothermia) interferes with normal blood coagulation.

Selective History and Chart Review

An actively bleeding patient requires immediate bedside evaluation. Have the RN bring the patient's chart to the bedside, and review the type of surgical procedure performed, the date of surgery, the known blood coagulation status and recent hematocrit, and any anticoagulant medication that the patient has been taking.

Selective Physical Examination

The goals of the selective examination are to assess the patient's hemodynamic stability and evaluate the site of bleeding.

VS:	Repeat now.
HEENT:	Look for sites of bleeding with the aid of good lighting and suction.
Resp/CVS:	Evaluate the drainage from chest tubes or mediastinal tubes. Ask the RN if the tubes are putting out a more bloody fluid. Is there frank blood draining from these tubes?
Wound:	Using sterile technique, remove any dressing from the wound site. Evaluate for frank bleeding, swelling or increase in girth, hematoma, or discoloration of the skin.

MANAGEMENT

Surgical Bleeding

Life-Threatening Postoperative Hemorrhage

Severe postoperative bleeding associated with hemodynamic compromise is a problem that must be dealt with quickly and emphatically. Follow a logical treatment plan, and obtain help from other physicians on duty immediately.

The first priority is to stabilize the patient hemodynamically. Intravascular fluid resuscitation is extremely important. For patients with hypotension, tachycardia, or other signs of impending circulatory shock, run a 500-mL bolus of NS or LR wide open. Have the RN take the vital signs every 2 minutes. Give more fluid or adjust the fluid rate based on the normalization of the patient's BP and HR. Some patients may require a bolus of several liters of IV fluid. Place a Foley to monitor the resuscitation.

Assess the airway and breathing. If bleeding is associated with severe hypotension and shock, consider intubation.

Control external hemorrhaging with direct pressure, if possible. Internal hemorrhaging is best treated in the operating room or the interventional radiology (IR) suite.

Trendelenburg's positioning may help maintain central perfusion in the presence of hemorrhaging and hypotension.

Consider immediate transfusion of packed red blood cells (PRBCs) in the presence of massive hemorrhage. Have a member of the team run to the blood bank to obtain O-type, Rh negative blood; crossmatched if available, uncrossmatched if no crossmatched blood is available. Begin transfusion immediately. While waiting for blood products, maintain BP with crystalloid or colloid infusion.

Have a team member set up suction and adequate lighting. Using sterile technique, try to visualize the source of bleeding. Sometimes, significant bleeding is superficial enough that it can be controlled directly and easily with a stitch or a Kelly clamp. If the bleeding is from an extremity, use a BP cuff or tourniquet to help slow the bleeding.

If the bleeding source appears to be internal, do not attempt to control bleeding at the bedside. Frequently, a large internal hematoma may tamponade bleeding. Disrupting this tamponade may exacerbate hemorrhaging. Treating the patient with fluid and PRBCs is the best support you can give at the bedside. Major internal bleeding requires control in the operating room. Consider emergent return and surgical reexploration for major internal bleeding. In some cases, angiography and embolization, or stenting, are appropriate in the IR/suite.

There are some cases in which widely opening a surgical wound at the bedside may be appropriate. If a patient develops airway compromise associated with bleeding after head and neck surgery, a hematoma may be compressing the trachea. This wound should be opened immediately to evacuate the hematoma. Direct pressure on the bleeding can be applied until surgical control can be achieved. If a patient is near arrest or has arrested at the bedside, it is also appropriate to widely open a surgical wound. A good example would be a cardiac surgery patient who has developed cardiac tamponade.

Always keep in mind that bleeding into large potential spaces (pleural, abdominal, pelvic, and thigh) can lead to exsanguination. Control of bleeding into these spaces may require immediate surgical exploration.

Minor Postoperative Bleeding

These calls are very common. Many postoperative patients will have minor oozing from surgical sites. These patients are hemodynamically stable and generally show blood spotting on outer dressings.

Consult the attending surgeon or chief resident before rendering any treatment. If the attending surgeon feels it is appropriate, and using proper lighting and sterile technique, remove the outer dressing, exposing the surgical incision line or wound. Evaluate the wound for evidence of direct bleeding. Frequently, skin bleeding will be easily visualized. A simple stitch or a figure eight stitch will usually stop bleeding.

If the wound is open and bleeding appears to be coming from very small vessels in a diffuse area, apply a pressure dressing to the area. If the wound is closed and bleeding is coming from the incision line, apply manual pressure for 10 minutes and apply a sterile pressure dressing to the area. Sterile gauze sponges, ABD pads, Elastoplast adhesive tape, and Ace wraps are very helpful in creating these dressings.

If a hematoma is present, apply a pressure dressing and contact the chief resident. Hematoma evacuation may require a nonemergent trip to the operating room.

Medical Bleeding

Medical bleeding is caused by coagulopathy. Bleeding tends to be diffuse from all cut surfaces. Normally, vasoconstriction and platelet action tend to stop bleeding by creating a platelet plug in cut vessels. In the presence of thrombocytopenia or platelet dysfunction, normal numbers of platelet plugs are not formed. In the absence of adequate soluble blood clotting factors, an organized clot cannot be formed. This also leads to continued, prolonged postoperative bleeding. To best manage medical bleeding, identify whether the bleeding problem is related to platelets, soluble blood clotting factors, or both.

Platelets

THROMBOCYTOPENIA

Platelet counts of less than 30,000/μL may cause prolonged bleeding in postoperative patients. Postoperative bleeding associated with a platelet count of less than 30,000/μL should be treated with a platelet transfusion. Thrombocytopenia may be caused by dilution, decreased marrow production, or increased peripheral destruction of platelets.

It is a good idea to give at least a six-pack of platelets if bleeding is significant. For dilutional thrombocytopenia, a general rule is that 8 units of platelets should be given for each 10 to 12 units of blood transfused. Although many of the platelets transfused are sequestered rapidly by the spleen, they usually act long enough to create a platelet plug.

PLATELET DYSFUNCTION

Many drugs including NSAIDs interfere with platelet aggregation. Other conditions including renal failure (uremia) and von Willebrand disease inhibit platelet function. Platelet function may be tested with a bleeding time. A normal bleeding time (Ivy bleeding time test) is less than 7 minutes.

Patients with significant postoperative bleeding who have a history of platelet dysfunction, a prolonged bleeding time, or known ingestion of drugs that interfere with platelet activity may require a platelet transfusion. Patients with known von Willebrand disease or uremia may be treated with cryoprecipitate, factor VIII, or desmopressin acetate (DDAVP). If possible, contact the chief resident or attending physician before giving platelet transfusions. Anticoagulation is sometimes desirable in vascular or microsurgical postoperative management.

Soluble Blood Clotting Factors

When blood clotting factor production or concentration is low, prolonged postoperative bleeding results. There are many causes of low clotting factor activity. However, in an acutely bleeding patient, most of these are treated by fresh frozen plasma (FFP) transfusion. Usually a minimum of 2 to 3 units of FFP is required to observe clinical improvement of the coagulopathy. Indications for the transfusion of FFP include the following:

1. Bleeding patients on warfarin (Coumadin) therapy

    Warfarin depletes the vitamin K-dependent blood clotting factors (Table 26–1). FFP reverses the effects of warfarin rapidly. Administration of vitamin K generally corrects the effects of warfarin slowly.

2. As an adjunct to massive blood transfusions

    A bleeding patient whose entire blood volume has been replaced over a short time generally will need FFP to have acceptable (<50% greater than normal) PT and PTT values. Frequently, these patients will also require platelet transfusions.

3. Bleeding patients with liver disease

4. Patients with dilutional coagulopathy

TABLE 26–1 **Vitamin K–Dependent Factors**

II
VII
IX
X
Protein S
Protein C

Hemodilution may lead to prolonged PT and PTT values. Bleeding patients with dilutional coagulopathy may require FFP and platelets. Patients with a history of congestive heart failure or who are already fluid overloaded can be given IV furosemide *(Lasix)* in conjunction with the FFP.

5. Patients with vitamin K deficiency

Vitamin K is a fat-soluble vitamin synthesized in the GI tract by bacteria. Deficient states may occur in setting of malabsorption, biliary obstruction, or following treatment with antibiotics. Treat with supplemental **vitamin K 10 mg SC/PO every day for 3 days.**

Postoperative bleeding associated with heparin therapy. Some postoperative patients will be maintained on IV heparin therapy. This is common practice in vascular surgery and microsurgery. If a patient develops postoperative bleeding on heparin therapy, check a PTT or anti-X_a level to assess for over treatment. Consider slowing the rate of heparin infusion or discontinuing heparin. Because the half-life of heparin is only 90 minutes, minor bleeding may resolve with this conservative approach. Patients with significant bleeding should be treated by discontinuing the heparin therapy. If necessary, heparin effect can be reversed with **protamine sulfate (1 mg/90 U heparin) given IV slowly.** You can estimate the circulating amount of heparin by calculating one-half of the previous hour's dose. For example, a patient on a heparin infusion of 1000 U/hour should be given 5 mg of protamine. No more than 50 mg of protamine should be given in a single dose. Furthermore, protamine should be given over 10 to 15 minutes. Side effects of protamine include bradycardia, hypotension, and flushing.

Postoperative bleeding in patients with known clotting factor deficiencies. Patients with a known clotting factor deficiency are best managed with specific factor replacement. Most of these factors are available as recombinant, purified proteins. If specific clotting factors are not available, FFP or cryoprecipitate (containing factor VIII) may be useful. A consulting hematologist may help with the management of these patients.

Disseminated intravascular coagulation. DIC is a poorly understood process in which diffuse bleeding is accompanied by a rapid consumption of blood clotting factors. DIC is seen after trauma, some types of surgery (lung, brain, or prostate), obstetric complications, and septicemia. DIC commonly presents with diffuse bleeding from surgical sites, IVs, and sites of recent needle puncture. The PTT is significantly prolonged, fibrinogen values are very low (<75 mg/dL), thrombin time is prolonged, and fibrin degradation products are elevated. Treatment includes FFP, cryoprecipitate, and platelet transfusions. Correction of the underlying cause is also mandatory.

In some cases, no known preexisting conditions are identifiable as the cause of intractable, life-threatening medical bleeding. For these patients, the use of recombinant Factor VIIa may be an option.

Seizures

Seizure activity is a synchronous discharge of electrical activity in the brain. The locus in the brain dictates what clinical symptoms are noted. Generalized tonic–clonic seizure activity is the major symptom for which you will be called. Seizure activity is frightening and disturbing to witness. Patients actively having seizures can harm themselves, and the underlying abnormalities are often serious.

Some patients will have epilepsy, and will occasionally have seizures, despite therapeutic levels of antiepileptic medication.

PHONE CALL

Questions

1. **Is the patient still having seizures?**
   This requires immediate attention. Patients who are actively having seizures are at risk for aspiration, for metabolic derangements, and for hypoxia.
2. **What is the type of seizure?**
   Is it a full-body tonic–clonic, a focal, or a petit mal seizure? Is the patient conscious or unconscious?
3. **Has the patient had a seizure before?**
   New-onset seizure activity is a medical emergency. An expected seizure such as in a patient with a known seizure disorder may need no specific evaluation other than ensuring the patient's safety and attention to specific injuries, if present. If the patient is being treated with antiseizure medication, therapeutic levels should be checked.
4. **Was there a change in the patient's mental status either before or after the seizure?**
   Be mindful that most tonic-clonic seizures are followed by an unconscious postictal period.
5. **Is the patient injured in some way?**
6. **Has the patient undergone a surgical procedure, and if so, how long ago?**
   Seizures are common after neurosurgical procedures, and they represent a significant change in mental status.
   It also may indicate malfunction in any shunting or drainage device present.

7. **Are there any other symptoms?**
8. **Are there any changes in vital signs?**

Orders

If the Patient Is Actively Having a Seizure

1. Order oxygen (O_2) and oximetry monitoring.
2. Confirm that intravenous (IV) access is available.

    An IV will be very difficult to place during an active seizure. If IV access is not established and the seizure is prolonged, some medications (including diazepam) may be given intramuscularly (IM), rectally, or via endotracheal tube.

3. Observe seizure precautions (Table 27–1).

    Make the environment safe for the patient.

4. Have suction available at the bedside to handle secretions.
5. Observe aspiration precautions.
   - Place the patient in a lateral decubitus position. Remove dentures and other oral objects if easily done.
   - Have a nasal trumpet or an oral airway at the bedside.
6. Have an IV insertion tray available at the bedside if an IV is not already started.

    Have 1 L normal saline (NS) available, and have the IV tubing preflushed.

7. Have the means to perform a finger stick glucose test at the bedside.
8. Have the following medications available at the bedside:
   - **Thiamine 100-mg vial for IM injection**
   - **50% dextrose in water 50 mL for IV injection**
   - **Diazepam** (*Valium*) **20-mg vial for IV injection**
   - **Lorazepam** (*Ativan*) **4-mg vial for IV injection**

If the Patient Is Postictal

1. Check oximetry and deliver O_2 as necessary.
2. Check finger stick glucose test.
3. Observe seizure precautions; the patient may have another seizure.
4. Observe aspiration precautions.

TABLE 27–1 **Seizure Precautions**

1. Put bed in lowest position.
2. Put oral airway or nasal trumpet at the head of the bed.
3. Pad side rails of the bed, and put rails up while the patient is in bed.
4. Make suction and oxygen available at the bedside.
5. Allow out-of-bed privileges (including bathroom visits, showers, and baths) with supervision only.
6. Take axillary temperatures only.
7. Provide supervision when patient uses potentially dangerous objects such as razors or scissors.

Degree of Urgency

Patients who have unexpected seizure activity require immediate attention, whether they are actively having a seizure or they are in a postictal state.

ELEVATOR THOUGHTS

What are the causes of seizure?

Central Nervous System

1. Tumor
   The type of seizure noted depends somewhat on the location of the mass.
2. Stroke
   Old scarring from a previous stroke or infarct may be a seizure focus. Ongoing stroke with active injury may cause seizure.
3. Head injury
   As with previous stroke, other causes of neural tissue scarring can be a seizure focus.
4. Recent cranial surgery
   Seizures are common after neurosurgical procedures; these may be because of injury to the brain or because of complicating bleeding or infection. Often neurosurgeons are quite specific regarding the treatment of patients with seizures. Do not give any medications until specifically told to do so by the resident or the attending physician. If the seizure activity is a new symptom, an immediate head computed tomographic (CT) scan without contrast is often required.
5. Infection
   Infection may be from meningitis, abscess, or other causes of encephalitis.
6. Primary epilepsy
   Primary epilepsy includes grand mal or petit mal seizures. **Remember patients with a history of seizure disorders tend to have seizures.**
   A. Metabolic (the "hypos")
      (1) Hypoglycemia
      (2) Hyponatremia
      (3) Hypocalcemia
      (4) Hypomagnesemia
      (5) Hypoxia
      (6) Acid–base derangements
   B. Medications
      (1) Inappropriately low levels of antiepileptic medication
      (2) Meperidine (Demerol) overdose
         This is common in elderly patients, especially in the postoperative period.

(3) Benzodiazepine intoxication or withdrawal
(4) Barbiturate withdrawal
(5) Alcohol withdrawal
(6) High-dose penicillins
(7) Lidocaine intoxication
(8) Aminophylline intoxication
(9) Neuroleptic intoxication
(10) Isoniazid
(11) Lithium carbonate or other antidepressants
(12) Insulin
> Note that overmedication of diabetes mellitus with resultant hypoglycemia can be more dangerous than undermedication.

C. Other
(1) Organ failure (e.g., hepatic and renal)
(2) Cerebral vasculitis
(3) Other encephalopathy or degeneration (e.g., hypertension and human immunodeficiency virus)
(4) Cerebral edema
(5) Nonseizure or pseudoseizure

MAJOR THREAT TO LIFE

- Hypoxia
- Aspiration
- Ongoing central nervous system (CNS) injury; for example, extension of a stroke or a worsening cerebral edema
- Status epilepticus

IF THE PATIENT IS ACTIVELY HAVING A SEIZURE

BEDSIDE

Quick Look Test

Don't Panic. A seizure is disturbing to witness, but the initial therapy follows common sense. Most seizures are self-limited and will resolve in 2 to 5 minutes. Bear in mind that many of those around you will also be fighting the urge to panic.

Airway and Vital Signs

Most at risk is the patient's ability to breathe. Evaluate the airway. Clear foreign bodies and secretions from the mouth, and confirm good aeration of the lungs. Insert an oral airway, if possible, to facilitate respiration and allow suctioning. Do not attempt to insert the airway if it is difficult to do so or if force is required. It is often safer and easier to insert a nasal trumpet.

Evaluate oxygenation by pulse oximetry. Deliver O_2 by nasal cannula or mask as necessary. Because of the high metabolic rate during seizure activity, do not rely on arterial blood gas (ABG) data. Many of the abnormalities noted on ABGs will resolve without additional treatment in the postictal state.

Confirm a femoral pulse. Do not attempt to restrain the patient (this includes application of blood pressure cuffs).

Initial Management

1. Have someone notify the resident.
   New-onset seizures are medical emergencies.
2. Place the patient into the lateral decubitus position.
3. Keep the airway clear, and maintain oxygenation.
4. Observe the seizure activity.
   Note if the whole body is involved or just a portion of it. Is the patient conscious? Has the patient lost bowel or bladder control? This should be well documented later.
5. Make a safe environment.
   Make sure bed rails are up and padded. Clear unnecessary items away.
6. Wait.
   No other therapy is initially required for seizures that last up to 3 minutes and then spontaneously resolve.

If the Seizure Lasts Longer Than 3 Minutes:

1. Reevaluate airway and oxygenation status.
2. Confirm IV access.
   If no IV access is available, this is the time to start it. It may take several holders to immobilize a limb long enough to establish an IV. Speed of access is important, so defer to the most experienced hands.
3. Draw up to 20 mL of blood for hematology and chemistries.
   See Selective Physical Examination below.
4. Give **thiamine 100 mg by slow IV push over 3 to 5 minutes.**
5. Give **50% dextrose in water by slow IV push.**
   If hypoglycemia is the cause of the seizure, the activity may suddenly cease. Stop the infusion and switch to a 5% dextrose in water infusion. (Thiamine is administered before the glucose to avoid exacerbation of Wernicke's encephalopathy.) **If the seizure activity continues:**
6. Administer **diazepam** *(Valium)* **at a rate of 2 mg/minute IV until the seizure activity stops, to a total dose of 30 mg.** Whenever diazepam is administered, have resuscitation equipment nearby, because it is a respiratory depressant.
   Lorazepam *(Ativan)* **in doses of 2 to 4 mg IV push over 3 to 5 minutes** may be used instead of diazepam. Lorazepam

also has the advantage of being rapidly absorbed rectally and may be administered by this route, via red rubber catheter followed by an NS flush, if no IV access is available. **If the seizure activity continues despite 10 mg diazepam (one-half the total dose):**

7. Begin to administer **phenytoin (Dilantin).**

An additional IV will be required, because diazepam and phenytoin are not compatible in the same IV line, nor is phenytoin compatible with dextrose-containing solutions. **Phenytoin loading dose is 18 mg/kg by slow IV push, no faster than 25 to 50 mg/minute.** Administration of phenytoin is associated with hypotension and cardiac dysrhythmias. If the patient is not on a cardiac monitor, keep a finger on the femoral pulse during the infusion. If dysrhythmias are noted or femoral pulse weakens, slow the infusion rate. If the seizure stops during the administration of phenytoin, stop the diazepam infusion but continue the phenytoin load until complete. The phenytoin derivative, fosphenytoin, may be administered more rapidly. See Management below for further care.

8. This is a medical emergency.

If the patient continues to have the seizure for more than 30 minutes:

Status epilepticus is best treated by an intensivist or neurologist. Renotify the resident and arrange transfer to the intensive care unit for comprehensive care.

IF THE PATIENT HAS STOPPED HAVING THE SEIZURE

BEDSIDE

Quick Look Test

Immediately after grand mal seizures, patients are generally in a postictal state (unconscious). Some focal seizures are also associated with loss of consciousness (i.e., complex seizures).

Airway and Vital Signs

Check vital signs and pulse oximetry, and treat with O_2 as necessary. It is not unusual for a patient to become acidotic during a seizure, so temporary compensatory tachypnea is common.

Initial Management

1. Observe seizure and aspiration precautions.

The initial seizure may have stopped, but another seizure is possible. Make sure that the patient is in the lateral decubitus position and that the airway is clear. Suction the oral cavity as

necessary. Confirm that an oral airway or nasal trumpet is at the bedside.
2. Make sure the patient has adequate IV access.
3. Draw blood for appropriate chemistries (see Selective Physical Examination below).
4. Check a finger stick glucose test.
    Treat significant hypoglycemia (<60 mg/dL) with **50 mL 50% dextrose in water by slow IV infusion** or by constant administration of **5% dextrose solution.**
5. Be sure the environment is safe.

Selective History and Chart Review

Is there a condition that would predispose to seizure activity?

See Elevator Thoughts.

What was the quality of the seizure?

Did it start as focal and then secondarily generalize?

Focal or partial complex seizures are more likely of primary CNS cause than other causes.

Review the patient's medications.

Review recent laboratory data with emphasis on electrolyte, Ca^{2+}, Mg^{2+}, and glucose levels.

Review recent antiepileptic medication levels if any.

Selective Physical Examination

VS:	Repeat now.
MS:	Assess level of consciousness; for example, response to pain and voice.
HEENT:	Examine for mouth lacerations, chipped teeth, and facial fractures.
	Remove dentures and other foreign objects from mouth.
Resp:	Check for adequate aeration and evidence of aspiration.
Skin:	Check for bruising or trauma.
Extrem:	Examine for fractures.
Neuro:	When the patient is awake, do a complete neurologic examination.
	Are there any focal neurologic findings?
Wound:	Are sutures intact? Is there any new bleeding or discharge?
Tubes:	Confirm that any necessary tubes are still in place and are well secured.
Additional tests:	1. Serum glucose
	2. Electrolytes
	3. Calcium

4. Magnesium
5. Blood urea nitrogen and creatinine
6. Albumin
7. Levels of appropriate antiepileptic medications
8. Complete blood count and differential

MANAGEMENT

1. Endeavor to find the cause.
   Seizures are a symptom and not a diagnosis.
2. Treat any reversible causes such as hyponatremia or medication overdose.
3. Treat any identifiable injuries.
4. Maintain seizure and aspiration precautions and IV access for at least 24 to 48 hours past the last seizure.
5. Many seizures are self-limited and are single events (especially following head trauma). They often do not require long-term antiepileptic medication therapy.
6. Give antiepileptic medications, if needed.
   If further seizure activity is suspected, or if the patient has a known seizure disorder, make sure ongoing antiepileptic medication is within therapeutic range. If the patient is not currently taking antiepileptic medication, load with phenytoin as described above (if not already done). Once loaded with phenytoin, continue the dosing at 300 mg orally or IV per day, and adjust according to serum levels.
7. Order head CT scan without contrast immediately.
   If a structural lesion is suspected or if the seizure follows a neurosurgical procedure or recent head trauma, a head CT scan without contrast is indicated.
8. If meningitis is suspected, a lumbar puncture should be performed and appropriate antibiotic started as indicated. Make sure to rule out cerebral herniation with a head CT scan or adequate fundi visualization before the lumbar puncture.
9. Follow up in the morning with appropriate laboratory and medication level checks.
10. Perform neurologic checks every hour. Then decrease the interval as the patient stabilizes. Instruct the bedside caregiver to notify you if any change occurs. Document any changes in neurologic status.

Special Surgical Considerations

Preoperative Considerations

New seizure activity is a medical emergency and preempts any elective procedure planned. Any metabolic derangements should be corrected before surgery.

Postoperative Considerations

Postoperative neurosurgical patients and patients with traumatic brain injury should be evaluated with an immediate head CT scan for any unexpected seizure activity or significant change in mental status. Always clear, the use of antiepileptic medication with the resident or attending physician. These medications alter the sensorium and may mask symptoms that indicate a serious change in mental status.

Shortness of Breath

It is common to be asked to assess problems with a patient's breathing. Shortness of breath (SOB) has many causes. Most at risk to develop respiratory distress are patients who have had thoracic or upper abdominal procedures, elderly patients, obese patients, and poorly nourished patients.

PHONE CALL

Questions

1. How long has the patient had SOB?
2. Was the onset slow or rapid?
   A rapid onset suggests pneumothorax or pulmonary embolus.
3. Is the patient cyanotic?
4. Is the patient already on oxygen (O_2)? What is the arterial hemoglobin saturation (SaO_2)?
5. Does the patient have a history of chronic obstructive pulmonary disease (COPD)?
   If the patient retains carbon dioxide (CO_2), the amount of oxygen that may be delivered is affected.
6. Has the patient undergone a surgical procedure, and if so, how long ago?
   Be especially mindful after placement of central lines.
7. Are there any other symptoms such as chest pain, cough, or fever?
8. Are there any changes in vital signs?

Orders

1. Measure SaO_2 by pulse oximetry if not already done.
   As an alternative, have an arterial blood gas (ABG) kit at the bedside. This will give a rapid indication of the arterial partial pressure of oxygen (PaO_2).
2. Deliver oxygen as necessary.
   If the patient does not retain CO_2, O_2 may be safely delivered at a rate that keeps the O_2 saturation at greater than or equal to 93%. See Table 28–1 for various regimens of O_2 delivery.

3. If the patient has a history of reactive airway disease (RAD) (COPD or asthma), order bronchodilator treatment if it has been more than 2 hours since the last treatment (Table 28–2).

TABLE 28–1 **Oxygen Delivery Techniques**

System	Recommended Flow	Maximum FiO_2	Humidification	Control of FiO_2
Room air	N/A	0.28	Poor	N/A
Nasal cannula	1–6 L/min	0.44	Poor	Poor
Open face mask	8–10 L/min	0.44	Good	Good
Venturi mask	10 L/min	0.45	Poor	Great
Tight face mask	8–10 L/min	0.60	Poor	Good
Non-rebreather mask	10 L/min	1	Poor	Good
Endotracheal tube	N/A	1	Great	Great

FiO_2, fraction of oxygen in inspired air.

TABLE 28–2 **Bronchodilator Therapies to Control Reactive Airway Disease**

Generic	Trade	Dosage	Interval
Beta-2 Agonists			
Albuterol	Proventil, Ventolin	2.5–5 mg in 3 mL NS	Every 4–6 hr
		2 puffs of MDI	Every 4–6 hr
		2–4 mg PO	Every 4–8 hr
Fenoterol	Berotec	0.5–1.0 mg in 3 mL NS	Every 4–6 hr
Isoetharine	Bronkosol	0.3 mg in 2.7 mL NS	Every 4–6 hr
		2 puffs of MDI	Every 4–6 hr
Metaproterenol	Alupent, Metaprel	0.3 mg in 2.7 mL NS	Every 4–6 hr
		2 puffs of MDI	Every 4–6 hr
		10 mg PO	Every 6 hr
Terbutaline	Brethaire, Bricanyl	0.25–0.5 mg in 2.6 mL NS	Every 6–8 hr
		2 puffs of MDI	Every 6–8 hr
		2.5–5 mg PO	Every 6–8 hr
Anticholinergics			
Ipratropium Bromide	Atrovent	0.5 mg in 3 mL NS	Every 6–8 hr
		2 puffs of MDI	Every 6 hr
Atropine		0.5–1 mg in 3 mL NS	Every 8 hr

Continued

TABLE 28–2 **Bronchodilator Therapies to Control Reactive Airway Disease–Cont'd**

Generic	Trade	Dosage	Interval
Injectable			
Terbutaline		0.25–0.5 mg IM	Every 6–8 hr
Epinephrine (1:1000)		0.25–0.5 mg IM	Every 8–12 hr
Aminophylline		5 mg/kg IV over 20–30 min	
Loading		0.6–0.9 mg/kg/hr IV (maintain levels at 10–20 mcg/mL)	
Maintenance		6 mg/kg every 12 hr of the long-acting preparation	
PO form			

Medication	IV Dose	PO Dose	Dose Equivalency*
Steroids			
Hydrocortisone	250 mg bolus, then 3–5 mg/kg divided every 6 hr	—	1
Methylpred-nisolone	1–1.5 mg/kg	—	5
Prednisone	—	1–1.5 mg/kg	4
Dexamethasone	0.1–0.2 mg/kg	5–10 mg	25–30

*Glucocorticoid potency compared with hydrocortisone milligram per milligram.
NS, normal saline; MDI, metered dose inhaler; PO, orally; IM, intramusculary; IV, intravenously.

Degree of Urgency

The patient must be evaluated immediately.

ELEVATOR THOUGHTS

What are the causes of shortness of breath?

Cardiovascular Causes

1. CHF
2. Pulmonary embolism
3. Cardiac tamponade

Pulmonary Causes

1. Atelectasis (usually 24 to 48 hours after a surgical procedure)

2. RAD (e.g., COPD, asthma, or gastroesophageal [GE] reflux)
3. Upper airway obstruction
4. Pneumothorax
5. Pleural effusion
6. Pneumonia
7. Aspiration of gastric contents

Miscellaneous Causes

1. Anxiety
2. Marked abdominal distention

MAJOR THREAT TO LIFE

- Hypoxia
- Myocardial infarction, as a cause of SOB or as a sequela of other causes of SOB
- Pulmonary embolism
- Cardiac tamponade

BEDSIDE

Quick Look Test

Hypoxia is evident by agitation and cyanosis. Patients with significant hypoxia will appear anxious and ill. CO_2 retention is evident by lethargy or obtundation.

Airway and Vital Signs

Confirm the patency of the upper airway. Remove any oral obstruction such as dentures or foreign bodies. Tachypnea (respiration rate [RR] >20 breaths/minute) will be present if hypoxia, anxiety, pain, or acidosis is present. Slow RRs (<12 breaths/minute) indicate a depression of the central nervous system (CNS) with medications (such as opiates) or primary cerebral lesion. If there is a cardiac cause, tachycardia or arrhythmia may also be present. Fever denotes an infectious cause but may also be present with atelectasis or pulmonary embolism. A drop in blood pressure (BP) may indicate pulmonary embolism, tension pneumothorax, congestive heart failure (CHF), or sepsis.

IF THE PATIENT IS HYPOXIC

Initial Management

1. Deliver adequate O_2.
     The delivery technique will vary by the situation. The factors that determine the delivery technique are as follows:
     - Amount of oxygen needed

- Need for precise control of fraction of oxygen in inspired air (FiO_2)
- Need for humidification
- Patient comfort

See Table 28–1. Remember that if the patient has a history of COPD and retains CO_2, the amount of O_2 delivered should be limited. Patients with baseline high partial pressure of carbon dioxide (PCO_2) levels do not have a hypercapnic drive for respiration and must rely on their hypoxic drive. FiO_2 levels at greater than 0.28 may decrease their drive to breathe.

2. Evaluate the O_2 delivery by following pulse oximetry and periodic ABGs.

Use the minimum amount of O_2 necessary to achieve the desired oxygenation. Pulse oximetry gives a good estimate of the arterial hemoglobin saturation (SaO_2), which is generally linked to the PaO_2 (Fig. 28–1).

Remember, however, that the pulse oximeter will not evaluate PCO_2, bicarbonate ion (HCO_3), or pH of the serum.

3. Be ready to resuscitate.

If the patient is severely hypoxic or in obvious distress, have a resuscitation cart nearby. Make sure the patient has a patent intravenous (IV) line.

Selective History and Chart Review

Cardiovascular Causes

1. Congestive heart failure

Are there symptoms of orthopnea or paroxysmal nocturnal dyspnea? Is there evidence of fluid overload from overzealous resuscitation or the mobilization of third-space fluids? CHF is a symptom, not a disease. **A cause must be sought.** Possible causes are listed in Table 28–3. Left-sided heart failure presents as pulmonary edema and SOB. Right-sided heart failure

Figure 28–1 Approximate relationship between PaO_2 and SaO_2.

TABLE 28–3 **Causes of Congestive Heart Failure**

Myocardial infarction
Hypertension
Valvular heart disease
Congenital heart disease
Pericardial disease
Cardiomyopathy
Pulmonary embolism
Fluid overload
Sodium retention or salt overload
Dysrhythmia
Beta-blockade or other cardiac depressant
Renal disease
Anemia
Fever and infection
Pregnancy
Noncompliance with medications or diet

presents as peripheral edema and organomegaly. Most often, components of both are present.

2. Pulmonary embolism

Is the patient postoperative? Most perioperative deep vein thromboses of significance form intraoperatively on the operating table and are best prevented by preoperative application of support (thromboembolic disease [TED]) stockings and sequential compression boots. Were support stockings and sequential compression boots in place during surgery? Are they in place now? Is there a history of prior thromboembolic phenomena?

Is the patient hypercoagulable (is there malignancy, inflammatory bowel disease, nephrotic syndrome, use of oral contraceptive pills, or deficiency of antithrombin III, protein C, or protein S)? Are there other risk factors for pulmonary embolism (prolonged bed rest, immobile limb, obesity, CHF, pregnancy, or vein trauma)? Do not expect to find the classic triad of chest pain, hemoptysis, and SOB. Rarely are they all present simultaneously.

3. Tamponade

Was there a recent central line placement? Is there a history of penetrating chest trauma? Did the patient have cardial surgery?

Pulmonary Causes

1. Atelectasis

This a very common cause of postoperative SOB, hypoxia, and fever. Is the patient postoperative or taking pain medication?

2. Reactive airway disease

Is there a history of COPD, asthma, or GE reflux? COPD may be present as chronic bronchitis (production of mucus on most days for 3 months of a year in 2 consecutive years) or as emphysema, or it may have components of both. Cigarette smoking is strongly linked with COPD. Is there a history of exposure to a specific asthma trigger (respiratory infection, irritant, allergen, or medication such as aspirin or beta-blocker)?

Is the patient taking steroids? Has the patient ever required mechanical ventilation in the past?

3. Upper airway obstruction

Is there a history of aspiration or sleep apnea? Causes include laryngeal edema, epiglottitis, vocal cord paralysis, recent extubation, and foreign body.

4. Pneumothorax

Was there a recent central line placement or thoracic surgery? Has a chest tube been removed recently?

Is there a history of penetrating chest trauma or spontaneous pneumothorax?

5. Pleural effusion

Is there a history of pulmonary infection or abscess? Other risk factors are listed in Table 28–4.

6. Pneumonia

Risk factors include advanced age, immunosuppression, prolonged hospitalization, mechanical ventilation, aspiration of foodstuffs or vomitus, and preexisting cardiac, pulmonary, or CNS disease.

7. Aspiration of gastric contents

This may lead to pneumonia or RAD symptoms. Is there decreased level of consciousness, hiatal hernia, vomiting, nasogastric (NG) tube in place, or history of chronic reflux?

TABLE 28–4 **Causes of Pleural Effusions**

Congestive heart failure
Organ failure (liver and kidney)
Nephrotic syndrome
Malignancy
Pulmonary infection
Abdominal abscess
Collagen vascular disease
Asbestos exposure
Chylothorax
Pancreatitis
Superior vena cava syndrome
Peritoneal dialysis
Dressler syndrome
Meigs syndrome

Miscellaneous Causes

1. Anxiety
   Is there a history of panic disorder?
2. Marked abdominal distention
   Is there a history of liver failure, other forms of ascites, or bowel obstruction? Has there been any recent gastrointestinal (GI) surgery? Is an NG tube in place? Is it properly functioning?

Selective Physical Examination

VS:	Repeat now; tachycardia (CHF and pulmonary embolus)
	Tachypnea (CHF)
	Fever/chills (atelectasis and pneumonia)
MS:	Agitation (hypoxia) and lethargy (hypercapnia)
HEENT:	Upper airway obstruction (foreign body)
	Elevated jugular venous distention (JVD) (tamponade, CHF, RAD, and pneumothorax)
	Deviated trachea (pneumothorax)
CVS:	Arrhythmia (CHF and pulmonary embolus)
	S_3 (this is the most specific finding for CHF)
	Loud P_2 (RAD)
	Cardiac murmur (CHF)
Resp:	Rales (CHF)
	Decreased aeration (pleural effusion or pneumothorax)
	Pleuritic chest pain (pneumonia)
	Pleural friction rub (pulmonary embolus)
	Pulmonary consolidation (pulmonary embolus or pneumonia)
	Pleural effusion (CHF, pulmonary embolus, and pneumonia)
	Use of accessory respiratory muscles (RAD)
	Wheezing (CHF, RAD, pneumonia, and pulmonary embolism)
	Prolonged expiratory phase (RAD)
Abd:	Distention and ascites (CHF and bowel obstruction)
	Use of abdominal musculature to breathe
	Hepatomegaly (CHF)
Skin:	Cyanosis (hypoxia and RAD)

Extrem:	Ankle or presacral edema (CHF) Tender or red calf (thromboembolism)
Tubes:	Chest tube in place or recent chest tube removal NG tube in place Recent central venous line placement
Special examinations:	Measurement of pulsus paradoxus may give an indication of the severity of airflow obstruction in RAD. To measure pulsus paradoxus, take a routine BP. Inflate the cuff to 30 mm Hg above the systolic pressure and slowly release. Note the BP at which Korotkoff's sounds are first noted. These sounds are initially heard only with exhalation. Then note the pressures at which the Korotkoff's sounds are audible during both inhalation and exhalation. The pulse will seem to double. If the difference between these two pressures is greater than 10 mm Hg (pulsus paradoxus), there is a significant obstruction to airflow. This is also seen in significant cardiac output obstruction such as pulmonary embolus or tamponade.
Additional tests:	1. CXR: This may be done at the bedside immediately if necessary; see Table 28–5 for significant findings 2. ABG: Gives rapid assessment of serum PaO_2, PCO_2, pH, and a calculation of HCO_3^- 3. CBC: Evaluate hemoglobin and hematocrit 4. ECG: Pulmonary embolism may give findings of tachycardia, dysrhythmia, or evidence of right ventricular strain: S1, Q3, right axis deviation, and right bundle branch block. Peaked or inverted T waves, or ST changes may indicate myocardial infarction.

MANAGEMENT

Congestive Heart Failure

1. Deliver oxygen as required.
2. Establish IV access.

TABLE 28-5 Radiographic Findings in Common Etiologies of Shortness of Breath

Congestive Heart Failure

Cardiomegaly
Perihilar congestion
Bilateral interstitial or alveolar infiltrates
Cephalization of flow (redistribution of lung markings)
Kerley's B lines
Pleural effusion

Atelectasis

Volume loss
Basilar streaking or infiltrates
(May be normal)

Pulmonary embolism

Atelectasis
Unilateral wedge infiltrate
Unilateral pleural effusion
Raised hemidiaphragm
(May be normal)

Pneumothorax

(Exhalation film most useful)
Mediastinal shift (with tension pneumothorax)
Unilateral hyperaeration
Loss of lung tissue in hemithorax

Pneumonia

Infiltrates (unilateral, bilateral, patch, and lobar)
Pleural effusion
(May be unremarkable until the patient is fully hydrated)

Reactive Airway Disease

Hyperinflation of the lungs
Flattened diaphragms
Increased anterior–posterior diameter
Occasional infiltrates (with associated pneumonias, atelectasis, pneumothorax, or pneumomediastinum)

Run 5% dextrose in water to keep the vein open.

3. Sit the patient up to allow maximum aeration of the lungs.
4. Give **morphine sulfate 2 to 4 mg IV every 5 to 10 minutes to 10 to 12 mg,** which will pool the blood in the splanchnic circulation and decrease pulmonary edema.

Hold morphine sulfate treatment if symptoms of decreased respiratory drive or hypotension are apparent. Reverse the effects of morphine sulfate as necessary with **naloxone hydrochloride 0.2 to 2 mg IV, intramuscularly (IM), or subcutaneously (SC) to a total of 10 mg.** Note that the half-life of naloxone is shorter than that of most narcotics and that repeat doses may be necessary.

5. Give nitroglycerin (NTG), as follows:
   - **Ointment:** 2.5 to 5 cm topically every 4 hours or
   - **Tablets:** 0.3 to 0.6 mcg sublingually (SL) every 5 minutes or
   - **Spray:** 1 puff SL every 15 minutes

   Hold NTG for systolic blood pressure (SBP) of less than 90 mm Hg. Adequate function of NTG is generally confirmed by a headache, which usually responds to **acetaminophen (Tylenol and others) 650 to 1000 mg orally (PO) or rectally (PR) every 4 hours as necessary.**

6. Give diuretic therapy, as follows:
   - **Furosemide** *(Lasix)* **20 to 80 mg IV over 2 to 5 minutes.**

   The dose may be doubled and administered **every hour as needed to a total dose of 400 mg** if no response is noted. Be cautious in giving large doses of furosemide. Doses of greater than 100 mg should be **given slowly** (<4 mg/minute) to avoid ototoxicity. Also use caution when used in conjunction with aminoglycoside antibiotics.
   - **Hydrochlorothiazide 25 to 50 mg PO** (a thiazide diuretic) or **metolazone** *(Zaroxolyn)* **5 to 10 mg PO** may be added once or twice a day to furosemide therapy (a loop diuretic) for more effective diuresis.

   If furosemide therapy is ineffective, consider use of **ethacrynic acid** *(Edecrin)* **50 mg IV every hour for 2 doses** or **bumetanide** *(Bumex)* **1 to 10 mg IV over 1 to 2 minutes.** Monitor diuretic therapy with intake/output measurements (I/Os), frequent weight checks, and serum electrolyte evaluations. Replace K^+ as necessary.

7. Restrict sodium in the diet and in the IV fluids.
8. Endeavor to find a cause. CHF is a symptom complex, not a diagnosis.

Pulmonary Embolism

1. Deliver oxygen as required
2. Confirm the diagnosis

   If the patient is stable, obtain a CT angiogram.

   A ventilation-perfusion (V/Q) scan may also be obtained. A **high-probability** V/Q scan confirms pulmonary embolism and indicates the need for anticoagulation. A **normal** V/Q scan eliminates the possibility of pulmonary embolism. An **intermediate** or **low-probability** V/Q scan is not as helpful, and anticoagulation must be started or continued based on the clinical condition of the patient. Pulmonary angiography is useful in settings of equivocal V/Q scans or to implement local thrombolytic therapy.

3. Anticoagulate

   Anticoagulation must be started immediately (i.e., before the CT angiography scan) if the clinical suspicion is high. It may always be stopped later if the scan is normal. Proceed as follows:

a. Ensure that the patient has no potential bleeding problem (other bleeding diathesis, tumor, peptic ulcer, fresh surgical wounds, or stroke).

   If contraindications to immediate anticoagulation are present, confirm the pulmonary embolus first with a CT angiogram. Options other than anticoagulation may be available, such as interruption of the inferior vena cava with a filter or by direct ligation or surgical removal of the existing clot.

   If there are no contraindications:

b. Draw blood for complete blood count (CBC), prothrombin time (PT), partial thromboplastin time (PTT), and platelets.

c. Bolus with **heparin 100 U/kg IV.**

   Follow with a maintenance administration of **heparin** at **1000 to 1600 U/hour IV.** Heparin orders should be written in very specific language (e.g., 25,000 U per 500 mL of 5% dextrose in water to run at 20 mL/hour so as to deliver 1000 U/hour). Make sure to double-check dosages and rates.

d. Maintain the PTT in a therapeutic range (generally 1.8 to 2.8 times normal, but the attending physician may have a specific PTT in mind; ask if you are unsure). Some hospitals follow anti-X_a levels.

e. Follow each change in the rate of heparin in 4 to 6 hours with a PTT or factor X_a level.

   When stable, PT, PTT, factor X_a levels, or international normalized ratios (INRs) may be checked daily. Platelet counts should be ordered at 2- to 3-day intervals to assess for heparin-induced thrombocytopenia. This generally occurs after 7 days of heparin therapy and is associated with the appearance of immunoglobulin G (IgG) in the serum. Treatment includes discontinuation of heparin and conversion to another form of anticoagulation (PO warfarin or IV dextran).

f. If tolerated, heparin should be continued for at least 5 days.

g. On the first or second day, begin **warfarin (Coumadin) therapy 10 mg PO.** Titrate the dose to achieve a therapeutic increase in the PT (generally 1.3 to 1.5 times normal, with an INR in the 2 to 3 range; again, check with the attending physician for a specific number). Decrease the daily warfarin dose as a therapeutic PT is reached.

h. Attainment of a therapeutic PT/INR range will take about 5 days. When therapeutic range has been maintained for 48 to 72 hours, the heparin may be discontinued.

    i. Review the patient's medication list for any possible interactions with warfarin or heparin.

    j. Avoid IM injections or nonsteroidal anti-inflammatory drug (NSAID)-containing medications, sulfinpyrazone, dipyridamole, or thrombolytic agents while taking anticoagulants.

    k. Anticoagulation with warfarin should be maintained for at least 6 to 12 weeks with PT/INR checks every 1 to 2 weeks when stable.

    l. Remember some basic rules when using anticoagulation:

        Heparin primarily prolongs the **PTT** but also prolongs the PT; a therapeutic PTT range due to heparin will also cause a 1- to 3-second increase in the PT.

        Warfarin primarily prolongs the **PT** but also prolongs the PTT; this effect is due to the effect on factors IX and X and prothrombin and is seen after a week of therapy.

        Always remember to order both PT and PTT when the patient is taking both warfarin and heparin.

    m. Low-molecular weight heparin in therapeutic doses may also be used.

4. Find the source.

    Most pulmonary emboli originate in the lower extremities. Deep vein clots may be present in the absence of thrombophlebitis. Clinical suspicion is heightened by the presence of *Homan's* sign (pain behind the knee with dorsiflexion of the foot) or a swollen, tender leg. Studies to evaluate the deep venous system include noninvasive techniques such as Doppler ultrasonography and impedance plethysmography. Doppler ultrasonography is good for completely occluded veins but is limited in its evaluation of partially occluded veins or in settings of venous collateralization or edema. Impedance plethysmography is especially good at evaluation of the iliofemoral and popliteal systems but is limited in its ability to localize disease. Invasive techniques include IV contrast or radioisotope venography.

5. Thrombolysis.

    In selected patients, thrombolysis with streptokinase or urokinase may be indicated. **Thrombolysis should not be done on a postoperative patient, because there is a significant risk of bleeding or anastomotic leak.** If appropriate, this technique should be done by those specifically trained in the technique, such as interventional radiologists.

Tamponade

1. Deliver oxygen as required.
2. Confirm the diagnosis.

This potentially fatal complication usually follows penetrating trauma to the chest, thoracic surgery, or, rarely, central line placement. It may also be slowly progressive in settings of pericarditis. Findings in tamponade include progressive cardiac outflow obstruction with *Beck's triad* of distended neck veins, muffled heart sounds, and decreased BP. *Kussmaul's* sign of a paradoxical increase in JVD with inspiration may also be present. Pulsus paradoxus should be present at 10 to 15 mm Hg. Chest x-ray (CXR) may not be helpful, as the average tamponade is only about 200 mL in volume and does not significantly increase the size of the heart silhouette. Occasionally the "water bottle" sign is present, which suggests pericardial effusion.

Electrocardiography (ECG) is also nonspecific. Emergency echo is the most specific for diagnosis of tamponade.

3. Volume load.

Increasing the preload is important to maintain adequate cardiac output. Give a 1-L bolus of NS.

4. Perform emergent pericardiocentesis.

If clinical suspicion is high, diagnosis and treatment may be affected by pericardiocentesis. This is a code situation and should be done at the bedside only if the patient has hemodynamic collapse. Notify your resident immediately. Defer to the most experienced person. Contact the intensive care unit (ICU) or cardiac care unit (CCU) for assistance in the procedure.

Emergency Pericardiocentesis Technique (Sterile)

1. Prepare the patient.
   In an emergency situation, perform the procedure first when medically necessary.
   a. Explain the procedure.
   b. Explain the risks and alternatives.
   c. Answer any questions.
   d. Have a consent form prepared and signed.
2. Position the patient.
   The patient should be on continuous ECG monitoring and is best placed in a 30-degree semi-Fowler position, if possible. Attach a V lead to the pericardiocentesis needle for greater sensitivity. An insulated wire with alligator clips at each end works well.
3. Prepare the skin.
   a. Use sterile technique, and wear sterile gloves, mask, and gown.
   b. Provide local skin preparation and draping over the xiphoid area.
   c. Perform local infiltration with 1% to 2% lidocaine into the skin at the entry site.

4. Insert the needle.
   a. Puncture the skin 2 cm below the costal margin to the left adjacent to the xiphoid with a blade (see Fig. 32–1).
   b. Direct the needle upward and posterior at a 45-degree angle for 4 to 5 cm.

      A good target at which to aim is the right or left scapular tip; the right is preferable because the risk of right ventricular penetration is lessened.
   c. Aspirate continuously as the needle is advanced.

      Continue to advance the needle until fluid is encountered, until cardiac pulsations are noticeable, or until ST elevation is noted on the ECG monitor. You may experience the sensation of entering a cavity.

5. Remove blood, if possible.
   a. Most blood in a hemopericardium is clotted, so only 5 to 10 mL usually is removable.
   b. If 20 mL or more is easily withdrawn, then the needle most likely is in the right ventricle.
   c. A small aspiration of fluid often makes a big difference in cardiac function.
   d. If blood is encountered and is clotted or if no hemodynamic change is apparent after aspiration, the patient may need a thoracotomy or local pericardial window excision.

6. If not frank blood, send fluid efflux to the laboratory.

   The following studies may be indicated (in trauma settings, where only blood is aspirated, no studies are indicated):
   a. Gram stain
   b. Culture (bacterial, fungal, and mycobacterial)
   c. Hematological cell count
   d. Cytology
   e. Protein
   f. Glucose
   g. Other studies as indicated (rheumatoid factor, antinuclear antibodies, or complement levels)

7. Document the procedure.

Complications of Emergency Pericardiocentesis

1. Lack of resolution of the problem

   If persistent hemodynamic compromise is present despite adequate attempt at pericardiocentesis
   a. Reconfirm the diagnosis.
   b. Perform an emergency thoracotomy or local pericardial window excision

2. Penetration of the myocardial wall
3. Myocardial infarction
4. Pneumothorax
5. Bowel perforation

Atelectasis

1. Deliver oxygen as required.
   Maintain the lowest FiO_2 necessary.
2. Alter the patient's pain medication as necessary to achieve a better balance between adequate relief and somnolence.
   The patient must be able to breathe deeply, ambulate, and cough effectively.
3. Order assisted ambulation.
   Make sure the patient is adequately mobilized. Order ambulation with assistance, if necessary.
4. Stimulate and encourage coughing.
   This requires adequate pain relief and instruction to the patient on how to support the wound to avoid undue discomfort. Encourage incentive spirometry.
5. Vigorous chest physiotherapy (CPT) may be useful in patients with copious secretions or COPD.
6. Bronchodilators may be useful for those patients with a component of RAD (see Table 28–2).
7. Order supplemental nutrition as necessary.
8. Consider bronchoscopy.
   On occasion, severe atelectasis responds to bronchoscopy, especially where there is segmental or large regions of collapse.

Reactive Airway Disease (Asthma and COPD)

1. Supply oxygen as necessary.
   Use the minimum FiO_2 required to maintain an SaO_2 at greater than 93%.
2. Order bronchodilators as outlined in Table 28–2.
   With adequate cardiac monitoring and precautions, the beta-2 agonists may be given as frequently as every 1 to 2 hours, as needed. Also, some benefit may be derived from alternating between different types of beta-2 agonists in a combined therapy approach. Note that steroids should be started early, as their effects may not be noticed for many hours after initiation of therapy. Steroid therapy in excess of 15 days should be slowly tapered over several days.
3. Mobilize secretions with CPT.
4. Maintain adequate hydration.
5. Look for medications that impair smooth muscle responsiveness to beta-2 agonists, such as beta-blockers or cholinergics.
6. Look for and treat triggers to asthma, as follows:
   - Respiratory infection (this is the most common)
   - Irritation (including cigarette smoke)
   - Drugs (aspirin and beta-blockers)
   - GE reflux
7. Order ventilator support as indicated for respiratory failure.

Pneumothorax

1. Confirm the diagnosis.

    Findings may include decreased breath sounds and hyper-resonance of the hemithorax, deviation of the trachea, hypoxia, and chest pain. In cases of tension pneumothorax, progressive cardiac outflow obstruction is apparent.

2. Give O_2 at 100%.

    Many small pneumothoraces will resolve spontaneously by increasing the FiO_2. This acts by replacing the air in the pleural space with oxygen, which is absorbed through the tissues much more rapidly than nitrogen.

3. Treat tension pneumothorax with immediate insertion of an 18-gauge needle into the second intercostal space anteriorly at the midclavicular line on the affected side.

    This will confirm the diagnosis and allow some relief of symptoms until adequate chest tube drainage can be implemented.

4. Place a tube thoracostomy.

    If the air leak is small, a small to moderately sized chest tube (12–24 Fr) may be placed in an anterior position from a high intercostal space in the midaxillary line. Occasionally, it is preferable to place the tube in the second intercostal space in the midclavicular line anteriorly to facilitate patient comfort.

    Placement and management of chest tubes is outlined in Chapter 30. Confirm tube placement by immediate bedside upright posterior-to-anterior and lateral CXR. Reposition as necessary. Daily CXRs are recommended to follow the course of therapy and to confirm continued adequate placement of the tube.

    The tube insertion site will remain uncomfortable until the tube is removed; make sure the patient has adequate pain relief.

    Pulmonary toilet is important in a patient with chest tubes. Make an incentive spirometer available, and instruct the patient as to its use and importance.

5. Know when to go to the operating room (OR).

    Pneumothoraces that do not respond to tube thoracostomy may require surgical repair.

Pleural Effusion

1. Deliver oxygen as required.

2. Confirm the diagnosis by CXR and thoracentesis. A lateral decubitus CXR will help confirm that the fluid is free flowing and not loculated.

3. Determine the cause.

    See Table 28–4. The treatment will include reversal of the underlying condition.

4. Perform thoracentesis.

    If the patient is in respiratory distress, a thoracentesis will significantly improve the patient's ability to oxygenate by increasing lung inflation. Do not remove (tap) more than 1500 mL of fluid in a single procedure to avoid reinflation pulmonary edema. A sample of the pleural fluid should be sent to the laboratory for the following studies as indicated:

Gram stain, cultures (aerobic and anaerobic bacterial, fungal, and mycoplasma), Ziehl–Neelsen (ZN) stain and TB culture, cell count and differential lactate dehydrogenase (LDH), protein glucose cytology for malignant cells, and other studies as appropriate (amylase, triglycerides, pH, rheumatoid factor, antinuclear antibodies, or complement levels).

A simultaneous serum LDH, protein, and glucose should be drawn to compare with the results of the pleural fluid.

5. Tube thoracostomy.

If frequent taps are required for recurrent accumulation of fluid, such as in chylothorax, consider placement of a moderately sized (25–28 Fr) chest tube (see Chapter 30). Pleurodesis may be necessary.

Pneumonia

1. Deliver oxygen as required.
2. Identify the organism.

Perform a Gram stain on the sputum and send for culture. Obtain special stains as necessary (ZN stain, TB culture, and immunofluorescence staining for *Pneumocystis carinii* in human immunodeficiency virus-positive patients). Sputum may be induced with nasotracheal suction if a sample is difficult to obtain.

3. Order blood cultures ×2.

Order CBC and differential.

4. Begin empirical antibiotic treatment if indicated (Table 28–6).

Focus the therapy based on Gram stain and culture results when available.

5. Order chest physical therapy.
6. Perform thoracentesis, if an effusion is present.

Evaluate the pleural fluid as described above.

Aspiration of Gastric Contents

Patients with impaired mental status or severe GERD or who are vomiting are at risk for aspiration of gastric contents. This results in chemical pneumonitis as well as bacterial pneumonia. Treat as in pneumonia (see earlier).

SPECIAL SURGICAL CONSIDERATIONS

Preoperative Considerations

Severe SOB indicates the new onset or exacerbation of a problem that may affect a scheduled procedure.

TABLE 28–6 **Empirical Treatment for Suspected Pneumonia**

Community Acquired

Streptococcus pneumoniae	Penicillin G 1–2 million U IV every 4–6 hr, or ampicillin 1 g PO or IV every 6 hr, or 1st-generation cephalosporin
Haemophilus influenzae *Mycoplasma pneumoniae* Legionella pneumophila	Erythromycin 500 mg PO or IV* every 6 hr

Complex Pneumonia

Complex pneumoniae include those acquired in the hospital or nursing homes, those associated with COPD, those occurring in the elderly or those previously treated with antibiotics. In addition to the community-acquired infection coverage listed above, consider treatment for Gram-negative organisms, mouth flora, and *Staphalococcus aureus*

Consider:	Ceftriaxone 1–2 gm IV each day, plus Erythromycin 500 mg PO or IV every 6 hr Levofloxacin 250–500 mg PO or IV daily Meropenem 500 to 1000 mg PO of IV every 8 hr

If *Pseudomonas aeruginosa* is cultured, or if multiple resistant organisms are present, consider any TWO of the following:

	Ceftazidime 1–2 g IV or IM every 8 hr Piperacillin 6–18 g/day in 4 to 6 divided doses Imipenem/cilastin 500 mg every 6–8 hr Meropenem 500–1000 mg PO or IV every 8 hr Gentamicin 5–7 mg/kg IV daily

Aspiration

Consider in patients who have decreased mental status or defective cough or gag reflex. Treat with antibiotics only if there are associated symptoms of bacterial disease (e.g., fever, leukocytosis, and purulent sputum)

Mouth anaerobes	Penicillin G 2 million U IV every 4 hr Clindamycin 300–600 mg PO or IV every 6 hr

Alcoholic Associated

In addition to organisms associated with aspiration pneumonia, alcoholic patients also have a high incidence of *Klebsiella pneumoniae*, which is treated with double antibiotic therapy as listed above for complex pneumoniae, according to the hospital flora sensitivities

HIV Positive

Patients with HIV may be infected with *Pneumocystis carinii*, and also with a variety of bacterial organisms such as *S. pneumonia* or *H. influenza*. In addition, mycobacteria and fungi may also require treatment

TABLE 28–6 **Empirical Treatment for Suspected Pneumonia—***Continued*

Pneumocystis carinii[†]	
	Trimethoprim sulfamethoxazole (TMP SMX) 15–20 mg/kg (based on TMP) IV every 6–8 hr
	Pentamidine isethionate[‡] 4 mg/kg IV or IM every day

[*]Administration of IV erythromycin is associated with severe venous burning and thrombophlebitis. Dilute the dose in 500 mL NS and run slowly over 6 hr.

Gentamicin and other aminoglycoside medications are nephrotoxic and ototoxic. They should have their maintenance doses adjusted based on serum peak and trough levels, with special care with their use in patients with renal insufficiency.

[†]If *Pneumocystis carinii* is suspected, then diagnosis should be made by bronchoscopy. Infectious disease consultation is advisable when managing the infections of HIV-positive patients.

[‡]Pentamidine administration is associated with hypotension, tachycardia, nausea, vomiting, and hyperemia. Side effects may be limited by dilution in 500 mL 5% dextrose in water and by administration over 2 to 4 hours. Other associated derangements include hyperkalemia, hypocalcemia, megaloblastic anemia, leukopenia, thrombocytopenia, hyperglycemia or hypoglycemia, increased LFTs, and dose-related nephrotoxicity.

IV, intravenously; PO, orally; COPD, chronic obstructive pulmonary disease; IM, intramuscularly; ICU, intensive care unit; CCU, cardiac care unit; HIV, human immunodeficiency virus; NS, normal saline; LFT, liver function test.

Steps that aid in the prevention of specific etiologies of postoperative SOB are as follows:

Pulmonary Embolism

1. All patients scheduled to undergo general anesthesia should have sequential compression devices in place before induction.
2. Patients with a history of thromboembolic phenomena may benefit from additional treatment with **low-dose heparin 5000 U SC every 8 hours before and after surgery** or **low-molecular-weight heparin.**

Discuss this with the attending surgeon before ordering this therapy.

As an alternative, low-dose warfarin may be given in doses sufficient to maintain the PT in the upper normal range (i.e., prolonged by 1 to 3 seconds) for 10 to 14 days before surgery. Immediately after surgery, the warfarin dose is doubled to maintain the PT in the 1.5 times normal range. This therapy decreases the incidence of postoperative thromboembolism and is not associated with a significantly increased risk of postoperative bleeding.

Atelectasis

The most important preventive measure is patient education. Make sure the patient understands the importance of ambulation, incentive spirometry, and cough. Treat postoperative pain adequately enough to support these activities. Encourage incentive spirometry use.

Reactive Airway Disease

1. Patients with known asthma or COPD must be stable and prepared for surgery. Review with the patient possible modalities for postoperative care such as nebulizer treatments, incentive spirometry, and medication use.
2. Patients who are on chronic steroid therapy may need stress doses of steroids perioperatively (see Table 24–4).
3. Preoperative pulmonary testing may be required in some patients with severely diminished pulmonary reserves.

Postoperative Considerations

Most susceptible to SOB are those patients who have undergone thoracic or abdominal procedures.

Thoracic Surgery

1. Think first of chest tube malfunction (see Chapter 30 for a complete discussion). If the chest tube was recently removed, evaluate the patient for possible replacement.
2. In patients after lung resection, think of a pulmonary staple line leak. This is mostly evident by a persistent air leak through the chest tube but may occur after chest tube removal.
3. Pneumothorax and hemothorax are frequent findings after thoracic surgery and are generally well controlled and monitored by tube thoracostomy. SOB will result from tube malfunction.
4. Chylothorax is an infrequent complication of thoracic surgery or penetrating chest trauma with injury to the thoracic duct. Findings include pleural effusion with high triglyceride content (generally right sided). This is controlled with tube thoracostomy. Be mindful that much of the patient's nutrition is draining into the Pleur-Evac tube, and IV lipids may be required if the leak is prolonged.

Abdominal Surgery

1. Respirations are painful after abdominal surgery, so splinting with poor lung expansion is the rule.
   Incentive spirometry and frequent coughing help avoid atelectasis and postoperative pneumonia.
   Make sure that the patient is alert and has adequate pain control.
2. Abdominal distention secondary to bowel obstruction may decrease the diaphragmatic excursion and may lead to hypoventilation. NG decompression may aid in decreasing the distention.

3. Rarely, dehiscence of diaphragmatic hernia repairs may result in herniation of abdominal contents back into the thoracic cavity. This is evident on CXR and requires immediate surgical repair.

Respiratory Failure

Respiratory failure is defined as inadequate effort to supply the existing oxygenation needs. It may result from any of the etiologies above and requires immediate treatment to correct hypoxia. Initial findings of hypoventilation may be RR of less than 12 breaths/minute and cyanosis, agitation, or lethargy. ABG results may show progressive hypoxia (PaO_2 of <60 mm Hg), hypercapnia (PCO_2 of >50 mm Hg), and acidosis (pH of <7.3). In settings of impaired gas exchange, such as adult respiratory distress syndrome, the RR may be greater than 20. Correct the cause if it is immediately evident. If not, act immediately to ensure adequate oxygenation, as follows:

1. Reverse narcotic medication.

   Use **naloxone hydrochloride** *(Narcan)* **0.2 to 2 mg IV** immediately. Pinpoint pupils may aid in the diagnosis of narcosis.

2. Ventilate the patient.

   Use bag-valve-mask ventilation to adequately oxygenate the patient until intubation may be performed.

   This is a **code** situation; notify the resident and get help immediately. Make sure the resuscitation cart is on hand and open.

3. Monitor oxygenation with pulse oximetry.

   Follow acidosis and hypercapnia with frequent ABGs.

4. Arrange for intubation of the patient and transfer to the ICU or CCU.

Do not panic if you are not skilled at endotracheal intubation. Bag-valve-mask ventilation is often adequate to oxygenate and ventilate a patient for long periods of time until a skilled individual arrives.

Syncope

Syncope is a brief loss of consciousness due to an interruption of cerebral blood flow. Causes range from benign processes such as vasovagal episodes to more serious conditions such as dysrhythmias. As the on-call physician, your job is to identify the cause of the syncopal episode, to stabilize the patient if necessary, and to identify any injuries resulting from falls secondary to the syncopal episode.

PHONE CALL

1. **Does the patient have a regular pulse and vital signs, and is there any history of syncope?**

   Patients who have a history of syncopal episode are more likely to have another syncopal event. These patients will often have had a prior syncopal workup, which makes it easier to identify the likely cause of the current syncopal event.

2. **Did the patient lose consciousness or just feel faint?**

   There is a difference between true syncope and presyncope. In presyncope, a patient feels on the verge of losing consciousness but actually does not.

3. **How long was the patient unconscious, and is the patient still unconscious?**

4. **Did the patient have a seizure before the loss of consciousness (LOC), and is there any history of epilepsy?**

   It is important to rule out seizures as a cause for LOC. If a patient had an unwitnessed seizure, it may be difficult to rule out seizure as a cause for an alteration in consciousness. Bites to the tongue, incontinence, and prolonged postictal period after regaining consciousness suggest seizure.

5. **What medical problems does the patient have?**

   Diabetes (hypoglycemia), cardiac disease (e.g., dysrhythmias, myocardial infarction [MI], aortic stenosis), and neurologic conditions (transient ischemic attacks [TIAs] and stroke) can cause syncope.

6. **Was the patient injured from a fall?**

   Elderly patients are most likely to have syncopal episodes. These patients are susceptible to fractures and soft-tissue injury.

Orders

If the patient is still unconscious or has any instability of vital signs, give the following orders to the RN:

1. Take vital signs.
2. Establish an intravenous (IV) line immediately. Run 5% dextrose in one-half normal saline to keep the vein open.
3. If the patient is still unconscious, turn the patient on the left side with the mouth in a slightly downward direction. This will minimize the risk of aspiration and will help the tongue move forward to avoid obstructing the airway.
4. Order 12-lead electrocardiogram (ECG) with rhythm strip immediately.
5. Check a Dextrostick.

Inform RN

Will arrive at the bedside in . . . minutes.

Syncope associated with prolonged unconsciousness or instability requires assessment of the patient immediately. This is especially true in neurosurgical patients or patients with a history of head trauma, in whom a significant change in mental status may be a harbinger of serious intracranial events.

ELEVATOR THOUGHTS

What are the causes of syncope?

Cardiovascular Causes

1. Rate and rhythm problems
   - Ventricular tachyarrhythmias
   - Sinus bradycardia
   - Atrioventricular block (secondary or tertiary)
   - Sick sinus syndrome
   - Pacemaker problems
2. Mechanical problems
   - Aortic stenosis
   - Mitral stenosis
   - Pulmonic stenosis
   - MI
   - Hypertrophic obstructive cardiomyopathy
   - Pulmonary embolism

Reflex-Vagal Causes

1. Vasovagal episodes (fainting)
2. Orthostatic hypotension
   Hypovolemia
   Drug related
3. Carotid sinus syncope

Neurologic Causes

1. TIAs
2. Costovertebral angle (CVA)
3. Seizure
4. Cervical spondylosis
5. Subclavian steal syndrome

Psychiatric Causes

1. Anxiety disorder (hysteria and panic attack)
2. Hyperventilation

MAJOR THREAT TO LIFE

Dysrhythmia

Dysrhythmias represent the most acute threat to life. Ventricular tachyarrhythmias often present with syncope. These rhythms may persist or deteriorate to ventricular fibrillation. If you believe that the patient has suffered a transient tachyarrhythmia, it is appropriate to transfer the patient to a monitored (ECG) hospital bed. A patient with ongoing tachyarrhythmia should be treated as outlined in Chapter 9.

Aspiration

It is important to protect an unconscious patient from airway obstruction and aspiration. When a patient is unconscious and supine, the tongue falls to the back of the oropharynx and may obstruct the airway. Furthermore, because emesis may be concurrent with syncope, it is important to minimize the risk of aspiration. Positioning of the patient in the left decubitus position, with the mouth turned slightly downward, helps maintain the open airway by moving the tongue anteriorly. If emesis occurs, this positioning allows vomitus to flow out of the mouth.

Intracranial Bleeding

Neurosurgical or trauma patients who develop intracranial bleeding after craniotomy or trauma may have an LOC. They will often develop a deteriorating LOC that progresses to a state of unconsciousness. Although this is not true syncope, it may be mistaken as syncope. These patients usually do not recover rapidly from the LOC. Computed tomographic (CT) scanning may be required to assess intracerebral or extracerebral collections of blood.

Falls

If a patient loses consciousness from a standing position, they may sustain injuries while falling. See Chapter 10 for a full discussion.

BEDSIDE

Quick Look Test

Does the patient look well (comfortable), sick (uncomfortable or distressed), or critical (about to die)?

Patients who have had a brief syncopal episode and have regained consciousness will often look well. Patients who have ongoing dysrhythmias, poor cerebral perfusion, or unstable vital signs will look sick or critical.

Airway and Vital Signs

Airway

Patients who have regained consciousness from a short-lived syncopal episode will generally have control of their airway. However, patients who are still unconscious should be placed on the left side as described earlier. Proper positioning will diminish the risk of airway obstruction and aspiration.

Heart Rate

Symptomatic bradycardia should be treated with atropine as discussed in Chapter 9. Supraventricular or ventricular tachyarrhythmias causing syncope should be documented by ECG and treated as outlined in Chapter 9. Consider transferring a patient with significant dysrhythmia and hemodynamic instability to the cardiac care unit (CCU) or the intensive care unit (ICU).

Blood Pressure

Hypotension may result in syncope. Evaluate the patient for hypovolemia, bradycardia, and signs of shock. Orthostatic hypotension should be treated as outlined in Chapter 17. Hypertension may result in CVA or subarachnoid hemorrhage. Although these conditions may not result in an interruption of blood flow to the brain, they may first present with an episode of LOC.

Temperature

A fever in the presence of syncope may indicate an infectious process of the central nervous system. Evaluate the patient carefully for meningitis. LOC and fever may also be seen in septic processes.

Selective History and Chart Review

Does the patient have a history of syncopal episode?

Patients who present with syncope frequently have had a prior syncopal episode. The cause of the prior episode may be known and documented in the medical record. If workup has been done previously, management will be much easier.

Does the patient have a history of heart disease?

Look for a history of coronary artery disease, valvular stenoses (especially aortic stenosis), and dysrhythmias.

Does the patient have a history of seizure disorder?

A patient with a seizure disorder who has a reported syncopal episode is likely to have had a seizure.

What does the patient recall just before losing consciousness?

A patient who recalls an aura (auditory, visual, or olfactory) is likely to have suffered a seizure. A patient who recalls that he or she suddenly changed position (supine or sitting position to standing position) just before losing consciousness may have had an orthostatic hypotensive syncopal episode. Chest pain or palpitations before syncope suggests a cardiac cause.

What medications or drugs is the patient taking?

Certain medications are known to increase the occurrence of syncope. Alpha blockers (e.g., prazosin), smooth-muscle relaxants (e.g., hydralazine), and angiotensin-converting enzyme inhibitors (e.g., enalapril) reduce afterload and may cause syncope in elderly or hypovolemic patients. Drugs that slow the heart rate, such as calcium channel blockers (e.g., nifedipine), digoxin, and beta-blockers (e.g., propranolol), may cause bradycardia and result in syncope. Sympathetic stimulants such as tricyclic antidepressants (imipramine) and cocaine may cause tachyarrhythmias and syncope.

Selective Physical Examination

As you examine the patient, try to ascertain the cause of the syncopal episode. First, make sure that the patient is stable. Then try to identify the cause of the syncopal episode. Finally, make sure that the patient has not suffered any injuries related to a fall.

VS:	Repeat now.
HEENT:	Examine tongue, cheeks, and lips for lacerations or bite injuries (seizure). Neck stiffness suggests meningitis.
	Examine face and scalp for traumatic injuries.
Resp:	Listen for crackles or wheezes secondary to aspiration.
CVS:	Irregularly irregular rhythm suggests atrial fibrillation.
	Note murmurs consistent with a valvular stenosis. Look for presence of a pacemaker (look for subcutaneous pocket on upper chest).
	Note jugular venous distention (volume depletion).
GU:	Urinary incontinence suggests seizure.
GI:	Incontinence of stool suggests seizure.
MSS:	Examine patient for evidence of contusions or fractures.
Neuro:	Complete neurologic examination is required. Look for focal findings suggestive of a distinct lesion.
	Focality suggests CVA, TIA, or space-occupying lesion.

MANAGEMENT

In many cases, it will be difficult to arrive at the cause of a syncopal episode. Many of the causes of syncope are transient events. It generally takes a fairly extensive workup to collect the information necessary to arrive at a likely cause. For this reason, definitive treatment for syncope is reserved for medical conditions that have been clearly defined and documented. As the on-call physician, your job is to assess the syncopal patient, to document the syncopal event, to stabilize the patient if necessary, and to arrange initial workup.

Syncope Due to Cardiac Events

1. Syncope can result from a dysrhythmia or a mechanical problem.
   Any patient who has a syncopal episode from a cardiac cause should be transferred to a continuous ECG monitored unit (transitional care unit, CCU, or ICU).
2. If dysrhythmia is likely, consider silent ischemia or MI as a possible cause of transient rhythm disturbances.
   Evaluate the 12-lead ECG carefully, and consider enzyme studies if indicated. Treat cardiac ischemia as outlined in Chapter 7.
3. If dysrhythmia is ongoing, treat specific rhythm disturbances as outlined in Chapter 9.
4. Holter monitoring may be helpful to evaluate the occurrence of transient rhythm disturbances in stable patients.
5. Pacemaker problems require cardiology consultation.
6. Mechanical problems such as aortic stenosis, obstructive cardiomyopathy, and pulmonic stenosis should be worked up with a nonemergent echocardiogram. Cardiology consultation is also advisable.

Syncope Due to Vagal Events

1. If the patient is bradycardic and symptomatic, consider **atropine 0.5 to 1 mg IV; the dose may be repeated every 5 minutes, for a maximum dose of 2 mg.**
2. If the syncopal episode is due to a simple vasovagal attack, place the patient supine with the legs elevated.
   Spontaneous resolution will generally occur. Vasovagal episodes are one of the most common causes of syncope.

Syncope Due to Orthostatic Hypotension

Syncope may occur in volume-depleted patients. Simple dehydration, inadequate fluid resuscitation after surgery or illness, or postoperative or posttraumatic bleeding will lead to states of volume depletion. These patients are susceptible to syncope when moving from supine to sitting or standing positions. Treatment consists of fluid resuscitation or transfusion as outlined in Chapter 12.

Orthostatic hypotension may also result from vasodilator drugs and autonomic dysfunction. When evaluating a patient with orthostatic hypotension, be sure to evaluate the medications a patient is taking. It is appropriate to hold medications that are vasodilators or antihypertensives.

Syncope Due to Psychological Factors

Patients can lose consciousness from sudden shock, anxiety, or stress. It is important to reassure anxious patients. Antianxiety medications may be appropriate (e.g., **diazepam [Valium] 5 to 10 mg orally**). Remind the anxious patient not to hyperventilate. Hypocapnia, resulting from hyperventilation, can lead to syncope.

Syncope Due to Neurologic Events

1. A patient who is believed to have had a stroke or a brain stem TIA should have a CT scan of the head.

    The CT scan is best performed without contrast. Neurologic consultation should be obtained if workup suggests that the patient has had a stroke.

2. If a patient is believed to have had a subarachnoid hemorrhage (SAH), CT scan is appropriate.

    More than 90% of patients will show blood in the subarachnoid spaces of the sulci and the cisternae in the first 24 hours after SAH. CT scan may also show evidence of aneurysm. Lumbar puncture should be performed if the clinical impression leads strongly to SAH but CT scan is negative.

3. Intracerebral hemorrhage is diagnosed by CT scan.

    Treatment consists of supportive care and control of blood pressure. Neurosurgical consultation should be obtained for cerebral and cerebellar hematomas.

4. Seizures are managed as outlined in Chapter 27.

Tubes and Drains

Many postoperative patients will have drainage devices to facilitate their care. The types used most often fall into the following broad categories:

Chest tubes

Urinary drainage tubes (urinary catheters)

Gastrointestinal (GI) tubes (nasogastric [NG] or mercury-weighted tubes for decompression, feeding tubes, and gastrostomy and jejunostomy tubes)

Biliary drainage tubes (T-tubes)

Wound drainage tubes (Jackson-Pratt, Penrose, and other suction drains)

Problems with these tubes are frequent but generally straightforward. This section is organized by the type of tube. Intravenous lines are covered in Chapter 19.

CHEST TUBES

Appropriate treatment of the problems associated with chest tubes begins with a fundamental knowledge of how the tubes work. The apparatus is a means to apply external suction to the pleural cavity to rid the space of unwanted air or fluid. The collection apparatus looks complicated but may be easily understood if the components are considered separately; the apparatus may be thought of as three separate interconnected bottles (Fig. 30–1), as follows:

1. Suction from the wall or from a vacuum device is connected to the suction control bottle (see Fig. 30–1A). The volume of water in this bottle *(F)* dictates the amount of suction that is transmitted to the patient. When suction is ordered, it is ordered in units of centimeters of water (cm H_2O), and additional suction pressure results in entraining air from the open tube, as indicated by bubbling in this chamber.

2. The suction control bottle *(A)* is connected to the underwater seal bottle *(B)*. This bottle allows separation of the patient from the suction if desired, and is the site of indication of an air leak. Continued air evacuation is noted as persistent bubbling in this chamber.

Figure 30–1 Chest tube apparatus. *A*, Suction control chamber; *B*, underwater seal; *C*, collection chamber; *D*, to suction; *E*, from patient; *F*, height equals amount of suction in units of cm H_2O; *G*, height equals underwater seal in units of cm H_2O.
(From Marshall SA, Ruedy J: On Call: Principles and Protocols, 2nd ed. Philadelphia, WB Saunders, 1993, p. 180.)

3. The underwater seal bottle *(B)* is connected to the collection bottle *(C)*, which is the site of fluid collection. Fluid draining from the chest tube is stored in this chamber for measurement and testing, if desired. The collection bottle *(C)* is then connected to the chest tube in the patient *(E)*. These bottles may be combined into a single box-type drainage apparatus (Pleur-Evac).

Some Pleur-Evacs are designed to allow retransfusion of drained blood.

Placement of a Tube Thoracostomy

Percutaneous drainage of the pleural cavity may be diagnostic and therapeutic. In the setting of dyspnea and hypoxia, the need for a chest tube is an emergent event. In the stable patient, take the extra time necessary to adequately prepare and sedate the patient.

Indications

1. Pneumothorax
2. Pyothorax
3. Hemothorax
4. Chylothorax
5. Persistent pleural effusion
6. Postoperative application after thoracic procedures

Precautions

1. Coagulopathy
   Abnormalities in platelet count or function or in clotting factor concentrations should be corrected before insertion of the tube.
2. Skin infection over the site of needle insertion may carry infection into the pleural cavity.
   Try to choose an uninvolved site.

Equipment Needed

1. Skin preparation supplies (iodine, chlorhexidine, or alcohol).
2. Local anesthetic (1% or 2% lidocaine, 0.5% marcaine, 25-gauge needle, 3-mL syringe).
3. Sterile gloves, eye protection.
4. Sterile towels or drapes.
5. Sedative medication, as necessary.
6. Pulse oximeter.
7. Chest tube of the appropriate diameter: small (20-24 French) for air removal and large (36-40 French) for fluid removal. The perforated end may be cut down to facilitate a smaller patient. Placing a bevel on the end is not recommended; it may facilitate placement, but it is a perforation risk once inside the patient.
8. A chest tube insertion tray that includes blades, gauze, hemostats, trochars, thick silk suture with needle, and drapes.
9. Petroleum gauze.
10. Wide, gas-impermeable, occlusive tape.
11. Suction device or wall suction.
12. Chest tube suction apparatus (Pleur-Evac), pre-filled with water, as necessary, and hooked to the suction device.

Anatomy and Approach

The size and placement of the tube depend on the indication. A larger tube (36-40 French) and posterior placement are indicated for drainage of fluid; a smaller tube (20-24 French) and anterior placement are necessary for the drainage of air. The most versatile approach is laterally at the sixth interspace midaxillary line, about the level of the nipples. From this site, the tube may be directed either anteriorly or posteriorly.

Anesthesia

Local, with optional IV sedation and narcotic pain medicine. Conscious sedation is recommended for elective tube placement (see Chapter 4).

Technique (Sterile)

Elective chest tube placement in a relatively stable patient may be done in a controlled and safe manner using adequate premedication of the patient with sedatives and local anesthesia. This technique describes a hemostat technique; some prefer a trochar-assisted placement. In an unstable patient, defer to the most experienced hands, do not take the time necessary to premedicate, and move as quickly and safely as possible.

1. Prepare the patient.
   a. Explain the procedure.
   b. Explain the risks and alternatives.
   c. Answer any questions.
   d. Have a consent form prepared and signed.
2. Position of the patient.
   Supine with the arm on the affected side extended upward
3. Premedicate the patient.
   a. Short-acting benzodiazepine such as **lorazepam** *(Ativan)* **1 to 5 mg IV.**
   b. Short-acting narcotic such as **fentanyl** *(Sublimaze)* **25 to 50 mcg IV** also may be necessary.
   c. Skip all premedication (both benzodiazepine and narcotic) if the patient is dyspneic or is at risk for respiratory depression.
4. Prepare the skin.
   a. Use sterile technique and sterile gloves, mask, and gown.
   b. Plan the incision.
      The midaxillary line is generally used, with anterior direction of the chest tube to remove gas and posterior direction of the chest tube to remove fluid. Plan to make the skin incision about 2 to 3 cm below the rib interspace to be entered so that there is an oblique skin channel. This usually facilitates skin closure on removal of the tube. On occasion, the anterior midcla-

vicular line is used to treat uncomplicated pneumothorax, generally with a very small (12 French) tube.

c. Sterilely prep and drape the skin.

d. Infiltrate with 1% to 2% lidocaine into the skin at the entry
site and over the rib at the selected interspace.

The periosteum of the top of the rib is very sensitive; do not
skimp on lidocaine. Infiltrate the subcutaneous tunnel
as well while removing the needle.

5. Make the skin incision over a rib.

Confirm adequate anesthesia. Cutting over the bone allows a
clean, deep cut and avoids the neurovascular bundle that
travels the underside of each rib. The incision should be
about 1.5 times the diameter of the chest tube. Control any
bleeding with pressure. Reinject with lidocaine, as necessary (see Fig. 30–2A).

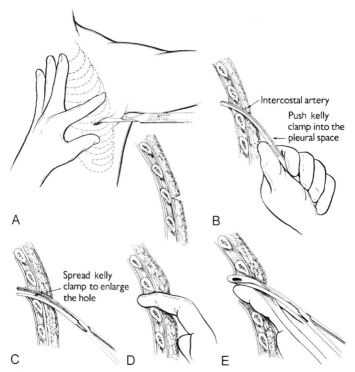

Figure 30–2 Thoracostomy tube placement. (From Dunmire SM, Paris
PM: Atlas of Emergency Procedures. Philadelphia, WB Saunders, 1995.)

6. Place a purse-string suture at the skin entry site.

   Position the tie such that the loose ends are positioned inferiorly to the tube exit site, and place a single throw loosely.

7. Bluntly dissect toward the pleura (see Fig. 30–2B).

   a. Using a hemostat, create a subcutaneous channel superiorly from the skin incision to over the top of the rib at the desired interspace.

   b. Using a fair amount of pressure, and with the hemostats closed, force the hemostats between the ribs through the intercostal muscles. Stay right on top of a rib to avoid the neurovascular bundle.

   c. You will notice a "pop" when the pleural cavity has been entered. Often, there is also a noticeable gush of air or fluid through the wound.

   d. Spread the hemostat tips to create sufficient space in the intercostal muscles to allow the tube to pass (see Fig. 30–2C).

   e. Remove the hemostat and insert a finger to confirm penetration into the pleural cavity (see Fig. 30–2D).

8. Insert the chest tube (see Fig. 30–2E).

   Using the hemostat, grasp the perforated end of the chest tube and place the tube through the subcutaneous channel and the intercostal muscle opening. This often is a difficult maneuver; it may take several passes to find the channel you created. (With trochar insertion, the tube is placed over the trochar and forced into the pleural cavity without hemostat perforation of the intercostal muscles.)

9. Position the chest tube.

   Note that the chest tube has a mark just beyond the last perforations. When the tube has been placed into the chest and directed in the appropriate direction, insert the tube to the desired length. Make sure the mark is either inside the chest wall or just visible at the skin incision line, or the tube will leak.

10. Secure the tube.

    Pull the purse-string suture snugly around the tube without adding throws. Wrap the loose ends around the tube several times to hold it in place. Make sure that several inches of suture are wrapped around the tube because this will be used to close the wound when the tube is removed. Once wrapped, the loose ends may be tied down securely (Fig. 30–3). Place additional sutures, as necessary, to close the skin incision. Wrap the long ends of each suture around the chest tube and tie securely.

11. Connect the chest tube to the Pleur-Evac and to wall suction.

    The suction pressure is defined by the volume of water (in cm of H_2O) in the suction control chamber of the Pleur-Evac. Bubbling in the underwater seal chamber will indicate

Figure 30–3 Purse-string ligature around chest tube site.

adequate suction to remove gas and will continue for as long as there is an air leak. If fluid is to be removed, it will collect in the collection chamber (Fig. 30–1C).

12. Tape the chest tube site.
   a. Wrap the tubing at the skin site with petroleum gauze.
   b. Apply occlusive tape in such a way that the tube site is relatively airtight and the tube is safe from being dislodged.
   c. Further secure the tube by applying an "umbilical" tape such that unexpected pulls on the tube will pull on the umbilicus instead of on the suture (Fig. 30–4).

13. Confirm tube placement by stat bedside upright AP chest x-ray (CXR).
   Reposition as necessary. Daily CXRs are recommended to follow the course of therapy and to confirm continued

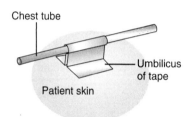

Figure 30–4 Tape umbilicus technique for securing chest tubes.

adequate placement of the tube. A lateral CXR may be helpful to find the exact location of the tube.

The most proximal hole in the chest tube interrupts the radio-opaque band on the tube, so it is easy to determine on CXR whether the tube is adequately placed. This most proximal hole should be well within the pleural space.

14. Control the patient's pain.

The tube insertion site will remain uncomfortable until the tube is removed, so make sure the patient has adequate pain relief.

15. Pulmonary toilet is important in a patient with a chest tube.

Make an incentive spirometer available, and instruct the patient as to its use and importance.

16. Send fluid efflux from the chest tube to the laboratory.

The following studies may be indicated:

a. Gram stain
b. Cultures (aerobic and anaerobic bacterial, fungal, mycoplasmal)
c. TB culture and acid-fast bacilli (AFB)
d. Cell count and differential
e. LDH
f. Protein
g. Glucose
h. Cytology for malignant cells
i. Other studies as appropriate (amylase, triglycerides, pH, rheumatoid factor, antinuclear antibodies or complement levels, and so on). Blood for simultaneous tests for serum LDH, protein, glucose, and so on should be drawn to compare with the results of the pleural fluid.

17. Document the procedure.

Complications/Problems

1. Lack of resolution of the problem
   Occasionally, more than one chest tube will be needed.
2. Perforation of the lung
   This is more likely with a trochar placement.
3. Perforation of abdominal viscera
   This may happen if the skin entry site is too far caudal on the chest wall.
4. Perforation of the heart
5. Persistent air leak
   a. Check the tubing between the drainage apparatus and the patient for loose connections.
   b. Untape the wound site and confirm that the chest tube is inserted properly.
      Check whether the chest tube is fully inserted and the line is at or inside the skin line.

   c. If the entry site is not well closed, or a "sucking" sound is noted at the site, it may be necessary to further close the site with 2-0 silk sutures. Be sure to adequately prep and anesthetize the area before repair.

   d. Reposition the chest tube if necessary, and redress the site using petroleum gauze.

   e. If the connections are intact and the site is dressed in an airtight manner, order a portable AP CXR to assess the patient's lungs and the tube position.

   f. If the CXR shows lack of resolution of pneumothorax, consider placement of a second tube.

6. Persistent fluid efflux
7. Bleeding at the entry site
8. Discomfort

Pleurodesis Through a Tube Thoracostomy

In settings of persistent pneumothorax or malignant effusion, it may be necessary to perform pleurodesis. This entails infusion of an irritant into the pleural space to create scarring between the visceral pleura and the parietal pleura. On removal of the tube, the lung will remain scarred to the chest wall. Table 30–1 shows the agents typically used for pleurodesis.

Indications

1. Persistent malignant effusion
2. Persistent pneumothorax

Contraindications

Hypersensitivity to lidocaine or the sclerosing agents.

Equipment Needed

1. Tube preparation supplies (iodine, chlorhexidine, or alcohol)
2. 40 mL 1% lidocaine
3. Sterile gloves, eye protection
4. Sedative medication, as necessary
5. Pulse oximeter
6. 60-mL syringes (2) with 18-gauge needles attached
7. Tubing clamps (2)
8. Pleur-Evac hooked to wall suction
9. Sclerosing agent as prepared above (see Table 30–1).

TABLE 30–1 **Agents Used in Pleurodesis**

Agent	Concentration
Talc	2 g/100 mL normal saline
Tetracycline	1 g/100 mL normal saline
Doxycycline	1 g/100 mL normal saline
Bleomycin	60 IU/100 mL normal saline

Anesthesia

Premedication of the patient with both a narcotic and an anxiolytic medication.

Technique (Sterile)

1. Prepare the patient.
   a. Explain the procedure.
   b. Explain the risks and alternatives.
   c. Answer any questions.
   d. Obtain informed consent, if necessary.
   e. Place the patient on continuous pulse oximetry.
2. Position of the patient.
   Supine
3. Premedicate the patient.
   a. Short-acting benzodiazepine such as **midazolam** *(Versed)* **1 to 5 mg IV** or **lorazepam** *(Ativan)* **1 to 5 mg IV**.
   b. Short-acting narcotic medication, such as **fentanyl** *(Sublimaze)* **25 to 50 mcg IV**, also may be necessary.
4. Prepare the tube.
   a. Clamp the chest tube on the soft rubber portion close to the patient.
   b. Sterilely prepare a portion of the rubber tubing proximal to the clamp.
5. Inject 40 mL 1% lidocaine into the tube.
6. Elevate the tube so that the entire volume enters the chest cavity.
7. Place a second clamp on the tube on the plastic portion just at the chest wall.
8. Position the patient as follows to distribute the lidocaine:
   a. 2 minutes supine Trendelenburg
   b. 2 minutes supine reverse Trendelenburg
   c. 2 minutes right lateral decubitus
   d. 2 minutes left lateral decubitus
   e. 2 minutes prone (optional)
9. Unclamp the tube at the site closest to the patient and inject the sclerosing agent into the tube.
10. Elevate the tube so that the entire volume enters the chest cavity.
11. Reclamp the tube on the plastic portion just at the chest wall.
12. Position the patient as follows to distribute the sclerosing agent:
    a. 15 minutes supine Trendelenburg
    b. 15 minutes supine reverse Trendelenburg
    c. 15 minutes right lateral decubitus
    d. 15 minutes left lateral decubitus
    e. 15 minutes prone (optional)
13. Unclamp the tube and allow the sclerosing agent to drain out.

14. Reconnect the chest tube to suction for 24 to 48 hours or until there is no persistent air leak.
15. Document the procedure.

Complications

1. If the patient becomes dyspneic or hypoxic at any time during the procedure, unclamp the chest tube and return it to suction.
2. Incomplete pleurodesis is common. If there are persistent symptoms, repeat application of pleurodesis or a surgical decortication may be necessary.
3. Successful pleurodesis requires the development of inflammation in the pleura. Do not administer anti-inflammatory medication, but be prepared to treat discomfort with a mild narcotic.

Removal of a Tube Thoracostomy

This is best done with an assistant.

1. Confirm that the patient is ready to have the chest tube removed.
   a. There should be no persistent air leak, or the patient should have been stable for at least 24 hours on water seal alone.
   b. Ongoing fluid leak or bleeding should have stopped.
   c. The lung should be inflated on CXR.
   d. There is no other reason to consider leaving the tube in place.
2. Have all equipment ready.
   a. Blade or scissors to cut the knot from the purse-string suture
   b. Petroleum gauze
   c. Wide, gas-impermeable occlusive tape
   d. Dry gauze sponges (4 in. × 4 in.)
   e. Pulse oximeter (as necessary)
   f. Gloves and eye protection.
3. Explain the procedure.
   Removal of the chest tube will require patient cooperation, and it is somewhat painful. Explain well what is to occur. Use the minimum effective amount of opiate pain medication necessary as high doses can depress respiratory function.
4. Position the patient: upright or supine.
5. Remove existing tape.
6. Cut the purse-string suture at the knot, leaving the long ends intact, and unwrap from the chest tube.
7. Tighten the purse-string suture such that the skin closes tightly around the tube.
   Confirm that the tube is free from the suture and tape.
8. Remove the chest tube.
   a. Have the patient inhale completely and hold his or her breath at the peak of inhalation.

This guarantees a positive pressure in the pleural cavity and does not leave room for an involuntary gasp by the patient when the tube is removed.

b. While the patient is holding his or her breath, the first person pulls the chest tube out.

The same individual should place the petroleum gauze over the skin site to avoid the influx of air.

c. At the same time as the tube is being removed, the second person pulls the ends of the purse-string suture such that the skin seals tightly underneath the petroleum gauze bandage.

d. Tie down the ends.

9. Apply dry gauze and occlusive tape to the site.

10. Obtain a CXR to assess for pneumothorax.

A small amount of air is common and may be treated with 100% O_2 therapy.

11. Observe the patient over the next few hours for adequate breath sounds and oxygenation.

12. Examine the patient in 24 hours and obtain a follow-up CXR.

If respiratory distress develops at any time, evaluate the patient for replacement of the chest tube.

Complications of Tube Thoracostomy

1. Lack of resolution of the problem
2. Perforation of the lung
3. Perforation of abdominal viscera
4. Perforation of the heart

Problems with Chest Tubes

1. Persistent air leak
2. Persistent blood leak
3. Bleeding at the entry site
4. Loss of underwater seal fluctuation
5. Shortness of breath (SOB)
6. Subcutaneous emphysema
7. Discomfort at the tube entry site

Persistent Air Leak

This is manifest by continuous bubbling in the underwater seal compartment of the drainage apparatus (see Fig. 30–1B). It may be present with or without the application of suction to the tube.

PHONE CALL

Questions

1. Why was the chest tube inserted?
2. How long ago was the tube inserted?

3. Is the patient short of breath?
4. Has the patient undergone a surgical procedure, and if so, how long ago?
5. Are there any other symptoms?
6. Are there any changes in vital signs?

Degree of Urgency

If there is a significant change in vital signs or symptoms, the patient must be evaluated immediately.

ELEVATOR THOUGHTS

What causes persistent air leak?
1. Loose tubing or connectors
2. Air leaking into the chest
   - From the entrance wound
   - From a new bronchial or pulmonary injury
3. Persistent bronchopleural fistula
   - After thoracic surgery (lobectomy and open biopsy)
   - After a closed chest procedure (needle biopsy and thoracentesis)
   - Due to ruptured bleb (asthma and emphysema)
   - After thoracic trauma

MAJOR THREAT TO LIFE

- Hypoxia, if the air leak is new or if it is associated with SOB
- Pneumothorax

BEDSIDE

Quick Look Test

If the air leak is small, the patient may look comfortable. A patient who has a new pneumothorax may look acutely distressed.

Selective History and Chart Review

- Review why the chest tube was placed.
- Discern if the air leak had ever resolved.

If the patient is recovering from a thoracic procedure, the air leak may persist for 2 to 5 days. A new air leak may indicate a complication derived from the procedure or from placement of the chest tube.

Selective Physical Examination

VS:	Increased respiratory rate (RR) (hypoxia)
Resp:	Unilateral decrease in aeration, and hyper-resonance (pneumothorax)

Tubes:	Are the connections secure?
Special intrapleural examination:	Some air leaks are small and will be noted only during increases in pressure such as coughing
Additional tests:	1. Pulse oximetry (hypoxia)

MANAGEMENT

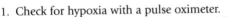

1. Check for hypoxia with a pulse oximeter.
2. Supply supplemental oxygen as required (see Chapter 28).
3. Check the tubing between the drainage apparatus and the patient for loose connections.
4. Untape the wound site and confirm that the chest tube is inserted properly.

   Each chest tube has a visible line a few centimeters away from the most distal holes. The tube must be inserted such that the line is at or inside the skin incision.
5. If the entry site is not well closed or if a sucking sound is noted at the site, it may be necessary to close the site further with 2-0 silk sutures.

   Be sure to adequately prepare and anesthetize the area before repair.
6. Reposition the chest tube if necessary, and re-dress the site using petroleum gauze.
7. If the connections are intact and the site is dressed in an airtight manner, order a portable AP CXR to assess the patient's lungs and the tube position.
8. If the CXR shows lack of resolution of pneumothorax, consider placement of a second tube.

Persistent Blood Leak Through the Chest Tube

PHONE CALL

Questions

1. Why was the chest tube inserted?
2. How long ago was the tube inserted?
3. Is the patient short of breath?
4. Has the patient undergone a surgical procedure, and if so, how long ago was it performed?
5. Are there any other symptoms?
6. Are there any changes in vital signs?
7. Does the patient have a history of trauma to the chest?

Orders

Order a hematocrit as a baseline if the bleeding is brisk.

Degree of Urgency

If there is a significant change in vital signs or symptoms, the patient must be evaluated immediately.

ELEVATOR THOUGHTS

What causes excess blood efflux?
1. Erosion of the tube into a bronchial artery or vein
2. Coagulopathy
3. Injury to an intercostal neurovascular bundle
4. The result of a blunt or penetrating trauma to the chest

MAJOR THREAT TO LIFE

- Hypotension and shock if the blood loss is great
- Disseminated intravascular coagulation (DIC)
- Hypoxia

BEDSIDE

Quick Look Test

Massive blood loss may result in shock. The patient may be lethargic or comatose. Hypoxia will result in agitation.

Airway and Vital Signs

Severe fluid loss may lead to tachycardia and hypotension. Hypoxia may be associated with tachypnea.

Selective History and Chart Review

- Review why the chest tube was placed.
- Is the patient taking an anticoagulant such as warfarin or heparin?
- Can the medication be safely reversed?
- Determine the amount of blood lost and whether the current efflux rate is a change.

MANAGEMENT

1. Check for hypoxia with a pulse oximeter.
2. Supply supplemental oxygen as required (see Chapter 28).
3. If tachycardia or hypotension is present, begin fluid resuscitation with normal saline (NS) or lactated Ringer's (LR) (see Chapters 12 and 17).
   - Start a large-bore IV.
   - Give **500-mL NS or LR quickly.**

- Send blood for a crossmatch for 4 to 6 units of packed red blood cells.
- Order a portable AP CXR immediately.
4. If coagulopathy is present, correct with fresh frozen plasma or cryoprecipitate as per Chapter 26.
5. If the rate of loss is greater than 30 mL/hour over 3–4 hours, consider returning to the operating room (or consult a thoracic surgeon, if the patient is not already a thoracic surgery patient).

Special Surgical Considerations

POSTOPERATIVE CONSIDERATIONS

1. Bleeding is common after open thoracic procedures.

    This generally tapers off by 24 hours after the operation. If the bleeding does not abate, consider evaluating the patient for coagulopathy (prothrombin time, partial thromboplastin time, fibrinogen, fibrin degradation products, and platelets) or continued surgical bleeding.
2. New onset of blood in the chest tube may indicate a complication of the tube.

Bleeding at the Entry Site

PHONE CALL

Questions

1. Why was the chest tube inserted?
2. How long ago was the tube inserted?
3. Is the patient short of breath?
4. Has the patient undergone a surgical procedure, and if so, how long ago was it performed?
5. Are there any other symptoms?
6. Are there any changes in vital signs?

Degree of Urgency

Brisk bleeding in a patient is a serious finding, and the patient must be seen immediately. If there is a significant change in vital signs or symptoms, the patient must be evaluated immediately.

ELEVATOR THOUGHTS

What causes bleeding around the entry site?

1. Inadequate hemostasis during insertion of the tube
2. Inadequate closure of the incision site after removal of the tube
3. Coagulation disorders

4. Trauma to intercostal vessels during insertion of the tube
5. Loss of patency of the chest tube
   Blood from the pleural space may drain around the tube.

MAJOR THREAT TO LIFE

- Hypotension and shock if the blood loss is great
- DIC

BEDSIDE

Quick Look Test

Most bleeding is mild and is not associated with changes in patient condition. Severe bleeding, however, may be associated with development of shock. The patient may be lethargic or comatose. Hypoxia will result in agitation.

Airway and Vital Signs

Severe fluid loss may lead to tachycardia and hypotension. Hypoxia may be associated with tachypnea.

Selective History and Chart Review

- Review why the chest tube was placed.
- Is the patient taking an anticoagulant such as warfarin or heparin?
- Can the medication be safely reversed?
- Determine the amount of blood lost and whether the current bleeding rate is a change.
- Note also the output through the chest tube lumen.

MANAGEMENT

1. Check for hypoxia with a pulse oximeter.
2. Supply supplemental oxygen as required (see Chapter 28).
3. Untape the wound site; inspect the wound.
   If the entry site is not well closed, it may be necessary to close the site further with 2-0 silk sutures. Be sure to adequately prepare and anesthetize the area before repair. Look for sites of active bleeding and ligate as necessary.
4. Re-dress the site using petroleum gauze.
   Apply a pressure dressing.
5. If the chest tube is clotted, milk the tube to attempt to clear it.
   Special chest tube stripper instruments are available for this purpose, or it may be accomplished by lubricating the tube with lotion and using your fingers to milk the tube toward the

drainage apparatus. If you are unable to clear the tube or if the tube size is inadequate to manage the amount of drainage, consider replacement of the tube through a different site.

Loss of Underwater Seal Fluctuation

PHONE CALL

Questions

1. Why was the chest tube inserted?
2. How long ago was the tube inserted?
3. Is the patient short of breath?
4. Has the patient undergone a surgical procedure, and if so, how long ago was it performed?
5. Are there any other symptoms?
6. Are there any changes in vital signs?

Degree of Urgency

Loss of fluctuation of the underwater seal is a common but potentially serious problem. It indicates that the chest tube is not functioning properly. The patient should be seen fairly soon. If there is a significant change in vital signs or symptoms, the patient must be evaluated immediately.

ELEVATOR THOUGHTS

What causes loss of underwater seal fluctuation?
1. Kink in the tubing
2. Occlusion of the tubing
3. Improper positioning of the chest tube within the pleural cavity

MAJOR THREAT TO LIFE

- Tension pneumothorax
- Accumulation of fluid within the pleural space due to inadequate drainage

BEDSIDE

Quick Look Test

A patient with a tension pneumothorax will appear acutely ill. Hypoxia, hypotension, and shock may follow.

Airway and Vital Signs

Hypotension and tachypnea are indications of pneumothorax.

Selective History and Chart Review

- Review why the chest tube was placed.
- How long has the tube been malfunctioning?
- What volume has been draining from the tube?

MANAGEMENT

1. Check for hypoxia with a pulse oximeter.
2. Supply supplemental oxygen as required (see Chapter 28).
3. Check the tubing between the drainage apparatus and the patient for loose connections. Look also for regions of clotting or kinking.
4. Confirm that the suction is appropriately applied.
5. Inspect the tube and drainage apparatus.

   There are two regions that give clues to the function of a chest tube (Fig. 30–5). The underwater seal chamber (see Fig. 30–1*B*) is a low-pressure, one-way valve. Gas will bubble through this chamber if there is a continuous flow of air through the chest tube from the patient (such as a persistent air leak). Fluctuations may also be observed if there is fluid present in the tubing itself between the patient and the drainage apparatus. Often fluid will collect in dependent regions of this tubing and will act as an additional underwater seal site. Fluctuations in this region indicate normal functioning of the chest tube between this site and the patient. Have the patient cough during your observation of this region.
6. Attempt to milk the tubing with strippers or your fingers to loosen a clot.
7. If these measures do not re-establish normal chest tube function, obtain a portable AP CXR immediately.

   Check for proper placement of the tube and for persistence or worsening of the intrapleural pathology. A new tube may need to be placed.

Shortness of Breath

See also Chapter 28.

PHONE CALL

Questions

1. Why was the chest tube inserted?
2. How long ago was the chest tube inserted?

Watch for fluctuation

Watch for bubbling here

Figure 30–5 Loss of fluctuation of the underwater seal. Ask the patient to cough, and observe for any fluctuation or bubbling. (From Marshall SA, Ruedy J: On Call: Principles and Protocols, 2nd ed. Philadelphia, WB Saunders, 1993, p 187.)

3. Is the patient short of breath?
4. Has the patient undergone a surgical procedure, and if so, how long ago was it performed?
5. Are there any other symptoms?
6. Are there any changes in vital signs?

Orders

1. Check for hypoxia with a pulse oximeter.
2. Supply supplemental oxygen as required (see Chapter 28).
3. Have a 16-gauge angiocatheter available at the bedside for use for diagnosis and to treat tension pneumothorax.

Degree of Urgency

The patient must be evaluated immediately.

ELEVATOR THOUGHTS

What causes of shortness of breath are associated with chest tubes?
1. Tension pneumothorax
2. Increasing pneumothorax
   - Inadequate suction
   - Misplaced tube
   - Kinked or occluded tube
   - Bronchopleural fistula
3. Subcutaneous emphysema
      This may cause upper airway obstruction if the emphysema extends to the neck and displaces the trachea.
4. Increasing pleural effusion or hemothorax
5. Re-expansion pulmonary edema
      This may occur after rapid expansion of a pneumothorax or drainage of pleural effusion.
6. Non-chest tube-related causes (see Chapter 28).

MAJOR THREAT TO LIFE

- Tension pneumothorax
- Upper airway obstruction

BEDSIDE

Quick Look Test

Confirm the patency of the upper airway. Remove any oral obstruction such as dentures or foreign bodies. Tachypnea (RR >20 breaths/minute) will be present if hypoxia, anxiety, pain, or acidosis is present. A drop in blood pressure may indicate a tension pneumothorax.
   Confirm the functioning of the chest tube.

Selective History and Chart Review

- Review why the chest tube was placed.
- Was there a recent central line placement or thoracic surgery?
- Has a chest tube been recently clamped, placed to water seal, or removed? Is there a history of penetrating chest trauma or spontaneous pneumothorax?

Selective Physical Examination

VS:	Repeat now; tachycardia, tachypnea, and hypotension (pneumothorax)
MS:	Agitation (hypoxia) and lethargy (hyper-capnia)
HEENT:	Upper airway obstruction (foreign body and subcutaneous emphysema)

Elevated jugular venous distention (pneumothorax)

Deviated trachea (pneumothorax)

Resp: Decreased aeration, and unilateral hyperresonance (pneumothorax)

Tubes: Chest tube functioning normally

Recent central venous line placement

Additional tests: 1. CXR Portable AP immediately (confirm tube placement)

2. ABG Assessment of serum arterial partial pressure of oxygen (PaO_2), partial pressure of carbon dioxide (PCO_2), and pH and calculation of serum bicarbonate levels ($[HCO_3^-]$)

MANAGEMENT

1. If there is significant upper airway obstruction due to subcutaneous emphysema or other cause, do the following:
   - Contact the resident.
   - Prepare for possible intubation.
   - Contact the intensive care unit (ICU) or cardiac care unit (CCU) for probable transfer.
2. For suspected pneumothorax, do the following:
   - Confirm the diagnosis

   Findings may include decreased breath sounds and hyperresonance of the hemithorax, deviation of the trachea, hypoxia, and chest pain. In cases of tension pneumothorax, progressive cardiac outflow obstruction is apparent.
   - Immediately insert a 16-gauge needle into the second or third intercostal space anteriorly at the midclavicular line on the affected side.

   Enter 2 to 3 fingerbreadths below the clavicle to avoid the subclavian vessels. This will confirm the diagnosis and allow some relief of symptoms until adequate chest tube drainage can be reimplemented.
   - Reinsert the chest tube, as necessary.
   - Confirm appropriate placement of the tube with a portable AP CXR immediately.
   - Pneumothoraces that do not respond to tube thoracostomy may require surgical repair.

Subcutaneous Emphysema

PHONE CALL

Questions

1. **Why was the chest tube inserted?**

2. How long ago was the tube inserted?
3. Is the patient short of breath?
4. Has the patient undergone a surgical procedure, and if so, how long ago was it performed?
5. Are there any other symptoms?
6. Are there any changes in vital signs?

Degree of Urgency

Subcutaneous emphysema is a potentially serious symptom and must be evaluated quickly. If there is a significant change in vital signs or symptoms, the patient must be evaluated immediately.

ELEVATOR THOUGHTS

What causes subcutaneous emphysema?
1. Inadequate suction for the size of the pneumothorax
   This may be a matter of too little suction applied by the chest tube or a tube size that is inadequate.
2. Misplacement of the tube, as in the chest wall or in the abdominal cavity
3. Gas-producing bacterial infection at the site of tube entry
4. A small amount of subcutaneous gas collection, not uncommon after chest tube placement
5. Mechanical ventilation with high pressures

MAJOR THREAT TO LIFE

* Upper airway obstruction due to accumulation of gas in the tissue around the trachea
* Necrotizing fasciitis

BEDSIDE

Quick Look Test

Upper airway obstruction will cause distress and agitation. Early symptoms of local wound infection may be mild.

Airway and Vital Signs

Confirm that the airway is clear and that the subcutaneous gas has not impinged on the trachea. Tachypnea may indicate respiratory distress; also note symptoms of stridor. Fever may indicate infection.

Selective History and Chart Review

Review why the chest tube was placed.

MANAGEMENT

1. If there is significant upper airway obstruction due to subcutaneous emphysema or other cause, do the following:
   - Contact the resident.
   - Prepare for possible intubation.
   - Contact the ICU/CCU for probable transfer.
2. Obtain a portable AP CXR immediately to confirm placement of the tube.
3. If there are continued symptoms of pneumothorax, do the following:
   - Increase the suction.
   - Consider repositioning the tube.
   - Consider replacing the tube with one of larger diameter.
4. Inspect the entry site, and confirm that all fenestrations are within the pleural cavity.

REMEMBER

1. Never push an extruding chest tube back into the pleural cavity. If the fenestrations are not shown to be inside the chest cavity by CXR and additional drainage of fluid or air is required, insert a new tube through a fresh site.
2. Many cases require the placement of more than one tube for adequate resolution of the problem requiring the thoracotomy. The existing tube must be removed only if it no longer functions.
3. A tube that has been placed on water seal (no suction) too soon may allow reaccumulation of air or fluid within the pleural space. Remember that a simple solution to this problem is the reintroduction of suction. This order may be given over the telephone before you see the patient.

URINARY DRAINAGE TUBES

There are a variety of types of urinary drainage tubes. They fall into two basic placement approaches, transurethral and suprapubic. The transurethral approach may be used to place a long-term drainage tube or may be used simply to gain access to the bladder to obtain a sterile urine sample. Periodic in-and-out catheterization may be used if a patient cannot spontaneously void. The suprapubic approach is indicated in a patient whose urethra is not competent to drain urine, such as in a patient with perineal trauma or urethral surgery.

Transurethral Catheters

Transurethral catheters come in single-, double-, or triple-lumen varieties. Their general shapes are shown in Figure 30–6.

Single-lumen tubes are used for sterile sample collection or acute relief of pressure. They are not meant to remain within the bladder

A **B** **C** **D**

Figure 30–6 Urethral catheters. *A*, Foley catheter; *B*, straight (Robinson) catheter; *C*, Coudé catheter; *D*, three-way irrigation catheter.
(From Marshall SA, Ruedy J: On Call: Principles and Protocols, 2nd ed. Philadelphia, WB Saunders, 1993, p. 194.)

for a long period of time. They include straight Robinson (often called red Robinson tubes) and Coudé tubes, which have a curved tip to facilitate passage through tight urethral obstructions.

Double-lumen tubes are the standard Foley catheters that allow urine drainage through the larger of the lumens. The smaller of the lumens leads to an intravesicular balloon that is filled with air or saline. This serves to anchor the tube within the bladder.

Triple-lumen catheters allow retrograde irrigation of the bladder to dilute active bleeding after urologic surgery. Each lumen is smaller in a triple-lumen catheter compared with a double-lumen tube. If large amounts of clots or sediment must be drained, a double-lumen tube may be preferable.

Indwelling catheters may also have stents passed through them that lead to individual ureters. These ureteral stents are placed cystoscopically or intraoperatively.

Placement of Transurethral Tubes (Foley Catheters)

Indications

1. Urinary retention
2. Neurogenic bladder
3. Monitoring of urinary output
4. Retrograde irrigation of the bladder
5. Sterile urinary sampling

Contraindications and Precautions

1. Ureteral stricture: known and severe
2. Traumatic ureteral tears or lacerations
3. Acute infections of the urethra or prostate
4. Always use sterile technique. The placement of a urinary catheter introduces a foreign body to the urinary system, which greatly increases the risk of infection.
5. Always use a lubricant when placing a urinary catheter to minimize urethral trauma. Most urinary catheter kits come with a water-soluble lubricant.
6. Avoid multiple passes in an attempt to pass a catheter. If urethral narrowing or prostatic enlargement is suspected, quickly attempt smaller catheter or Coudé catheter placement.
7. Be careful when placing urinary catheters in anticoagulated patients.
   These patients tend to bleed easily. Use copious amounts of lubricants and nontraumatic technique.
8. Never inflate the Foley balloon without good urinary return and certainty of catheter placement in the urinary bladder. Inflation of a Foley balloon in the urethra will likely traumatically tear the urethra.

Equipment Needed

1. Catheterization kit
   a. Skin preparation supplies (povidone-iodine solution)
   b. Sterile gloves, eye protection
   c. Sterile gauze sponges
   d. Sterile towels
   e. Urinary catheter, usually 16 or 18 French Foley catheter
   f. Water-soluble lubricant (may use Lidocaine 2% jelly)
   g. Syringe (10-mL)
   h. Sterile water or saline (5 mL)
   i. Adhesive tape
   j. Urinary drainage system with tubing and collection bag
2. Additional urinary catheters, as necessary

Anesthesia

No anesthesia is necessary for most patients. Lidocaine 2% jelly can be used as both a lubricant and topical anesthetic agent. It can be injected into the urethra before catheter insertion.

Placement Technique

Male Patient

1. Prepare the patient.
   a. Explain the procedure.
   b. Explain the risks and alternatives.
   c. Answer any questions.
   d. Make sure all equipment is available. Pretest the balloon by inflating it with saline and then withdrawing the saline again.
2. Position of the patient.
   Supine
3. Prepare the skin.
   a. Don sterile gloves and place sterile towels.
   b. Retract the foreskin, if present.
   c. Thoroughly prepare the entire penis with at least three applications of povidone-iodine solution. Include the urethral meatus.
4. Keep one hand sterile while the other holds the penile shaft.
5. Lift the penis straight upward.
6. Insert the catheter.
   a. Lubricate the catheter tip and catheter shaft.
   b. Insert the catheter into the urethral meatus.
   c. Continue upward penile traction to straighten the urethra and ease catheter passage.
   d. Advance the catheter slowly. Note the return of urine.
   e. Only if urine drains, inflate the balloon with 5–10 mL of saline.
      If urine does not drain and the catheter is fully inserted, press on the bladder to start the flow of urine.

    f. Gently pull back on the catheter until gentle resistance is appreciated.

    g. Passage through the prostatic urethra may be facilitated by retracting the penis caudally.

7. Tape the catheter to the thigh with slight catheter slack, protecting the catheter from traction.

8. Return the foreskin over the penis tip, if present.

Female Patient

1. Prepare the patient.
   a. Explain the procedure.
   b. Explain the risks and alternatives.
   c. Answer any questions.
   d. Make sure all equipment is available. Pretest the balloon by inflating it with saline and then withdrawing the saline again.

2. Position of the patient.
   Supine in frog-leg position

3. Prepare the skin.
   a. Don sterile gloves and place sterile towels.
   b. Expose the urethra using one hand by spreading the labia. Look for the vaginal orifice. The urethral meatus is anterior to the vagina and posterior to the clitoris.

      There is some minor variation in both appearance and location of the urethral meatus in female patients, so retraction of the labia and good visualization are critical to identify the urethra.

    c. Thoroughly prepare the entire periurethral area with at least three applications of povidone-iodine solution. Include the urethral meatus.

4. Lubricate the catheter tip and catheter shaft.

5. Insert the catheter into the urethral meatus.

6. Advance the catheter slowly; note the return of urine.

7. Only if urine drains, inflate the balloon with 5–10 mL of saline. If urine does not drain and the catheter is fully inserted, press on the bladder to start the flow of urine.

8. Gently pull back on the catheter until gentle resistance is appreciated.

9. Tape the catheter to the thigh with slight catheter slack, protecting the catheter from traction.

Suprapubic Tubes

Suprapubic tubes are placed in settings of urethral trauma or surgery or in any other case in which urethral drainage is undesirable. Placement is under local anesthesia by the Seldinger technique. Specific kits are available. Once in place, they may remain long term but are subject to the same complications as transurethral catheters. Additional complications include misplacement of the tube into the abdominal cavity, entry site infection, and vesiculo-cutaneous fistula formation. In most hospitals, this procedure is performed by a urologist.

Indications

1. Collection of accurate urine output data
2. Inability to spontaneously void
   - Relief of acute distention
   - Ongoing drainage
3. Collection of sterile urine, if a clean-catch or transurethral specimen is unobtainable or inaccurate
4. Maintenance of a lumen during the healing process after urethral trauma or surgery
5. Immobilized or incontinent patients

Complications of Urinary Drainage Tubes

1. Infection, especially with indwelling catheters of greater than 3 days' duration
2. Misplacement of a catheter. Occasionally, false lumens may be created during the placement of a nonpliable tube.
3. Bladder or urethral trauma.

Problems with Urinary Drainage Tubes

1. Blocked urethral catheter
2. Inability to place or replace catheter
3. Gross hematuria

Blocked Urethral Catheter

PHONE CALL

Questions

1. Why was the urinary drainage tube inserted?
2. How long ago was the tube inserted?
3. How long has the catheter been blocked?
4. Does the patient have suprapubic pain?
   Differentiate whether this may be due to acute bladder distention or to postoperative pain.
5. Has the patient undergone a surgical procedure, and if so, how long ago?
6. Are there any other symptoms?
7. Are there any changes in vital signs?

Orders

Have a catheter insertion tray and sterile gloves available at the bedside.

If not already done, have the bedside caregiver flush the catheter gently with 30 to 40 mL sterile saline. If the patient is newly postoperative from a urologic procedure involving the bladder, prostate, or urethra, do this irrigation yourself. Clear this with the resident first.

Degree of Urgency

Patients with acute bladder distention with symptoms of pain must be seen immediately. Likewise, if there is a significant change in vital signs or symptoms, the patient must be evaluated immediately. If the patient is stable and without symptoms of acute pain or distention, the evaluation may wait for an hour or two.

ELEVATOR THOUGHTS

What causes blockage of urinary catheters?
1. Blood clots
   - Postoperatively
   Early active bleeding is generally brisk, especially after transurethral resection of prostate. This is treated by intraoperative placement of a triple-lumen catheter and continuous bladder irrigation. This generally resolves within 24 to 48 hours.
   - Acute bladder trauma
   In addition to abdominal trauma, this may be iatrogenic due to a misplaced tube or to attempted removal of the catheter before deflating the balloon.
2. Urinary sediment
   - Urinary tract infection
   - Lysis of bladder tumor
   - Urolithiasis
3. Catheter dysfunction, including clamped or kinked catheter

MAJOR THREAT TO LIFE

- Bladder rupture
  This is preceded by very painful symptoms of increased bladder pressure in those patients who can identify and communicate these symptoms. Be careful with patients who are paraplegic or unconscious.
- Progressive renal failure
  This is secondary to long-term obstruction.

BEDSIDE

Quick Look Test

Most patients will appear comfortable. If there are symptoms of acute distention, the patient will be in distress.

Airway and Vital Signs

Pain may be associated with tachypnea or tachycardia.

Selective History and Chart Review

Review why the urinary drainage tube was placed and whether it is still necessary.

Look for underlying causes (see Elevator Thoughts).

Selective Physical Examination

GU:	Palpate the abdomen for bladder distention.
Tubes:	Confirm that there are no kinks in or clamps on the tubing.
	Confirm that the drainage bag is not full.
	Examine the tubing for evidence of blood or sediment.
Additional tests:	UA rule out infection.

MANAGEMENT

1. Reattempt to flush the catheter.
   a. Obtain a sterile irrigation tray or catheter insertion kit.
   b. Wear sterile gloves and eye protection.
   c. Have someone immobilize the distal end of the catheter as you clean it with chlorhexidine or iodine.
   d. Disconnect the catheter from the drainage bag, and have your assistant hold the bag end of the connection up, to maintain sterility.
   e. Using a catheter tip syringe, aspirate vigorously, and remove any resultant clots or debris.
   f. Gently flush the catheter with 30 to 40 mL sterile saline.
   g. Repeat previous two steps if not initially successful.
   h. Reconnect the catheter to the bag.
2. If not successful in restoring adequate drainage, replace the existing catheter with a new one.
   a. Confirm that the patient still requires a catheter.
   b. If the patient is freshly postoperative from a urologic procedure, check first with the resident.
   c. If bladder irrigation will be required, replace the tube with a triple-lumen catheter. Otherwise, simply replacing the tube with a larger catheter may be sufficient.

Inability to Place Catheter

PHONE CALL

Questions

1. **Why was the urinary drainage tube ordered?**

2. Has one been in place previously?
3. Does the patient have suprapubic pain?
4. How many attempts have been made to place the new catheter?
5. Has the patient undergone a surgical procedure, and if so, how long ago was it performed?
6. Are there any other symptoms?
7. Are there any changes in vital signs?

Orders

Have a catheter insertion tray and sterile gloves available at the bedside.

Degree of Urgency

Patients with acute bladder distention with symptoms of pain must be seen immediately. Likewise, if there is a significant change in vital signs or symptoms, the patient must be evaluated immediately. If the patient is stable and without symptoms of acute pain or distention, the evaluation may wait for an hour or two.

ELEVATOR THOUGHTS

What causes the inability to pass a catheter?
1. Urethral edema
   - Multiple insertion attempts
   - Urethral infection
   - Inadvertent removal of the old catheter without first deflating the balloon
2. Urethral obstruction
   - Benign prostatic hypertrophy
   - Carcinoma of the prostate
   - Urethral stricture
   - Other anatomic abnormality (diverticulum and false lumen)
   - Urethral transection due to trauma

MAJOR THREAT TO LIFE

- Bladder rupture
  This is preceded by very painful symptoms of increased bladder pressure in those patients who can identify and communicate these symptoms. Be careful with those patients who are paraplegic or unconscious.
- Progressive renal failure
  This is secondary to long-term obstruction.

BEDSIDE

Quick Look Test

Most patients will appear comfortable. If there are symptoms of acute distention, the patient will be in distress.

Airway and Vital Signs

Pain may be associated with tachypnea or tachycardia.

Selective History and Chart Review

Review why the urinary drainage tube was ordered and whether it is still necessary.

Is there a history of previous attempts to place a catheter?

Is there a history of traumatic removal of a catheter?

Is there a history of abdominal or pelvic trauma?

Is there evidence of obstruction? (see Elevator Thoughts)
  Look for a history of benign prostatic hypertrophy, carcinoma of the prostate, or anatomic abnormalities.

Selective Physical Examination

GU: Palpate the abdomen for bladder distention

MANAGEMENT

1. Attempt to place the catheter.
2. If urethral swelling is the problem, consider using a tube with smaller diameter.
3. If obstruction is the problem, consider using a Coudé catheter.
4. If the catheter cannot be placed by the transurethral approach, consider the suprapubic approach.

Consult with your urology colleagues before attempting this procedure. They may have other transurethral options to try.

Gross Hematuria

Hematuria is covered in Chapter 31.

REMEMBER

1. Transurethral catheters in immediately postoperative urology patients require very gentle care; contact your resident before flushing, manipulating, or replacing them.

2. In patients who have perineal trauma, do not attempt to place a transurethral tube until the patency of the urethra is demonstrated with a retrograde contrast urethrogram. A rectal examination demonstrating a "high-riding prostate" is an indication for the test.

GASTROINTESTINAL DECOMPRESSION TUBES

Adynamic ileus or intestinal obstruction can lead to accumulation of gases and liquids in the GI tract. Unless these are removed, a significant aspiration risk is present.

Indications

1. Adynamic ileus
2. Small-bowel or gastric outlet obstruction
3. Severe burns or polytrauma
4. After intestinal surgery with anastomosis
5. Gastric lavage for bleeding or poison ingestion
6. Endotracheal intubation with positive pressure ventilation

Contraindications and Precautions

1. Known or suspected facial fracture; the tube may be placed via the mouth
2. Known or suspected cervical spine injury

Equipment Needed

1. 16 to 18 Fr NG tube; these tubes may be sumped with a side arm port
2. Lubricant jelly; K-Y jelly is sufficient, but lidocaine jelly may be used
3. Topical nasal vasoconstrictors such as phenylephrine or cocaine (optional)
4. Topical anesthetic, such as Hurricaine spray (optional)
5. Emesis basin
6. Catheter tip syringe
7. Suction apparatus (i.e., wall suction or portable apparatus), tonsil tip suction tube
8. Gloves and eye protection
9. A small cup with water, with a straw for the patient to sip through
10. Benzoin and tape to secure the tube, once placed

Anatomy/Approach

It is safer to place an NG tube in a conscious patient who can cooperate with the procedure. The risk of placement in an unconscious or a paralyzed patient is misplacement into the lungs.

Anesthesia

None, or topical lidocaine administered to the nares.

Placement

1. Prepare the patient.
   a. Explain the procedure.
   b. Explain the risks and alternatives.
   c. Answer any questions.
2. Position the patient.
   Upright or decubitus, neck flexed
3. Estimate the tube length.
   Measure the distance from the patient's ear to the umbilicus; this is a good estimate of the needed length.
4. Premedicate the patient.
   a. Choose a nostril. Select the most patent one.
   b. Spray topical anesthetic to the back of the throat (optional).
   c. Apply vasoconstrictor and topical anesthetic to the nasal mucosa.
   d. Apply lubricating jelly liberally to the tip of the tube and along the length of the tube as well.
5. Have the suction apparatus turned on with the tonsil tip attached.
6. Insert the tube.
   a. With the patient's neck flexed (confirm that there is no cervical spine injury), insert the tube into the nostril.
   b. Aim straight back toward the occiput.
   c. Apply firm, constant pressure to the tube.
   d. Have the patient hold the cup of water and take small sips and swallow as you apply pressure (Fig. 30–7).
   e. Continue to advance the tube to the desired length.
   A good guideline is to advance the tube until two black lines on the tube are visible out of the nares.
   The nose should be between the second and third black lines.
   f. Anticipate some gagging during placement.
   This may be decreased by spraying additional topical anesthetic to the back of the throat.
7. If the tube does not pass easily
   a. If the tube coils in the mouth or esophagus, chill the tube in some ice to stiffen it.
   b. If the tube does not pass at all, try the other nostril.
   c. If, during advancement, the patient begins to cough, withdraw immediately. This indicates misplacement into the lung.
8. Once the tube is inserted
   a. Hold it firmly in place close to the nostril (often, this requires steadying your hand against the patient's nose).
   b. Attach the catheter tip syringe to the tube, and inject 30 to 60 mL of air into the tube. Listen over the epigastrium for the rumbling of the air into the stomach (Fig. 30–8).

Figure 30–7 Position of patient while inserting a nasogastric tube. (From Rakel RR: Saunders Manual of Medical Practice. Philadelphia, WB Saunders, 1996, p. 314.)

    c. Aspirate back on the syringe to confirm the efflux of gastric fluid. Normal stomach contents pH should be less than 5.

    d. Secure the tube to the nose with benzoin and tape.

        Avoid taping the tube in such a way that pressure is applied to the nostril; this is a common cause of necrosis of the nares.

    e. Be sure to attach the tube to a second site, such as the patient's forehead or shoulder, so that inadvertent traction on the tube does not dislodge it.

    f. Radiographic confirmation of the placement is not necessary if suction is to be applied.

        The tube may be used for decompression immediately. NG tubes have radio-opaque marker tape incorporated into their design so they are visible on routine abdominal x-ray.

Figure 30–8 Technique for confirming nasogastric tube placement. (From Rakel RR: Saunders Manual of Medical Practice. Philadelphia, WB Saunders, 1996, p. 314.)

     g. You may want to place a mark on the tube near the nose, to mark proper placement.
9. Document the procedure.
10. Routine care
     a. Record suction output volume and character.
     b. If the output is of a large volume, consider replacement of NG output: use 0.5 to 1 mL lactated Ringer's or normal saline (NS) + 30 mEq KCl/L per mL of output; replace intravenously each shift.
     c. If the tube becomes blocked, attempt to irrigate it with 30 to 40 mL of NS.
       If the block does not resolve, reposition the tube. Check with the nursing staff to see whether there are protocols regarding routine irrigation of NG tubes. If not, have the tube routinely irrigated at least every shift and PRN with 30 to 40 mL of NS.
     d. If routine x-rays are taken for other reasons, examine them for appropriate placement of the NG tube.
     e. An indwelling NG tube often is very uncomfortable.

Make sure the patient has some throat lozenges at the bedside for PRN use.

Complications of Nasogastric Tubes

1. Aspiration pneumonia
2. Trauma to nasal mucosa or external nasal skin
3. Trauma to lung or esophagus
4. Sinusitis

Indwelling catheters can cause trauma and swelling around sinus orifices, leading to acute sinusitis. Think of this as a possible cause of fever in a patient with an NG tube.

Problems with Nasogastric Tubes

1. Blocked tube
2. Dislodged tube

Blocked Nasogastric Tube

PHONE CALL

Questions

1. Why was the nasogastric tube inserted?
2. How long ago was the tube inserted?
3. What type of tube is in place?
4. How long has the tube been blocked?
5. Has the patient undergone a surgical procedure, and if so, how long ago was it performed?
6. Are there any other symptoms?
7. Are there any changes in vital signs?

Orders

Have a 60-mL catheter tip syringe, sterile NS, an emesis basin, gloves, and eye protection at the bedside.

Degree of Urgency

Evaluating a patient with a nonfunctioning NG tube may be delayed for several hours if there are more urgent issues. If there is a significant change in vital signs or symptoms, the patient must be evaluated immediately.

ELEVATOR THOUGHTS

What causes blockage of a nasogastric tube?

1. Debris within the tube lumen
   This includes food or medications. This generally results from failure to irrigate the tube routinely.
2. Clotted blood

3. Kinked tube
     A tube that is folded within the esophagus will appear clogged.
4. Clogged vent (blue part)

MAJOR THREAT TO LIFE

Aspiration pneumonia
A nonfunctioning tube does not adequately empty the stomach, thus increasing the risk of aspiration of gastric contents.

BEDSIDE

Quick Look Test

Nausea and vomiting may be present.
Abdominal distention is possible.

Airway and Vital Signs

Tachypnea with or without fever may indicate aspiration.

MANAGEMENT

1. Flush the tube with 30 to 40 mL sterile saline. Listen over the epigastrium to hear if the fluid is audible entering the stomach. If the NG tube is vented, push a small amount of air into the vent with the catheter-tip syringe.
2. Remove the tape and reposition the tube a few centimeters in or out. Do not replace a guide wire into the tube for repositioning. This could cause perforation of the esophagus or the stomach.
3. If the above maneuvers are not effective in restoring function, replace the tube. The same tube may be used if it is patent, or use a new one. Make sure that the indication for the tube still exists.
4. Confirm that the tube is being flushed routinely (30 mL NS every 4 hours and PRN).

Dislodged Nasogastric Tube

PHONE CALL

Questions

1. **Why was the nasogastric tube inserted?**
2. **How long ago was the tube inserted?**
3. **What type of tube is in place?**
4. **Has the patient undergone a surgical procedure, and if so, how long ago was it performed?**

5. Are there any other symptoms?
6. Are there any changes in vital signs?

Degree of Urgency

Evaluating a patient with a misplaced NG tube may be delayed for several hours if there are more urgent issues. If there is a significant change in vital signs or symptoms, the patient must be evaluated immediately.

ELEVATOR THOUGHTS

What causes a dislodged nasogastric tube?
1. Inadvertent traction
   This may be caused accidentally by the medical staff or by a confused or uncooperative patient.
2. Failure to secure the tube appropriately.

MAJOR THREAT TO LIFE

Aspiration Pneumonia
A nonfunctioning tube does not adequately empty the stomach, thus increasing the risk of aspiration of gastric contents.

Hypoglycemia

If the tube is used for feeding, be sure to arrange a way to deliver calories, especially in diabetic patients who have had their insulin administered.

BEDSIDE

Quick Look Test

Nausea and vomiting may be present.
Abdominal distention is possible.

Airway and Vital Signs

Tachypnea with or without fever may indicate aspiration.

MANAGEMENT

1. Inspect the tube. Has the tube been marked to indicate proper placement? Has the tube moved from that position?
2. Flush the tube with 30 to 40 mL sterile saline. Listen over the epigastrium to hear if the fluid is audible entering the stomach.

3. Remove the tape and reposition the tube a few centimeters in or out. Do not replace a guide wire into the tube for repositioning. This could cause perforation of the esophagus or stomach.

4. If the above maneuvers are not effective in restoring function, replace the tube. The same tube may be used if it is patent, or use a new one. Make sure that the indication for the tube still exists.

5. Confirm that the tube is being routinely flushed (30 mL NS every 4 hours and PRN).

REMEMBER

1. NG tubes may be used for GI decompression or for enteral feeding. Generally, if a feeding tube is used, it is of smaller diameter and is made of softer material. Some feeding tubes are so flexible they require a guide wire for adequate placement.

2. Longer tubes with distal mercury weights are available for decompression of more distal aspects of the small bowel.
   These may take several days to pass into the desired region of the small bowel.

3. If a gastrostomy or a jejunostomy tube becomes dislodged, it may be safely replaced if the enterocutaneous tract is well healed, that is, it is greater than 6 weeks since the placement. Placement must take place within 12 to 24 hours of dislodgment and may be confirmed radiographically by injection of a small volume of water-soluble contrast material into the tube during the x-ray. More recently placed tubes must be reinserted with great care so as to not disturb the fistulizing tract. Use of a guide wire or repeat surgery may be necessary.

BILIARY DRAINAGE TUBES (T-TUBES)

T-tubes are placed intraoperatively into the common bile duct after reconstruction or exploration of the duct. They are also placed after procedures involving choledochoenteral anastomoses. The tube allows external drainage of bile while the bile duct heals. Seven to 10 days after a procedure, a contrast T-tube cholangiogram is performed to assess the patency of the bile duct. T-tubes are generally left in place for 4 to 6 weeks to allow a tract to form. If the T-tube cholangiogram is normal, the tube is then removed. If it is abnormal (because of stricture, retained stones, or occlusions), the T-tube is left in place. Normal outputs range from 300 to 750 mL/day.

Problems with Biliary Drainage Tubes

1. Blockage of the tube, that is, loss of spontaneous flow
2. Dislodged tube

Blocked T-Tube

PHONE CALL

Questions

1. How long has the tube been blocked?
2. Has the tube been dislodged?
3. What was the surgical procedure, and how long ago was it performed?
4. What had the normal output been?
5. Are there any other symptoms?
6. Are there any changes in vital signs?

Orders

Have a pair of sterile gloves, eye protection, skin preparation supplies, and clean dressing materials available at the bedside.

Degree of Urgency

If the T-tube has not been displaced, the patient may be evaluated in 1 to 2 hours. If there is a significant change in vital signs or symptoms, the patient must be evaluated immediately.

ELEVATOR THOUGHTS

What causes blockage of T-tubes?

1. Debris within the tube
2. Blood clots
3. Inadvertent clamping

MAJOR THREAT TO LIFE

Sepsis from cholangitis
Abscess formation

BEDSIDE

Quick Look Test

Patients will tend to look well, unless their underlying condition is serious.

Airway and Vital Signs

No alteration is anticipated with blockage of T-tubes unless the patient is beginning to exhibit signs of sepsis.

MANAGEMENT

1. Confirm that the tubing is not clamped or kinked, and confirm that the drainage bag is not full.
2. Aspirate and irrigate the tubing as follows (always confirm with the chief resident before aspirating or flushing a biliary tube):
   - Ask an assistant to hold the distal end of the T-tube close to the connection with the drainage bag.
   - Using sterile technique, wearing sterile gloves, clean the connection site with chlorhexidine or Betadine.
   - Disconnect the tubing from the drainage bag. Take care to maintain the sterility of both ends.
   - Using a 5-mL syringe, aspirate gently. If aspiration is insufficient to dislodge the obstruction, fill a second 5-mL syringe with sterile saline and irrigate the tube gently.
3. If successful in dislodging the occlusion, reconnect the tube with the drainage bag.
4. If the aspiration and irrigation is not successful:
     Do not attempt to reirrigate. Notify your resident. Consider a contrast T-tube cholangiogram. If an intraluminal obstruction is noted in the tube, this often may be removed using a Fogarty balloon catheter. Manipulation of the tube should be done only by someone familiar with the tube. For example, many operators remove the back wall of the top of the T to facilitate removal of the tube. This may make passage of a Fogarty catheter a potentially dangerous procedure.

Dislodged T-Tube

PHONE CALL

Questions

1. How long has the tube been dislodged?
2. What was the surgical procedure, and how long ago was it performed?
3. What had the normal output been?
4. Are there any other symptoms?
5. Are there any changes in vital signs?

Orders

Have sterile gloves, skin preparation supplies, and clean dressing materials available at the bedside.

Degree of Urgency

A patient with a dislodged T-tube needs to be evaluated immediately. Likewise, if there is a significant change in vital signs or symptoms, the patient must be evaluated immediately.

ELEVATOR THOUGHTS

What causes a dislodged T-tube?
1. Failure to adequately secure the tube
2. Inadvertent traction on the tube
   - Accidentally by the medical staff
   - Accidentally by a confused or an uncooperative patient

MAJOR THREAT TO LIFE

- Sepsis from cholangitis
- Abscess formation

BEDSIDE

Quick Look Test

Patients will tend to look well, unless their underlying condition is serious.

Airway and Vital Signs

No alteration is anticipated with a dislodged T-tube.

MANAGEMENT

1. A T-tube cholangiogram should be obtained. If the cholangiogram demonstrates a dislodged tube in a newly postoperative patient, repeat surgery may be required. Contact your resident.
2. If the tract is fairly well healed and T-tube drainage is still required, interventional radiology can often place the T-tube or a similar drainage tube back into the common bile duct without subjecting the patient to another operation.

3. Check with your resident; occasionally, the T-tube may simply be left out.

WOUND DRAINAGE TUBES

(Penrose, Jackson-Pratt, Blake, and Davol)

These drains are placed intraoperatively to facilitate drainage of fluids from a surgical site. This may include abscess material, serosanguineous fluid, or fluid resulting from anastomotic insufficiency. The output and character of the fluid draining from the wound should be monitored. The drains themselves usually exit from a site different from the incision, but occasionally they exit through the incision. Removal of these drains is dependent on the output and specific circumstances. Changes in output may indicate new infection, significant postoperative bleeding, or anastomotic leak. There are several types, as follows:

Penrose: This is a flat rubber tube of graded sizes that simply acts to keep a drainage tract open.

Closed suction: These include Jackson-Pratt, Blake, and Davol drains. These are placed in large spaces deep within a cavity. Drainage of these spaces postoperatively decreases the risk of abscess or seroma formation and facilitates healing.

Problems with Wound Drainage Tubes

1. Blockage of a drain
2. Dislodged drain

Blocked Wound Drainage Tube

PHONE CALL

Questions

1. What type of drain is in place?
2. How long has the drain been blocked?
3. Has the drain been dislodged?
4. What was the surgical procedure, and how long ago was it performed?
5. What has the normal output been?
6. Are there any other symptoms?
7. Are there any changes in vital signs?

Orders

Have sterile gloves, eye protection, skin preparation supplies, and clean dressing materials available at the bedside.

Degree of Urgency

If there is a significant change in vital signs or symptoms, the patient must be evaluated immediately.

ELEVATOR THOUGHTS

What causes blockage of wound drains?
1. Debris within the tube
2. Blood clots
3. No further fluid to drain

MAJOR THREAT TO LIFE

- Sepsis
- Abscess formation

BEDSIDE

Quick Look Test

Patients will tend to look well, unless their underlying condition is serious.

Airway and Vital Signs

No alteration is anticipated with blockage of wound drains.

MANAGEMENT

1. Confirm that the wound drain is still necessary.
2. Attempt to milk debris or clots into the collection chamber.
3. Do not attempt to reposition the drain, except to remove it if necessary. Reintroduction of the drain into the body will result in bacterial contamination of the surgical bed.
4. If these maneuvers are not sufficient to dislodge an obstruction, contact your resident to see if it is a reasonable time to remove the drain.
5. Do not irrigate through the drain unless specifically asked to by your resident.

Dislodged Wound Drainage Tube

PHONE CALL

Questions

1. What type of drain is in place?
2. How long has the drain been dislodged?
3. What was the surgical procedure, and how long ago was it performed?
4. What has the normal output been?
5. Are there any other symptoms?
6. Are there any changes in vital signs?

Orders

Have sterile gloves, skin preparation supplies, and clean dressing materials available at the bedside.

Degree of Urgency

If there is a significant change in vital signs or symptoms, the patient must be evaluated immediately.

ELEVATOR THOUGHTS

What causes a dislodged wound drain?
1. Failure to adequately secure the tube
2. Inadvertent traction on the tube
   - Accidentally by the medical staff
   - Accidentally by a confused or an uncooperative patient

MAJOR THREAT TO LIFE

- Sepsis
- Abscess formation

BEDSIDE

Quick Look Test

Patients will tend to look well, unless their underlying condition is serious.

Airway and Vital Signs

No alteration is anticipated with a dislodged wound drain.

MANAGEMENT

1. Confirm that the wound drain is still necessary.
2. Do not attempt to reposition the drain, except to remove it, if necessary. Advancement of the drain will introduce bacterial contamination into the surgical bed.
3. Secure the drain in its present position with silk suture.
4. Contact your resident to see if it is a reasonable time to remove the drain.

Urine Output Changes

Changes in urine output (UO) encompass a variety of complaints, the most common being a decrease in UO in a postoperative patient because of changes in intravascular volume. Also considered in this chapter are other causes of decreased UO, increased UO, and blood in the urine. Components of these evaluations are also covered in other chapters where indicated. The function of the kidney may be divided into two major categories: fluid management and solute management.

DECREASED URINE OUTPUT

UO is considered one of the three major indicators of end-organ perfusion (remember from Chapter 12: UO, mental status, and skin temperature). In postoperative patients, a decreased UO must be considered a decrease in intravascular volume until proved otherwise because of the frequency of this occurrence and because of the seriousness of underestimating fluid resuscitation in a sick patient. Remember that the postoperative or gravely ill patient has undergone neuroendocrine changes that help to retain fluid and that third spacing of intravascular fluid is to be expected.

PHONE CALL

Questions

1. **How is the UO being measured?**
   Indwelling urinary catheters give the most reliable estimates of hourly output but are not always clinically appropriate. Routine intake and output (I/O) measurements without catheters can overestimate or underestimate UO volumes by a factor of close to 100%.
2. **What are the current trends over the last 2 to 3 hours, and what is it over the last 24 hours?**
   Oliguria is defined as less than 400 mL/day (<20 mL/hour). Anuria is defined as less than 50 mL/day. Great variances in hourly output suggest collection errors or postrenal obstruction.

3. Have there been recent changes in laboratory studies including those for potassium, creatinine, blood urea nitrogen (BUN), and urinalysis (UA).

4. Has the patient undergone a surgical procedure, and if so, how long ago was it performed?

   Pay special attention to surgeries involving bladder, ureters, or kidneys, including renal transplants.

   Also be mindful that ureters may be damaged in any pelvic or extra peritoneal surgery.

5. Are there any other symptoms, including abdominal pain, fever, or dysuria?

6. Are there any changes in vital signs?

Orders

1. If an indwelling urinary catheter (Foley) is present, it may be flushed gently with 20 to 30 mL normal saline (NS) to dislodge sediment or clots. Check with the chief resident or the attending physician before flushing a catheter in place after surgery on the bladder or urinary tract.

2. Take steps to evaluate the hydration status of the patient. Repeat taking the vital signs and order orthostatic blood pressure (BP) measurements.

3. If the patient is immediately postoperative, and fluid shifts out of the intravascular space are clinically apparent, a fluid bolus of 500 mL crystalloid is appropriate; note that the fluid status of a patient must be evaluated (see Chapter 12).

Degree of Urgency

If the patient is stable and comfortable, 30 to 60 minutes is appropriate. If there is a significant change in vital signs or symptoms, the patient must be evaluated immediately.

ELEVATOR THOUGHTS

What are the causes of decreased UO?

   In the postoperative patient, intravascular fluid deficit is such a common cause of decreased UO that there is a tendency to believe that this is always the case. The fluid status should be quickly assessed, but do not forget to evaluate for other causes of oliguria. Decreased UO may be conveniently divided into three categories. **Prenal** causes of oliguria are often due to poor kidney perfusion. **Renal** causes of oliguria include the major renal pathologies and result in poor kidney function (i.e., urine formation). **Postrenal** causes of oliguria are often due to external forces that block the flow of urine anywhere along the tract from the kidney to the outside world. These are listed in Table 31–1.

   Remember that renal and prolonged prerenal and postrenal causes of oliguria can all lead to azotemia.

TABLE 31–1 Common Causes of Oliguria

Prerenal	Renal	Postrenal
Volume Depletion	**Glomerular Nephritides**	**Ureteral Obstruction (must be bilateral)**
Third spacing	Acute glomerulonephritis	Retroperitoneal mass
Hemorrhage	Vasculitis	Sloughed papillae
Gastrointestinal losses	Malignant hypertensive nephropathy	Strictures/valves
Renal losses	Renal thrombosis	Stones, clots
Poor Cardiac Output	**Tubular Interstitial**	**Bladder Neck Obstruction**
Congestive heart failure	Pyelonephritis	Prostatic hypertrophy
Tamponade	Hypercalcemia	Tumor
Myocardial infarction	Multiple myeloma	Sphincter spasm
Pulmonary embolus	Acute interstitial nephritis	Strictures/valves
	Acute Tubular Necrosis	**Urethral Obstruction**
Shock/Sepsis	Postischemic injury	Strictures/valves
Hepatorenal Syndrome	Prolonged vasopressor use	**Bladder Rupture**
	Nephrotoxic Agents	**Blocked Catheter**
	Antibiotics	
	Contrast dye	
	Anesthetics	
	Nonsteroidal anti-inflammatory drugs	
	Chemotherapeutic agents	
	Vascular Problems	
	Emboli	
	Renal vessel thrombosis	

MAJOR THREAT TO LIFE

- Hypotension and shock
- Acute renal failure
  This may require dialysis for treatment
- Hyperkalemia

BEDSIDE

Quick Look Test

Physical obstruction may be associated with abdominal discomfort, agitation, and sensation of needing to urinate. A serious deterioration of clinical status including neurologic changes or metabolic derangements may indicate hypotension or acute renal failure.

Airway and Vital Signs

Look for evidence of dehydration. Resting tachycardia or postural changes in pulse rate (a drop of 15 beats/minute) or BP (a drop in systolic BP [SBP] of 15 mm Hg or any fall in diastolic BP) indicate decreased intravascular volume. This is most likely due to under-resuscitation, but be mindful of early sepsis or cardiogenic shock.

Initial Management

1. Support cardiac output and perfusion.
   A fluid bolus is indicated for patients who are intravascularly depleted.
2. Determine cause of decreased UO.
   Once this is determined, the management is more clear.

Selective History and Chart Review

Is there a condition that would predispose a patient to decreased UO? (See Elevator Thoughts.)
- Review trends in UO and I/Os, and review changes in weight.
- Review recent laboratory studies trends.

Selective Physical Examination

VS:	Tachycardia or postural BP changes (dehydration)
MS:	Decreased mental status (decreased perfusion)
HEENT:	Dry or sticky mucous membranes and flat neck veins (dehydration)
	Full neck veins (tamponade)
Resp:	Rales and decreased aeration (fluid overload and congestive heart failure [CHF])
Abd:	Pain and distention (obstruction of urinary tract and urinary tract infection [UTI])
GU:	Dysuria (UTI)

Skin:	Decrease in warmth or turgor, and dry axillae (dehydration)
	Itching (azotemia)
Rectal:	Enlarged prostate or mass
Tubes:	Blocked urinary catheter
Additional tests:	1. UA: White blood cells (WBCs) indicate UTI, high specific gravity supports dehydration, and red blood cells (RBCs) indicate UTI or urolithiasis
	2. Electrolytes: To assess for metabolic derangement, elevations in BUN, and creatinine
	3. Urine Na^+: Assessment of renal function (Table 31–2)
	4. ECG: Assess for peaked T waves, indicating hyperkalemia

To differentiate renal causes from prerenal causes, calculate the fractional excretion of sodium (FENa) as follows:

$$FENa = UNa \times V/PNa \times UCr \times V/PCr$$

U	Urine
P	Plasma
Cr	Creatinine
V	Urine volume

As the urine volume cancels out, a simplified formula is:

$$UNa \times PCr/PNa \times UCr$$

This is the ratio of Na^+ excreted over Na^+ filtered. A FENa less than 1% is indicative of prerenal causes of renal failure. A FENa greater than 1% is indicative of renal causes of failure.

TABLE 31–2 **Comparison of Laboratory Findings in Various Urine Output Change Conditions**

| | Blood | | | Urine | | | |
	Na	BUN	BUN/Cr	Output	SG	Urine Na	FENa
Prerenal	—	Incr.	>10:1	Decr.	>1.020	<40	<1%
ATN	—	Incr.	<10:1	—	<1.020	>40	2–3%
SIADH	Decr.	Decr.	>50:1	Decr.	Incr.	>100	Varies
DI	Incr.	Incr.	<5:1	Incr.	Decr.	<10	

Na, sodium; BUN, blood urea nitrogen; Cr, creatinine; SG, serum glucose; Incr., increased; Decr., decreased; ATN, acute tubular necrosis; SIADH, syndrome of inappropriate antidiuretic hormone secretion; DI, diabetes insipidus.

MANAGEMENT

Prerenal

This is the most common etiology.

Fluid Deficit

1. Confirm with physical examination and laboratory studies.
2. Fluid bolus with 500 mL crystalloid; may repeat if not effective.
    If, after two fluid boluses, no effect is noted, reevaluate fluid status. Add invasive monitoring (central venous pressure, indwelling urinary catheter, and Swan-Ganz catheter), as necessary.
3. Monitor rehydration, as needed, with frequent vital sign checks, urine output, and electrolyte evaluations.
4. Order daily weights and strict I/O measurements.

Normal or Increased Fluid Status

1. Rule out myocardial infarction, as necessary.
2. If CHF, evaluate as directed in Chapter 28; evaluate oxygen status, and begin diuresis, as follows:
    Furosemide *(Lasix)* **20 to 80 mg intravenously (IV)** over 2 to 5 minutes. The dose may be doubled and administered every 1 hour as needed to a total dose of 400 mg if no response is noted. Doses of greater than 100 mg should be given slowly (<4 mg/minute) to avoid ototoxicity. Also use caution when used in conjunction with aminoglycoside antibiotics.
    Hydrochlorothiazide 25 to 50 mg orally (PO) (a thiazide diuretic) or **Metolazone** *(Zaroxolyn)* **5 to 10 mg PO** may be added once or twice a day to furosemide therapy (a loop diuretic) for more effective diuresis.
    If furosemide therapy is ineffective, consider use of **Ethacrynic acid** *(Edecrin)* **50 mg IV every hour × 2 doses or Bumetanide** *(Bumex)* **1 to 10 mg IV over 1 to 2 minutes.**
3. Monitor diuresis, as needed, with frequent checks of vital signs and evaluations of electrolytes.
    Supplemental K+ may be necessary with massive or prolonged diuresis.

Postrenal

This is most likely if UO is absent or is fluctuating widely.

1. Place a urinary catheter if one is not already in place.
    Note the postvoid residual. If the residual volume is greater than 400 mL and the discomfort is relieved, leave the catheter in place and reassess in 1 to 2 days. This will give the distended bladder muscles a chance to recover function.

Always consider subacute bacterial endocarditis prophylaxis when inserting a urinary catheter in a patient with a cardiac murmur. Current recommendations include treatment of patients with valvular abnormalities such as mitral valve prolapse with a persistent systolic murmur. Acceptable antibiotics include **ampicillin 2 g intramuscularly (IM)** or **vancomycin 1 g IV over 1 hour, plus gentamicin 1.5 mg/kg IM or IV 30 minutes** before a urinary procedure and repeat in 8 hours.

2. If a urinary catheter is already in place, flush with 20 to 30 mL sterile NS.

   This must be done with extreme caution in the setting of recent bladder or kidney surgery. If the catheter will not flush, replace with a new catheter.

   Make sure the catheter is not clamped for some reason (as after an abdominal or pelvic CT scan).

3. Look for nonbladder causes of postrenal oliguria such as stones or mass externally obstructing the urinary tract.

4. Order daily weights and strict I/O measurements.

Renal

1. Confirm with physical examination and laboratory studies.
2. Consult specialists, as necessary.
3. Order daily weights and strict I/O measurements.
4. Manage associated problems.
   a. Hyperkalemia
      i. Limit exogenous K^+. Place on continuous cardiac monitoring. Treat severe hyperkalemia as outlined in Chapter 12.
      ii. **Calcium gluconate 5 to 10 mL of a 10% solution IV over 2 minutes.**

         This is symptomatic relief only to stabilize neuromuscular and cardiac effects of hyperkalemia and does not alter the concentration of potassium in the serum. Its effects last only 1 hour.
      iii. **50% dextrose in water, 50 mL IV** followed by **regular insulin 5 to 10 U**, effects a shift of the extracellular potassium to intracellular. Its effects last 1 to 2 hours.
      iv. **Sodium bicarbonate 1 ampule (44.6 mmol) IV** also effects a shift of potassium from the extracellular to the intracellular space.
      v. The glucose/insulin/bicarbonate therapies, as follows, may be combined in an IV bag.

         1000 mL 10% dextrose in water + 3 ampules of sodium bicarbonate + 20 U regular insulin to run at 75 mL/hour until the desired K^+ level is reached.
      vi. **Sodium polystyrene sulfonate** *(Kayexalate)* **15 to 30 g (4 to 8 tsp) in 50 to 100 mL of 20% sorbitol PO every 3 to 4 hours** or **in 200 mL 20% sorbitol of 20%**

dextrose in water rectally (PR) by retention enema for 30 to 60 minutes every 4 hours.

This is chelation therapy and is the only treatment listed here that will actually remove potassium from the body. In the absence of functioning kidneys, the only other option is hemodialysis, which can remove up to 25 to 30 mEq/hour.

b. Metabolic acidosis

Evaluate with arterial blood gas and serum bicarbonate levels ($[HCO_3^-]$) and treat as necessary (see Chapter 12), as follows:

Mild: pH = 7.30 to 7.35
Moderate: pH = 7.20 to 7.29
Severe: pH = <7.20

Mild and moderate acidosis generally requires no specific therapy short of reversal of the underlying cause. Severe acidosis that results in decreased mental status, hyperventilation, cardiac abnormalities, and hypotension is treated with sodium bicarbonate as determined by the following formula:

$$\text{Bicarbonate required (in mmol)} = (\text{wt in kg})\,(0.4)\,(\text{desired } [HCO_3^-]) - (\text{measured } [HCO_3^-])$$

Replace bicarbonate slowly, over 24 hours; i.e., one-half to one-third of the deficit in the first 6 to 12 hours with the remaining deficit replaced in the remaining 12 to 18 hours. The usual desired $[HCO_3^-]$ is generally 15 mE/L. Remember that the goal of bicarbonate therapy is not to normalize the pH but rather to reverse the physiologic effects of acidosis. This usually occurs when the pH is greater than 7.20. Remember also that severe acidosis is also associated with hyperkalemia, as intracellular K^+ is exchanged with extracellular hydrogen ions.

c. Fluid overload

Treat with diuretics as listed above. If the kidneys are not sufficiently excreting free water despite diuretic therapy, there are only two ways to decrease the total body water:

i. Decrease the input by restricting oral and IV intake of fluid to minimums

ii. Fluid reduction by dialysis

Make sure the patient is oxygenating well. Treat symptoms of CHF as outlined in Chapter 28.

- Sit the patient up to allow maximum aeration of the lungs.
- **Morphine sulfate 2 to 4 mg IV every 5 to 10 minutes up to 10 to 12 mg** will pool the blood in the splanchnic circulation and decrease pulmonary edema.

Hold morphine sulfate treatment if symptoms of decreased respiratory drive or hypotension are apparent.
- Reverse the effects of morphine sulfate as necessary, with **naloxone hydrochloride 0.2 to 2 mg IV, IM, or subcutaneously (SC) to a total of 10 mg.** Note that the half-life of naloxone effect is shorter than that of most narcotics and that repeat doses may be necessary.

   iii. **Nitroglycerin ointment 2.5 to 5.0 cm topically every 4 hours.**

     Nitroglycerin tablets 0.3 to 0.6 mcg sublingually (SL) every 5 minutes or nitroglycerin spray 1 puff every 15 minutes may be used if ointment is not available. Hold nitroglycerin for SBP of less than 90 mm Hg.

     Adequate function of nitroglycerin is generally confirmed by a headache that usually responds to **acetaminophen** *(Tylenol* **and others)** **350 to 1000 mg PO every 4 hours as needed.** Diuretic therapy as outlined earlier.

  d. Uremia

    This is manifested by elevated BUN with symptoms of decreased mental status, pericarditis, or seizures. It is treated with hemodialysis.

5. Stop any nephrotoxic medications (nonsteroidal anti-inflammatory drugs and aminoglycosides), and adjust the doses of renally excreted medications.
6. Limit magnesium- and aluminum-containing medications.
7. Determine if the patient requires dialysis. The following are indications for dialysis:
   a. Fluid overload unresponsive to diuretics and resulting in CHF or edema
   b. Hyperkalemia, severe and symptomatic, with serum K^+ at 6 to 8 mmol/L
   c. Metabolic acidosis, severe, acute, and symptomatic, pH of less than 7.2
   d. Uremia, severe with symptoms of decreased mental status, pericarditis, or seizure, and BUN at greater than 35 mmol/L
      A nephrologist should be consulted to confirm the need for dialysis and to arrange the therapy.

SPECIAL SURGICAL CONSIDERATIONS

Preoperative Considerations

A serious decrease in UO in a preoperative patient is an indication of a serious problem and may require changing plans for a scheduled procedure.

Postoperative Considerations

1. The most common cause of decreased UO in immediately postoperative patients is insufficient resuscitation and intravascular volume deficit.
2. Expect low UO in patients with prolonged procedures.
   Postoperative IV fluid rates should routinely be at 100 to 150 mL/hour until adequate fluid hydration is ensured and UO is normal. Take care not to overhydrate.
3. Increased secretion of antidiuretic hormone (ADH) is a normal response to stress. Expect fluid retention following major operative procedures. In uncomplicated cases, the sequestered fluid will remobilize and be excreted in 3–4 days.
4. The syndrome of inappropriate antidiuretic hormone (SIADH) secretion is the condition of high ADH secretion in the absence of the normal stimulus of high serum osmolarity.
   It is diagnosed as outlined in Table 31–2 and treated initially with maintenance of intravascular volume, and then with fluid restriction until physiologic diuresis ensues.

REMEMBER

1. Azotemia may present with oliguria, but it may also occur with normal or increased UO.
2. Review all medications in oliguric patients, and adjust doses as necessary.

INCREASED URINE OUTPUT

PHONE CALL

Questions

1. **How is the urine output measured?**
   Indwelling urinary catheters give the most reliable estimates of hourly output but are not always clinically appropriate. Routine I/O measurements without catheters can overestimate or underestimate UO volumes by a factor of close to 100%.
2. **What are the current trends over the last 2 to 3 hours, and what is it over the last 24 hours?**
   Polyuria is defined as greater than 3 L/day. Great variances in hourly output suggest collection errors or resolution of an obstruction. Make sure that the volume is reported and not just the patient's sensation of frequency or urgency.
3. **Have there been recent changes in laboratory studies, including serum glucose, potassium, creatinine, BUN, and UA?**
4. **Has the patient undergone a surgical procedure, and if so, how long ago was it performed?**

This concerns especially neurosurgical or renal procedures.
5. **Are there any other symptoms?**
   A change in mental status may indicate decreased intravascular volume or a primary intracranial problem.
6. **Are there any changes in vital signs?**
7. **Differentiate whether the UO is increased or if the patient is just incontinent, making any UO(or measurement of UO) inconvenient.**

Orders

1. Establish an IV to replace ongoing fluid losses, if necessary.
2. Serum and urine electrolytes may be ordered at this time, if indicated.
3. If the patient is becoming more ill, order an indwelling urinary catheter if not already in place.

Degree of Urgency

A stable patient may be evaluated in an hour or so. If there is a significant change in vital signs, mental status changes, or symptoms of dehydration, the patient must be evaluated immediately.

ELEVATOR THOUGHTS

What are the causes of increased UO?
1. Diabetes mellitus
   New-onset or undertreated diabetes mellitus results in increased blood sugar. When the glucose concentration is greater than 300 mg/dL, the kidney's ability to reabsorb sugar may be overwhelmed and glucose is passed into the urine, causing an osmotic diuresis.
2. Diabetes insipidus (DI)
   This is a loss of normal secretion of ADH (or vasopressin) from either neurologic or nephrogenic causes.
   This occurs in settings of head trauma, cerebral edema (a late finding), pituitary tumors, and occasionally after neurosurgical procedures. Symptoms include massive UO at 5 to 10 L/day, polydipsia, and progressive dehydration. It is differentiated from other diuretic states by analysis of urine electrolytes. As listed in Table 31–2, the urinary sodium in DI is very low, as is the specific gravity because the kidney is unable to reabsorb water from the distal tubule. It is treated with intranasal **vasopressin 5 to 10 U three times per day** and treatment of fluid deficits.
3. High-output renal failure
4. Diuretic therapy
   This includes treatments for CHF or therapies to treat increased intracranial pressure.
5. Postobstructive diuresis
6. Diuretic phase of acute tubular necrosis

7. Salt-wasting nephritis
8. Physiologic diuresis
     This results from increased PO or IV intake during the res-
     olution phase of a major illness or during recovery from major
     surgery.

MAJOR THREAT TO LIFE

- Dehydration leading to hypovolemic shock
- Cerebral edema resulting in DI
- High-output renal failure

BEDSIDE

Quick Look Test

Patients tend to look well, unless significant dehydration is present.
If a serious illness is present, such as new-onset diabetes mellitus,
other problems (e.g., ketoacidosis) may be present.

Airway and Vital Signs

Look for evidence of dehydration. Resting tachycardia or postural
changes in pulse rate (a drop of 15 beats/minute) or BP (a drop in
SBP of 15 mm Hg or any fall in diastolic BP) indicate decreased
intravascular volume.

Initial Management

1. Support cardiac output and perfusion.
     A fluid bolus is indicated for patients who are intravascu-
     larly depleted.
2. Determine cause of increased UO.
     Once this is determined, the management is more clear.

Selective History and Chart Review

*Is there a condition that would predispose a patient to increased UO?
(See Elevator Thoughts.)*
     Review trends in UO and I/Os, and review changes in weight,
     which is a good indicator of whole body fluid status.
     Review recent laboratory studies trends, especially BUN, cre-
     atinine, and Na^+.
     Review current medications and whether the patient is taking
     diuretics.

Selective Physical Examination

VS:	Tachycardia or postural BP changes (dehydration)
MS:	Decreased mental status (decreased perfusion and intracranial problem)
HEENT:	Dry, sticky mucous membranes and flat neck veins (dehydration)

	Visual field defects (pituitary tumor)
	Papilledema (increased intracranial pressure)
Resp:	Rales and decreased aeration (fluid over load and CHF)
	Kussmaul's respirations (rate of 25 to 30 per minute, continuous and sonorous, an indication of acidosis, i.e., in diabetic ketoacidosis)
	Fruity breath (diabetic ketoacidosis)
Abd:	Pain (an occasional finding in diabetes mellitus)
Skin:	Decrease in warmth or turgor, and dry axillae (dehydration)
	Itching (azotemia)
Neuro:	Any change, especially lateralizing signs (intracranial process)
Tubes:	Presence of urinary catheter
Additional tests:	1. UA: High specific gravity supports dehydration; low specific gravity supports DI RBCs indicate UTI or urolithiasis
	2. Electrolytes: To assess for metabolic derangement and elevations in BUN and creatinine
	3. Urine Na^+: Assessment of renal function (see Table 31–2)

MANAGEMENT

1. Major management is directed at correcting the cause.
2. Replace depleted intravascular volume with crystalloid (see Chapter 12).
3. Maintain ongoing losses with crystalloid by supplying insensible losses (400 to 800 mL/day in addition to replacement of urinary and other measurable losses, e.g., nasogastric [NG] suction and drain output).

    The usual rate is 0.5 to 1 mL/mL of measurable output. Make sure to replace the type of fluid lost. When replacing ongoing losses of fluids, it is advisable to check electrolytes frequently to assess electrolyte balance.
4. Order daily weights and strict I/O measurements.
5. Stop or alter the dose of all diuretic medications.

SPECIAL SURGICAL CONSIDERATIONS

Preoperative Considerations

1. A serious decrease in UO in a preoperative patient is an indication of a serious problem and may require changing plans for a scheduled procedure.

2. In a patient with increased intracranial pressure, DI is a very late finding, and a patient with this manifestation is likely to die soon.

Postoperative Considerations

1. There is a normal diuresis of third-spaced fluid 3 to 4 days after an uncomplicated procedure or during the resolution phase of a serious illness.

    Be mindful of the patient's preoperative weight, and do not be alarmed if the patient who is well or improving, and is still above the preoperative weight, begins a normal diuresis.

2. Massive increases in UO in a postoperative neurosurgical patient are an indication for a computed tomographic scan of the head immediately.

HEMATURIA

Blood in the urine is always abnormal. When it is brought to your attention on call, it generally represents gross hematuria (bleeding that is noticeable without a microscope). A volume as small as 1 mL of blood/L of urine is noticeable as red. Although it is infrequent for hematuria to cause significant blood loss, occasionally an ill or unstable patient will be further stressed by what small blood loss is present. After a urologic procedure, urinary bleeding with clot formation is common and may be a cause of urinary obstruction.

PHONE CALL

Questions

1. *When did the hematuria start?*
    Has there been prolonged blood loss?

2. *What is the urine output?*
    Make sure that clots have not stopped the flow of urine.

3. *Is there a urinary catheter in place?*
    This is a common cause of microscopic hematuria but is also an avenue through which the bladder may be irrigated to treat occlusion caused by clots.

4. *Is the patient anticoagulated?*
    These patients must be evaluated immediately and have their anticoagulation reversed, as necessary.

5. *Has the patient undergone a surgical procedure, and if so, how long ago was it performed?*
    Procedures on the bladder or the kidney are associated with some transient bleeding but not generally with prolonged symptoms.

6. *Are there any other signs and symptoms?*

Signs and symptoms such as fever, dysuria, or flank pain may suggest an infection or stone disease.

7. *Are there any changes in vital signs?*

Significant loss of blood may be associated with tachycardia, tachypnea, and hypovolemic shock.

Orders

For Significant Bleeding

1. Order a hematocrit and UA.
2. Make sure IV access is in place for fluid replacement if necessary.
3. If the last hematocrit was low or if clinical symptoms of anemia are present, make sure blood is available for this patient.

If Urinary Obstruction Is Present

See Decreased UO section earlier.

Degree of Urgency

Loss of small amounts of blood does not require immediate attention. However, if the bleeding is severe, if urinary obstruction is evident, or if there is evidence of symptomatic anemia, the patient must be seen immediately. Likewise, if there is a significant change in vital signs or symptoms, the patient must be evaluated immediately.

ELEVATOR THOUGHTS

What are the causes of hematuria?

1. Trauma to the urinary tract

This is usually from the presence of a urinary catheter. Improper or traumatic placement can cause transient bleeding, as can attempted removal before the balloon is completely deflated. A large indwelling catheter occasionally causes some bladder or urethral irritation and may result in small amounts of blood in the urine or at the meatus. Abdominal or pelvic trauma can affect the urinary tract.

2. Coagulation abnormalities

If the patient is anticoagulated and symptomatically anemic, reversal of the anticoagulation is indicated.

Primary bleeding diatheses such as disseminated intravascular coagulation (DIC), thrombocytopenia, or hemophilia can also cause hematuria.

3. Infection

Cystitis, prostatitis, or pyelonephritis is a frequent cause of hematuria, if an indwelling catheter is in place.

Look for the presence of WBCs with bacteria to make a diagnosis, as catheters in place for greater than or equal to 3 days are often chronically colonized with bacteria. Chronic colonization is not associated with WBCs and does not require antibiotic treatment.

4. Medications

These include anticoagulants such as heparin or warfarin; thrombolytics such as streptokinase, urokinase, and tissue plasminogen activator; and chemotherapeutic agents such as cyclophosphamide.

5. Genitourinary (GU) surgery

Postoperative bleeding is common after bladder and prostate surgery, such as transurethral resection of the prostate and transurethral resection of a bladder tumor, and is generally treated preemptively with bladder irrigation. This bleeding is often associated with passage of blood clots and may be obstructing.

6. Renal calculi

Stones may be present anywhere in the urinary tract. They irritate the lumen wall and cause bleeding. This is usually associated with renal colic when flow is obstructed.

7. GU cancer

This is commonly of the bladder or the kidney. Hematuria may be a presenting symptom.

8. Abdominal or pelvic trauma

Blunt or penetrating injuries to the abdomen or pelvis may cause hematuria. Gross hematuria must be evaluated immediately with a retrograde urethrogram, then CT scan with IV contrast. Microscopic hematuria may be present after a renal contusion.

9. Other kidney disease, such as glomerulonephritis, severe hypertension, or benign familial hematuria.

MAJOR THREAT TO LIFE

- Anemia with associated hypoxemia
- Hypovolemic shock
- Urinary obstruction and bladder rupture

BEDSIDE

Quick Look Test

Patients tend to look well but are distressed about the symptoms. They may be agitated if urinary obstruction is present.

Airway and Vital Signs

Hypovolemia is associated with tachycardia and hypotension. Hypoxia is associated with tachypnea and agitation. Elevated temperature may indicate an infectious cause.

Initial Management

1. Take steps to ensure the comfort of the patient and to reassure the patient.
2. Evaluate the severity.
   If urine is slightly pink and flowing well, identification of the problem and vigilance may be all that is required.
3. If symptoms are more severe
   • Support hemodynamics, as necessary.
   • Treat hypoxia with O_2.
   • Relieve urinary obstruction.
   • Reverse anticoagulation, if necessary (check with resident first).

Selective History and Chart Review

• Causes of hematuria (see Elevator Thoughts)
• History of bleeding diathesis
  Does the patient have a history or a family history of bleeding problems? Have there been any recent bleeding symptoms? Note that while bleeding disorders may indeed be present and contributing to the hematuria, in more than one-third of the cases, an additional coexistent cause for bleeding will also be found.
• History of renal stones
  Risk factors include dehydration, hypercalcemia, hypercalciuria, hyperoxaluria, cystinuria, and recent UTI (especially with urease-producing bacteria such as *Proteus, Klebsiella, Serratia,* and *Pseudomonas* spp.). Loss of the normal diurnal pH variances in the urine can also cause stones. Consistent acid pH supports formation of uric acid stones, and persistent alkali conditions support precipitation of calcium phosphate salt.
• Risk factors for GU neoplasm
  These include occupational exposure to aniline dyes or rubber compounds, cigarette smoking, history of analgesic abuse, or prior pelvic irradiation.
• Evaluation of the need for a urinary catheter, if present
  If it was recently inserted, look for evidence of trauma. If it has been in place for more than 3 days, consider infection. Catheters often get pulled or misplaced during their use; the resultant trauma often causes bleeding, but it is usually transient. If use of the catheter is unnecessary, consider discontinuing it.
• Review of recent laboratory studies and UO trends
  How stable has the hematocrit been? Are the platelets adequate?

Selective Physical Examination

VS:	Repeat now if evidence of hypovolemia or hypoxia
MS:	Confusion or delirium (hypoxia and early urosepsis)
CVS:	Tachycardia and orthostatic hypotension (hypovolemia)

Resp:	Tachypnea (hypoxia and early urosepsis)
Abd:	Bladder distention or discomfort to palpation (obstruction)
GU:	Flank pain (pyelonephritis and renal stone)
Skin:	Pale (anemia); clammy and cool (hypovolemia)
Tubes:	Urinary catheter in place, and if so, length of time
Special examinations:	Other sites of bleeding, e.g., wounds, gingival, and IV sites
Additional tests:	1. Urinalysis: If not already done
	2. Urine culture and sensitivities: If fever or pyuria is present
	3. Urinary protein: May indicate a primary kidney disease
	4. Hematocrit and coagulation studies: As clinically indicated
	5. CT scan with IV contrast or IVP: If obstruction is suspected, CT scan or IVP may be ordered to visualize the renal collecting system; except for acute traumas, this is a nonurgent test. If the study is normal, future tests may include cystoscopy and urine cytology to rule out neoplastic cells.

MANAGEMENT

1. Management is directed at correcting the underlying cause.
2. Replace depleted intravascular volume with crystalloid (see Chapter 12).
3. Evaluate carefully the need for blood replacement.
     This is rarely necessary. Always consult the resident before transfusing, and check to see if the patient has autologous blood available.
4. Recheck UA in the morning, hematocrit as necessary.

SPECIAL SURGICAL CONSIDERATIONS

Preoperative Considerations

1. Gross hematuria noted on the initial acute trauma evaluation requires further study to assess patency of the urinary tract. Do not place a urinary catheter until the patency of the urethra has been documented with a retrograde urethrogram.

2. Significant hematuria or hypotension indicates an underlying condition that would affect a scheduled procedure. Check with the attending physician or chief resident to see if the case should be canceled.

Postoperative Considerations

Postoperative urologic patients often have transient bleeding with clot formation. Prophylactic treatment often includes continuous bladder irrigation with NS through a multilumen urinary catheter. The efflux of NS generally clears with time. If the efflux does not begin clearing within one shift, further evaluation is warranted. These patients are likely to form clots and are at the greatest risk for significant blood loss. Many, especially after radical prostatectomy, start off with a significant intraoperative blood loss and may be anemic as a baseline. Transfusions are not infrequent. If clots obstruct the urinary tract or catheter, first try to unplug the catheter by flushing gently with 20 to 30 mL NS. If this is ineffective, replacement of the urinary catheter is often necessary. Err toward a larger catheter if possible, as these are less likely to become clogged. Triple-lumen catheters add the advantage of being able to irrigate with NS but do not have as large a drainage tube as double-lumen catheters of the same outer diameter. Always consult with a resident or attending physician before flushing or replacing the catheter in a recent postoperative urology patient.

REMEMBER

1. In crush injury patients, it is important to differentiate between rhabdomyolysis and RBCs in the urine.

   Both read positive on the orthotoluidine test of a urine dipstick, which does not differentiate between RBCs (hematuria), free hemoglobin (hemolysis), and myoglobin (rhabdomyolysis). Rhabdomyolysis and hemolysis may also be rapidly differentiated by looking at a spun vial of blood; clear plasma supports rhabdomyolysis, and red plasma suggests hemolysis. In cases where muscle breakdown is present.
   - Maintain UO with adequate hydration and furosemide.
   - Confirm the diagnosis by checking urine for myoglobin.
   - Check serial creatine phosphokinase levels.
2. Any bleeding in a very ill patient may indicate DIC.
   Look for other sites of bleeding.

32

Wounds

The on-call physician for a surgical service should feel comfortable managing wound problems. Usually, most of these problems are straightforward. However, some calls about wound problems lead to the diagnosis of a serious problem. For this reason, it is important that you examine the patient. What may appear as a benign process to the patient or the RN may appear as a more significant process to you.

PHONE CALL

Questions

1. **What operation did the patient have, and when was the operation performed?**

It is important to consider the nature of the operation performed and the important anatomy in the surgical region. This helps you think about the possible causes of the wound problem. For example, consider a draining abdominal wound. If the patient had a small-bowel resection, you may consider a draining enteric fistula. On the other hand, if the patient had an operation limited to the abdominal skin and the fascia, you would probably consider a draining seroma or wound infection.

The number of days a patient is postoperative is also an important piece of information. For example, if you are asked to evaluate a wound with erythema, recall that early *streptococcus* and anaerobic infections may present at postoperative days 1 and 2. Typical wound infections with *Staphylococcus aureus* and other flora are most common between postoperative days 4 and 5.

2. **What are the vital signs?**

It is important to know if the patient is hypotensive, tachycardic, or febrile.

3. **What is the presenting problem, e.g., is there pain, fever, swelling, drainage, or bleeding?**

4. **What medical problems does the patient have?**

A patient who has wound healing problems due to steroids, diabetes, malnutrition, advanced malignancy, or chronic disease is more likely to have wound dehiscence and infection. Diabetic patients and patients taking steroids are immunosuppressed and often have few symptoms until they present with a serious wound problem.

5. **What medications is the patient taking, e.g., anticoagulants, antibiotics, or steroids?**

It is important to know if a patient is anticoagulated. You should be careful when manipulating a wound in an anticoagulated patient. If the patient has significant bleeding from the wound and is anticoagulated, platelets or fresh frozen plasma may be indicated. If a patient is taking intravenous (IV) antibiotics and develops a wound infection, consider the possible organisms responsible and adjust antibiotic therapy accordingly.

Orders

1. Have dressing supplies, sterile gloves, eye protection, and proper lighting and suction available at the bedside.
2. If the patient has significant bleeding from the wound or evidence of hematoma, have the RN draw a hematocrit immediately.

Inform RN

"Will arrive at the bedside in . . . minutes."

Wound problems represent a variety of postsurgical complications, ranging from benign to life-threatening processes. Examine the patient expeditiously.

ELEVATOR THOUGHTS

What causes wound problems?

For common causes of wound problems, see Table 32–1.

MAJOR THREAT TO LIFE

- Sepsis secondary to wound infection
- Necrotizing fasciitis
- Postsurgical bleeding
- Wound dehiscence or evisceration
- Intracranial hematoma

An unrecognized or an untreated wound infection can rapidly become a life-threatening process. In addition, bleeding from a wound may indicate that there may be bleeding into an undrained portion of the wound or bleeding into a body cavity. A patient can easily bleed to death if postsurgical or posttraumatic wounds bleed internally into large body cavities such as the pleural space, the abdomen, the retroperitoneum, or the deep compartment of the thigh. Intracranial bleeding after a neurosurgical procedure or a traumatic injury may lead to brain herniation and death.

TABLE 32–1 **Common Causes of Wound Problems**

Presenting Sign or Symptom	Potential Process
Wound erythema	Posttraumatic inflammation
	Cellulitis
	Fasciitis
	Abscess
Wound drainage (clear or cloudy)	Seroma
	Draining abscess
	Fistula (enteric, salivary, or urinary)
	Ascites
Wound drainage (bloody)	Draining hematoma (darker red)
	Active bleeding (lighter red)
Wound opening	Wound dehiscence
	Evisceration
Foul odor	Anaerobic wound infection
	Wound abscess
	Necrotic tissue
Wound swelling	Postsurgical inflammation
	Seroma
	Hematoma

BEDSIDE

Quick Look Test

Does the patient look well (comfortable), sick (uncomfortable or distressed), or critical (about to die)?

Most patients with small fluid collections in wounds look well. These collections may represent seromas or hematomas. When these collections become infected or represent an ongoing bleeding problem, the patient appears sick. Patients with cellulitis, abscess, or early fasciitis often present with fever and pain in the area of the wound. These patients are often uncomfortable and distressed. Patients with a rapidly progressive infection of a wound may present with fever, hypotension, and sepsis. These patients may look critically ill.

Airway and Vital Signs

What is the temperature?

Fever associated with a wound problem may represent infection. However, recall that the most common cause of fever in a postoperative patient is atelectasis, not infection.

What is the blood pressure and heart rate?

Hypotension, tachycardia, and fever may represent sepsis. In the presence of wound erythema, tenderness, or purulent drainage, suspect the wound as the source of infection.

Selective History and Chart Review

1. Ask the patient when he or she noticed that the wound had changed.

    When did the wound begin to swell, drain, hurt, or become erythematous? Understanding when the problem began helps you think about how to best manage the wound.

2. Ask the patient if the wound problem is new, recent, or chronic.

    A patient who has been having drainage from a wound for days may have a fistula or a chronic draining infection or an abscess. A patient who has just developed drainage from a wound may have a more benign problem, such as a draining seroma. A sudden-onset, rapidly spreading erythema extending from a wound may represent a *Streptococcus* or *Clostridium* infection, whereas a chronically erythematous wound often represents a chronic infection and a less emergent problem.

3. Ask the patient if he or she has wound healing problems.

    Patients who have had past problems with wounds are likely to have similar problems when you are on call.

    Learn about the past management by asking the patient how the wounds were treated and what the outcome was.

4. Ask the patient if he or she is diabetic, is on steroids, or if he or she has other medical problems.

    Although the RN may have told you that the patient was diabetic or had other medical problems, it is wise to ask the patient about his or her medical history yourself.

5. Review the chart briefly, paying special attention to medical history, current drugs, and recent surgical procedures.

    A thorough evaluation of the medical record and of the patient is indicated to provide the best diagnosis and the best treatment.

Selective Physical Examination

VS:	Repeat now. Note any change in temperature.
HEENT:	Evaluate scalp and facial wounds with the aid of gauze (to blot bleeding) and adequate lighting.
	Note the deepest layer exposed (fat, muscle, or bone). Look for drainage or bleeding.
	Look at oral wounds carefully with the aid of a tongue retractor and light.
	Note the deepest structures exposed.
	Evaluate any wounds in the ear canal with the aid of fine suction and an otoscope.
Chest:	Evaluate midline sternotomy wounds. Note skin redness, bleeding, drainage, and dehiscence.
	Check for sternal stability.
	Evaluate thoracotomy wounds. Note skin redness, bleeding, air leak, or dehiscence.

Abd: Evaluate abdominal wounds. If the wound is closed, note skin redness, drainage (serous, sanguineous, purulent, or fecal), swelling or fullness, and tenderness. If the wound is open, consider removing the dressing.

Note the deepest closed layer (fascia, muscle, or fat), the presence of any granulation tissue, evidence of fascial dehiscence, evidence of early evisceration, and drainage from the abdominal cavity. Inspect any suction drains for the amount and the quality of fluid in the drainage system.

Extrem: Examine wounds of the extremities carefully. Note any skin redness, bleeding, and drainage. Note the type of drainage (serous, serosanguineous, bloody, or purulent). Look for the deepest layer of tissue exposed at the base of the wound (fat, muscle, or bone). Note any nerves, vessels, or tendons exposed.

MANAGEMENT

Erythematous Wounds

Closed wounds that are erythematous outside the immediate edges of the wound may be infected. The skin may appear brawny red or reddish brown. These areas are usually indurated and tender. Wound cellulitis is best treated with elevation of the infected area, bed rest, and IV antibiotics. Common organisms include *S. aureus* and *streptococci* species. The classic antibiotics used for simple cellulitis are **cefazolin 1 g IV every 8 hours** or **nafcillin 1 to 2 g IV every 4 hours.** If the patient is already taking IV antibiotics and develops cellulitis, the organisms responsible for the infection may not be covered adequately by the antibiotic or the organisms are resistant to the antibiotic. Discuss adding a second drug or changing the primary antibiotic with the chief resident or the attending physician.

Rapid-Onset Cellulitis

Streptococci species or *Clostridium* may produce cellulitis in a wound within 12 to 24 hours. **Penicillin G potassium 2 to 4 million U IV every 4 hours** is usually effective if the infection is limited to the skin. If there is crepitus of the wound, skin discoloration (brown, blue, or black), and odor, the process may represent a severe infection involving mixed flora or clostridia. These infections require wound exploration and emergent surgical debridement. If you suspect a rapid, necrotizing process, call the chief resident or the attending physician before either opening the wound or arranging an emergent trip to the operating room (OR). In fulminant *streptococcal* infections such as those that can lead to toxic shock, **clindamycin** is a better antibiotic choice, as it is more active against the bacteria during a relatively penicillin-resistant growth phase.

Invasive or Gangrenous Wound Infection

These soft-tissue infections are usually caused by *Clostridium* species. The infection that may appear initially as a rapid-onset cellulitis, however, becomes rapidly progressive and invasive. Organisms initially invade superficial to the deep fascia but may move deeper into the muscle plane. Infected muscle tissue becomes necrotic. The skin appears discolored, edematous, and crepitant. A brown seropurulent exudate containing bubbles may drain from the wound or the involved area. The patient generally has significant pain, fever, and signs of toxemia. Treatment involves wide wound debridement, fascial compartment release if there are signs of compartment syndrome, local wound care, and IV antibiotics. **Penicillin G potassium 20 to 40 million U/day divided into every-4-hour dosing** is used. In patients allergic to penicillin or in whom double coverage is desired, consider **clindamycin 450 to 600 mg IV every 6 hours** or **metronidazole 1-g loading dose followed by 500 mg IV every 6 hours.**

Necrotizing Fasciitis

This is an invasive infection of the fascia caused by a mixed infection. Infection begins in proximity to a wound. Organisms may include *streptococci, staphylococci,* Gram-negative organisms, *bacteroides*, and *clostridia*. The skin adjacent to the wound first shows hemorrhagic bullae, followed by skin death. Crepitus of the involved skin is common as well as fever, tachycardia, and toxemia. At surgery, necrotic skin, fascia, and fat are seen. Thrombosis of blood vessels also occurs "dishwater fluid may be present." Necrotizing fasciitis usually begins in an extremity or in the perineal area and is more common in diabetic and immunocompromised patients. If you suspect that a patient may have necrotizing fasciitis, call the chief resident or the attending physician immediately. Arrange for emergent surgical debridement in the OR. Type and crossmatch the patient for 2 units of packed red blood cells and order IV antibiotics. Triple IV antibiotics are appropriate. Commonly used combinations include penicillin, metronidazole *(Flagyl)*, and gentamicin. Clindamycin may be added for severe infections. Give IV antibiotics after cultures are taken in the OR. Remember that management of these patients includes both surgical debridement and IV antibiotics. These patients may need several trips to the OR.

Wound Swelling

Wounds tend to swell postoperatively. However, closed wounds should not generally "bulge" or be fluctuant. A closed wound that appears abnormally swollen may have a trapped fluid collection.

The fluid may be serum and lymph (seroma), blood (hematoma), or another bodily fluid. If the suspicion is high that the swelling represents a fluid collection, it is often appropriate to aspirate with a 20-gauge needle and syringe using sterile technique. However, it is safe to aspirate the wound only if you know that there is no vital structure or organ below the skin surface. Discuss the case with a supervising surgical resident or the attending physician before proceeding with aspiration. He or she will generally be familiar with the surgical anatomy of that patient. For example, a swelling under an abdominal wound could represent a hernia. Aspiration of such a wound could lead to perforation of the bowel or another abdominal organ. Seromas are common after repair of abdominal hernias and are often just observed.

Draining Wounds

A draining wound could represent wound infection, seroma, hematoma, or fistula. Carefully examine the patient and the wound. Does the drainage appear serous, serosanguineous, bloody, or purulent? Does the drainage have an odor (infection or fistula)? If you suspect infection, obtain a wound culture and Gram stain using a sterile culture swab. These wounds may need to be opened to allow adequate drainage. If the wound appears to be draining a serous or a serosanguineous drainage and there is no sign of infection, either reinforcing the wound with sterile gauze or gently packing any open area of the wound with sterile Nu-Gauze is appropriate. If you suspect a fistula, contact your resident. Consult the supervising resident or the attending physician in cases of any significant wound drainage.

Wounds with Exposed Deep Structures

If called to evaluate a wound that has exposed deep structures, it is important to keep these deep structures moist. Deep wounds may have bone, muscle, fascia, nerve, or other structures exposed. These tissues are best kept viable by placing sterile gauze moistened with saline on the structure. Use sterile technique and make sure that the moist gauze is in gentle contact with the deep structure. Remember that when tissues desiccate, they die. Contact the appropriate surgical resident or the attending physician who can help with wound evaluation and closure.

Wound Dehiscence or Evisceration

Wounds may dehisce at any point in the postoperative period. You will likely be called to evaluate a wound that is opening spontaneously. Sutures may or may not still be in place. Usually, wounds dehisce because the fascial closure of a deep wound has broken down. The wound may have been closed with tension, or the tissues may be of poor quality. There may be a wound infection or a fluid collection. If the fascia and the skin break down, evisceration of abdominal organs may occur. The small bowel is the most common structure to eviscerate. In cases of wound dehiscence or evisceration, cover the wound and any exposed structures with sterile gauze moistened with saline. Place a sterile OR towel over the area. Call the supervising resident or the attending physician. These wound problems are best dealt with in the OR.

Superficial Wounds

Fresh wounds involving the skin may be easy to repair at the bedside. If a patient falls out of bed and suffers a simple laceration without other injury, you can clean the wound and repair it yourself. After anesthetizing the wound with a lidocaine 1% injection, clean the wound with large volumes of sterile saline. Use sterile technique. Wounds contaminated with dirt or debris will need some mechanical debridement with a sterile iris scissors, a scalpel, and a forceps. One-half strength hydrogen peroxide is often helpful in mechanically cleaning wounds. Prepare the skin adjacent to the wound with povidone-iodine (Betadine). Using sterile technique, place interrupted sutures of nylon or Prolene to approximate the skin edges. For the face, use 6-0 sutures. For the extremities or the trunk, usually 3-0 or 4-0 sutures are appropriate. On the scalp, staples may be used. Closure of the superficial fascia is often not necessary and may lead to increased risk of infection.

Actively Bleeding Wounds

Wounds that demonstrate bleeding may be difficult to manage. If the bleeding is from a superficial structure or from the wound edge, the bleeding structure can be seen and controlled. Have sterile gloves, eye protection, adequate lighting, and gauze or suction available. Carefully visualize the bleeding structure. Frequently, you will see a small blood vessel in the wound or at the edge of the wound that is causing bleeding. Apply pressure to the area for 5 to 10 minutes. If bleeding persists, you can use silver nitrate sticks (for very small vessels or bleeding granulation tissue), bedside cautery, or carefully placed suture ligature (for almost any bleeding structure) to stop the bleeding. If there is significant or massive bleeding from a wound, obtain a hematocrit immediately, type and crossmatch the patient for 2 units of blood, and apply pressure to the bleeding area, if possible. Use IV fluids to maintain hemodynamic stability. Call for help. You may need an emergent trip to the OR to explore the wound and to control the bleeding.

Adult Emergency Cardiac Care Algorithms

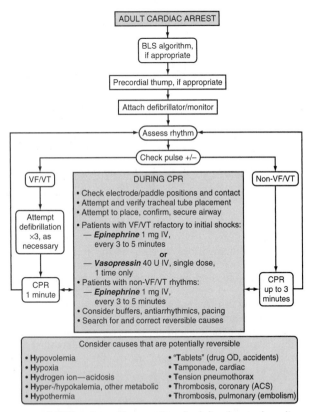

Figure A–1 ILCOR universal/international adult advanced cardiovascular life support algorithm. ACS, acute coronary syndrome; BLS, basic life support; CPR, cardiopulmonary resuscitation; IV, intravenous; OD, overdose; VF/VT, ventricular fibrillation/ventricular tachycardia. (Redrawn with permission from ACLS Provider Manual, 2002, Copyright American Heart Association.)

Figure A–2 Algorithm for ventricular fibrillation/pulseless ventricular tachycardia (VF/VT). CPR, cardiopulmonary resuscitation; IV, intravenous. (Redrawn with permission from ACLS Provider Manual, 2002, Copyright American Heart Association.)

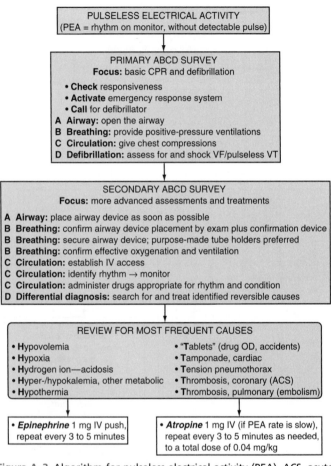

PULSELESS ELECTRICAL ACTIVITY
(PEA = rhythm on monitor, without detectable pulse)

PRIMARY ABCD SURVEY
Focus: basic CPR and defibrillation

- **Check** responsiveness
- **Activate** emergency response system
- **Call** for defibrillator
A **Airway:** open the airway
B **Breathing:** provide positive-pressure ventilations
C **Circulation:** give chest compressions
D **Defibrillation:** assess for and shock VF/pulseless VT

SECONDARY ABCD SURVEY
Focus: more advanced assessments and treatments

A **Airway:** place airway device as soon as possible
B **Breathing:** confirm airway device placement by exam plus confirmation device
B **Breathing:** secure airway device; purpose-made tube holders preferred
B **Breathing:** confirm effective oxygenation and ventilation
C **Circulation:** establish IV access
C **Circulation:** identify rhythm → monitor
C **Circulation:** administer drugs appropriate for rhythm and condition
D **Differential diagnosis:** search for and treat identified reversible causes

---

REVIEW FOR MOST FREQUENT CAUSES

- Hypovolemia
- Hypoxia
- Hydrogen ion—acidosis
- Hyper-/hypokalemia, other metabolic
- Hypothermia

- "Tablets" (drug OD, accidents)
- Tamponade, cardiac
- Tension pneumothorax
- Thrombosis, coronary (ACS)
- Thrombosis, pulmonary (embolism)

- **Epinephrine** 1 mg IV push, repeat every 3 to 5 minutes

- **Atropine** 1 mg IV (if PEA rate is slow), repeat every 3 to 5 minutes as needed, to a total dose of 0.04 mg/kg

Figure A–3 Algorithm for pulseless electrical activity (PEA). ACS, acute coronary syndrome; CPR, cardiopulmonary resuscitation; OD, overdose; VF, ventricular fibrillation; VT, ventricular tachycardia. (Redrawn with permission from ACLS Provider Manual, 2002, Copyright American Heart Association.)

Figure A–4 Algorithm for asystole: the silent heart. CPR, cardiopulmonary resuscitation; IV, intravenous; VF, ventricular fibrillation; VT, ventricular tachycardia. (Redrawn with permission from ACLS Provider Manual, 2002, Copyright American Heart Association.)

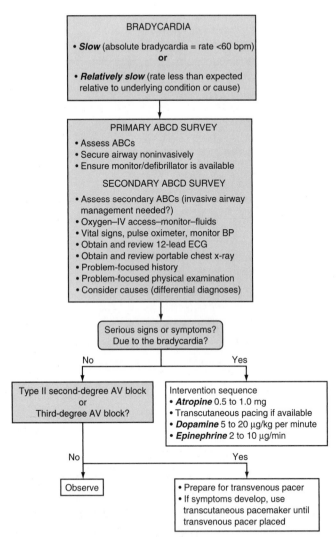

Figure A–5 Algorithm for bradycardia (patient not in cardiac arrest). AV, atrioventricular; BP, blood pressure; bpm, beats per minute; ECG, electrocardiogram; IV, intravenous. (Redrawn with permission from ACLS Provider Manual, 2002, Copyright American Heart Association.)

Figure A–6 Overview algorithm: the tachycardias. bpm, beats per minute; CHF, congestive heart failure; DC, direct current; ECG, electrocardiogram; SVT, supraventricular tachycardia; VT, ventricular tachycardia; WPW, Wolff–Parkinson–White syndrome. (Redrawn with permission from ACLS Provider Manual, 2002, Copyright American Heart Association.)

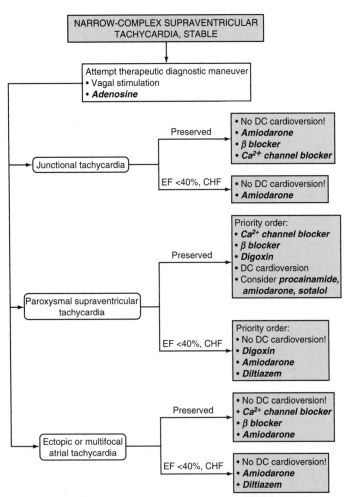

Figure A–7 Algorithm for narrow-complex tachycardia. CHF, congestive heart failure; DC, direct current; EF, ejection fraction. (Redrawn with permission from ACLS Provider Manual, 2002, Copyright American Heart Association.)

Figure A–8 Algorithm for stable ventricular tachycardia (VT)-monomorphic and polymorphic. IV, intravenous. (Redrawn with permission from ACLS Provider Manual, 2002, Copyright American Heart Association.)

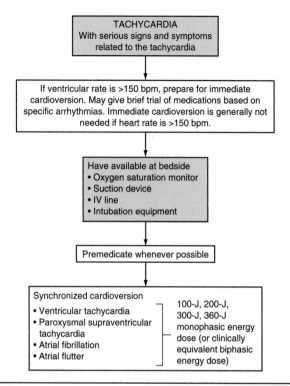

TACHYCARDIA
With serious signs and symptoms
related to the tachycardia

If ventricular rate is >150 bpm, prepare for immediate
cardioversion. May give brief trial of medications based on
specific arrhythmias. Immediate cardioversion is generally not
needed if heart rate is >150 bpm.

Have available at bedside
• Oxygen saturation monitor
• Suction device
• IV line
• Intubation equipment

Premedicate whenever possible

Synchronized cardioversion
• Ventricular tachycardia
• Paroxysmal supraventricular
  tachycardia
• Atrial fibrillation
• Atrial flutter

100-J, 200-J,
300-J, 360-J
monophasic energy
dose (or clinically
equivalent biphasic
energy dose)

Notes:
1. Effective regimens have included a sedative (e.g., *diazepam,
   midazolam, barbiturates, etomidate, ketamine, methohexital)* with
   or without an analgesic agent (e.g., *fentanyl, morphine, meperidine)*.
   Many experts recommend anesthesia if service is readily available.
2. Both monophasic and biphasic waveforms are acceptable if documented
   as clinically equivalent to reports of monophasic shock success.
3. Note possible need to resynchronize after each cardioversion.
4. If delays in synchronization occur and clinical condition is critical,
   go immediately to unsynchronized shocks.
5. Treat polymorphic ventricular tachycardia (irregular form and rate) like
   ventricular fibrillation: see ventricular fibrillation/pulseless ventricular
   tachycardia algorithm (see Fig. A–6).
6. Paroxysmal supraventricular tachycardia and atrial flutter often
   respond to lower energy levels (start with 50 J).

Figure A–9 Algorithm for electrical cardioversion. bpm, beats per minute;
IV, intravenous; VF, ventricular fibrillation. (Redrawn with permission from
ACLS Provider Manual, 2002, Copyright American Heart Association.)

TABLE A–1 Tachycardia: Atrial Fibrillation and Flutter

	1. Control Rate		2. Convert Rhythm	
	Heart Function Preserved	Impaired Heart EF <40% or CHF	Duration <48 Hours	Duration >48 Hours or Unknown
Normal cardiac function	**Note:** If AF >48 hr duration, use agents to convert rhythm with extreme caution in patients not receiving adequate anticoagulation because of possible embolic complications. Use only 1 of the following agents* ❏ Calcium channel blockers (class I) ❏ Beta-blockers (class I)	N/A	**Consider** DC cardioversion Use only 1 of the following agents* ❏ Amiodarone (class IIa) ❏ Ibutilide (class IIa) ❏ Flecainide (class IIa) ❏ Propafenone (class IIa) ❏ Procainamide (class IIa)	**No DC cardioversion! Note:** Conversion of AF to NSR with drugs or shock may cause embolization of atrial thrombi unless patient has adequate anticoagulation Use antiarrhythmic agents with extreme caution if AF >48 hr duration (see note above) **or** **Delayed cardioversion** ❏ **Anticoagulation × 3 wk at proper levels** ❏ Cardioversion, then ❏ Anticoagulation × 4 wk more **or Early cardioversion** ❏ Begin IV heparin at once ❏ TEE to exclude atrial clot

Continued

TABLE A–1 Tachycardia: Atrial Fibrillation and Flutter—cont'd

	1. Control Rate		2. Convert Rhythm	
	Heart Function Preserved	Impaired Heart EF <40% or CHF	Duration <48 Hours	Duration >48 Hours or Unknown
Impaired heart (EF <40% or CHF)	N/A	**Note:** If AF >48 hr duration, use agents to convert rhythm with extreme caution in patients not receiving adequate anticoagulation because of possible embolic complications **Use only 1 of the following agents*** ❑ Digoxin (class IIb) ❑ Diltiazem (class IIb) ❑ Amiodarone (class IIb)	**Consider** DC cardioversion or amiodarone (class IIb)	**then** ❑ Cardioversion within 24 hr **then** ❑ Anticoagulation × 4 wk more **Anticoagulation,** as described above, followed by **DC cardioversion**

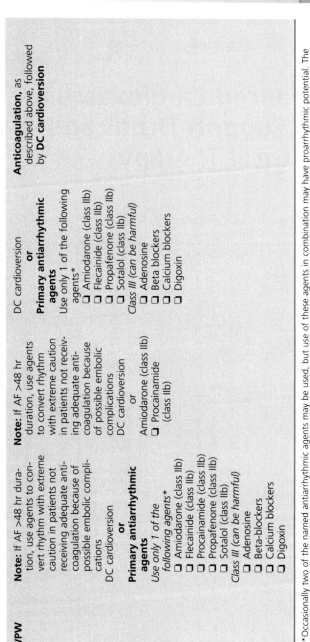

WPW			Anticoagulation, as described above, followed by DC cardioversion
	Note: If AF >48 hr duration, use agents to convert rhythm with extreme caution in patients not receiving adequate anticoagulation because of possible embolic complications DC cardioversion **or** **Primary antiarrhythmic agents** *Use only 1 of the following agents** ❑ Amiodarone (class IIb) ❑ Flecainide (class IIb) ❑ Procainamide (class IIb) ❑ Propafenone (class IIb) ❑ Sotalol (class IIb) *Class III (can be harmful)* ❑ Adenosine ❑ Beta-blockers ❑ Calcium blockers ❑ Digoxin	**Note:** If AF >48 hr duration, use agents to convert rhythm with extreme caution in patients not receiving adequate anticoagulation because of possible embolic complications DC cardioversion **or** Amiodarone (class IIb) ❑ Procainamide (class IIb)	DC cardioversion **or** **Primary antiarrhythmic agents** Use only 1 of the following agents* ❑ Amiodarone (class IIb) ❑ Flecainide (class IIb) ❑ Propafenone (class IIb) ❑ Sotalol (class IIb) *Class III (can be harmful)* ❑ Adenosine ❑ Beta blockers ❑ Calcium blockers ❑ Digoxin	

*Occasionally two of the named antiarrhythmic agents may be used, but use of these agents in combination may have proarrhythmic potential. The classes listed represent the Class of Recommendation rather than the Vaughn–Williams classification of antiarrhythmics.

AF, atrial fibrillation; CHF, congestive heart failure; DC, direct current; EF, ejection fraction; IV, intravenous; N/A, not applicable; NSR, normal sinus rhythm; TEE, transesophageal echocardiogram; WPW, Wolff–Parkinson–White syndrome.

B

Advanced Cardiovascular Life Support Drugs and Electrical Therapy

TABLE B–1 **Advanced Cardiovascular Life Support Drugs and Electrical Therapy**

Drug/Therapy	Adult Dosage	Indications/Precautions
ACE Inhibitors	**Approach**	**Indications**
	ACE inhibitor therapy should start with low-dose oral administration (with possible IV doses for some preparations) and increase steadily to achieve a full dose within 24–28 hr	ACE inhibitors reduce mortality and improve LV dysfunction in post-AMI patients. They help prevent adverse LV remodeling, delay progression of heart failure, and decrease sudden death and recurrent MI.
Enalapril	• PO: Start with a single dose of 2.5 mg; titrate to 20 mg PO BID • IV (enalaprilat): 1.25 mg IV initial dose over 5 min, then 1.25–5 mg IV q6hr	They are of greatest benefit in patients with the following conditions: • Suspected MI and ST segment elevation in 2 or more anterior precordial leads • Hypertension • Clinical heart failure without hypotension in patients not responding to digitalis or diuretics
Captopril	• Start with a single dose of 6.25 mg PO • Advance to 25 mg TID and then to 50 mg TID as tolerated	• Clinical signs of AMI with LV dysfunction • LV ejection fraction <40% **Precautions/ contraindications for all ACE inhibitors**

TABLE B–1 **Advanced Cardiovascular Life Support Drugs and Electrical Therapy—cont'd**

Drug/Therapy	Adult Dosage	Indications/Precautions
Lisinopril	• 5 mg within 24 hr of onset of symptoms, then • 5 mg given after 24 hr, then • 10 mg given after 48 hr, then • 10 mg once daily for 6 wk	• Contraindicated in pregnancy (may cause fetal injury or death) • **Contraindicated** in angioedema • Hypersensitivity to ACE inhibitors • Reduce dose in renal failure (creatinine >3 mg/dL); avoid in bilateral renal artery stenosis
Ramipril	Start with a single dose of 2.5 mg PO; titrate to 5 mg PO BID as tolerated	• Avoid hypotension, especially following initial dose and in relative volume depletion Generally not started in ED but within first 24 hr after fibrinolytic therapy has been completed and blood pressure has stabilized
Adenosine	**IV Rapid Push** • Place patient in mild reverse Trendelenburg's position before administration of drug • Initial bolus of 6 mg given rapidly over 1–3 sec followed by NS bolus of 20 mL; then elevate the extremity • Repeat dose of 12 mg in 1–2 min, if needed • A third dose of 12 mg may be given in 1–2 min, if needed **Injection Technique** • Record rhythm strip during administration • Draw up adenosine dose and flush in two separate syringes	**Indications** • First drug for most forms of narrow-complex PSVT; effective in terminating those due to re-entry involving AV node or sinus node • Does not convert atrial fibrillation, atrial flutter, or VT **Precautions** • Transient side effects include flushing, chest pain or tightness, brief periods of asystole or bradycardia, ventricular ectopy • Less effective in patients taking theophyllines; avoid in patients receiving dipyridamole • If administered for wide-complex tachycardia/VT, may cause deterioration (including hypotension)

Continued

TABLE B–1 **Advanced Cardiovascular Life Support Drugs and Electrical Therapy—cont'd**

Drug/Therapy	Adult Dosage	Indications/Precautions
Adenosine (cont'd)	• Attach both syringes to the IV injection port closest to patient • Clamp IV tubing above injection port • Push IV adenosine as quickly as possible (1–3 sec) • While maintaining pressure on adenosine plunger, push NS flush as rapidly as possible after adenosine • Unclamp IV tubing	• Transient periods of sinus bradycardia and ventricular ectopy are common after termination of SVT • Contraindication: poison/drug-induced tachycardia
Amiodarone	**Cardiac Arrest** 300 mg IV push; consider repeating 150 mg IV push in 3–5 min (maximum cumulative dose: 2.2 g IV/24 hr) **Wide Complex Tachycardia (Stable)** *Maximum cumulative dose:* 2.2 g IV/24 hr May be administered as follows: • Rapid infusion: 150 mg IV over first 10 min (15 mg/min); may repeat rapid infusion (150 mg IV) q10min as needed • Slow infusion: 360 mg IV over 6 hr (1 mg/min) • Maintenance infusion: 540 mg IV over 18 hr (0.5 mg/min)	**Indications** Used in a wide variety of atrial and ventricular tachyarrhythmias and for rate control of rapid atrial arrhythmias in patients with impaired LV function when digoxin has proved ineffective **Recommended for** • Treatment of shock-refractory VF/pulseless VT • Treatment of polymorphic VT and wide-complex tachycardia of uncertain origin • Control of hemodynamically stable VT when cardioversion is unsuccessful; particularly useful in the presence of LV dysfunction • Use as adjunct to electrical cardioversion of SVT, PSVT • Acceptable for termination of ectopic or multifocal atrial tachycardia with preserved LV function

TABLE B–1 **Advanced Cardiovascular Life Support Drugs and Electrical Therapy—cont'd**

Drug/Therapy	Adult Dosage	Indications/Precautions
Amiodarone (cont'd)		• May be used for rate control in treatment of atrial fibrillation or flutter when other therapies are ineffective
		Precautions
		• May produce vasodilatation and hypotension
		• May have negative inotropic effects
		• When multiple doses are administered, cumulative doses >2.2 g/24 hr are associated with significant hypotension in clinical trials
		• May prolong QT interval; do not routinely administer with other drugs that prolong QT interval (e.g., procainamide)
		• Use with caution if renal failure is present
		• Terminal elimination is extremely long (half-life up to 40 days)
Amrinone	**IV Loading Dose and Infusion**	**Indications**
	• 0.75 mg/kg, given over 10–15 min	Severe CHF refractory to diuretics, vasodilators, and conventional inotropic agents
	• Follow with infusion of 5–15 mg/kg/min titrated to clinical effect	**Precautions**
	• Optimal use requires hemodynamic monitoring	• Do not mix with dextrose solutions or other drugs
		• May cause tachyarrhythmias, hypotension, or thrombocytopenia
		• Can increase myocardial ischemia

Continued

TABLE B–1 **Advanced Cardiovascular Life Support Drugs and Electrical Therapy—cont'd**

Drug/Therapy	Adult Dosage	Indications/Precautions
Aspirin • 160- or 325-mg tablets • Chewable tablets more effective in some trials	• 160–325-mg tablet taken as soon as possible (chewing is preferable to swallowing) and then daily • May use rectal suppository for patients who cannot take PO • Give within minutes of arrival • Higher doses (1000 mg) interfere with prostacyclin	**Indications** • Administer to all patients with ACS, particularly reperfusion candidates, unless hypersensitive to aspirin • Blocks formation of thromboxane A_2, which causes platelets to aggregate, arteries to constrict; this reduces overall AMI mortality, reinfarction, nonfatal • Any person with symptoms ("pressure," "heavy weight," "squeezing," "crushing") suggestive of ischemic pain **Precautions** • Relatively contraindicated in patients with active ulcer disease or asthma • Contraindicated in patients with known hypersensitivity to aspirin
Atropine Sulfate Can be given via tracheal	**Asystole or Pulseless Electrical Activity** • 1 mg IV push • Repeat every 3–5 min (if asystole persists) to a maximum dose of 0.03–0.04 mg/kg • 0.5–1 mg IV every 3–5 min as needed, not to exceed total dose of 0.04 mg/kg • Use shorter dosing interval (3 min) and higher doses (0.04 mg/kg) in severe clinical conditions **Tracheal Administration** 2–3 mg diluted in 10 mL NS	**Indications** • First drug for symptomatic sinus bradycardia tube (class I) • May be beneficial in presence of AV block at the nodal level (class IIa) or ventricular asystole; **will not be effective when infranodal (Mobitz type II) block is suspected (class IIb)** • Second drug (after epinephrine or vasopressin) for asystole or bradycardic pulseless electrical activity (class IIb) **Precautions** • Use with caution in presence of myocardial ischemia and hypoxia; increases myocardial oxygen demand

TABLE B–1 **Advanced Cardiovascular Life Support Drugs and Electrical Therapy—cont'd**

Drug/Therapy	Adult Dosage	Indications/Precautions
Atropine Sulfate (cont'd)		• Avoid in hypothermic bradycardia • Will not be effective for infranodal (type II) AV block and new third-degree block with wide QRS complexes (in these patients, may cause paradoxical slowing; be prepared to pace or give catecholamines)
Beta Blockers		**Indications**
Metoprolol	• Initial IV dose: 5 mg slow IV at 5-min intervals to a total of 15 mg • Oral regimen to follow IV dose: 50 mg BID for 24 hr, then increase to 100 mg BID	• Administer to all patients with suspected MI and unstable angina in the absence of complications; these are effective antianginal agents and can reduce incidence of VF • Useful as an adjunctive agent with fibrinolytic therapy; may reduce nonfatal reinfarction and recurrent ischemia • To convert to normal sinus rhythm or to slow ventricular response (or both) in supraventricular tachyarrhythmias (PSVT, atrial fibrillation, or atrial flutter); beta-blockers are second-line agents after adenosine, diltiazem, or digitalis derivative • To reduce myocardial ischemia and damage in AMI patients with elevated HR, BP, or both • For emergency antihypertensive therapy for hemorrhagic and acute ischemic stroke

Continued

TABLE B–1 **Advanced Cardiovascular Life Support Drugs and Electrical Therapy—cont'd**

Drug/Therapy	Adult Dosage	Indications/Precautions
Beta Blockers (cont'd)		**Precautions**
Atenolol	• 5 mg slow IV (over 5 min) • Wait 10 min, then give second dose of 5 mg slow IV (over 5 min) • In 10 min, if tolerated well, may start 50 mg PO; then give 50 mg PO BID	Concurrent IV administration with IV calcium channel blocking agents such as verapamil or diltiazem can cause severe hypotension • Avoid in bronchospastic diseases, cardiac failure, or severe abnormalities in cardiac conduction
Propranolol	• Total dose: 0.1 mg/kg by slow IV push, divided into 3 equal doses at 2- to 3-min intervals, do not exceed 1 mg/min • Repeat after 2 min, if necessary	• Monitor cardiac and pulmonary status during administration • Contraindicated in presence of HR <60 beats/min, systolic BP <100 mm Hg, severe LV failure, hypoperfusion, or second- or third-degree AV block
Esmolol	• 0.5 mg/kg over 1 min, followed by continuous infusion at 0.05 mg/kg/min • Titrate to effect; esmolol has a short half-life (2–9 min)	
Labetalol	• May cause myocardial depression • 10 mg labetalol IV push over 1–2 min • May repeat or double labetalol every 10 min to a maximum dose of 150 mg, or give initial dose as a bolus, then start labetalol infusion at 2–8 mg/min	
Calcium Chloride	**IV Slow Push**	**Indications**
100 mg/mL in 10 mL vial (total = 1 g; a 10% solution)	• 8–16 mg/kg (usually 5 to 10 mL) IV for hyperkalemia and calcium channel blocker overdose; may be repeated as needed	• Known or suspected hyperkalemia (e.g., renal failure) • Hypocalcemia (e.g., after multiple blood transfusions)

TABLE B–1 **Advanced Cardiovascular Life Support Drugs and Electrical Therapy—cont'd**

Drug/Therapy	Adult Dosage	Indications/Precautions
Calcium Chloride (cont'd)	• 2–4 mg/kg (usually 2 mL) IV for prophylaxis before IV calcium channel blockers	• As an antidote for toxic effects (hypotension and arrhythmias) from calcium channel blocker overdose or beta-adrenergic blocker overdose • May be used prophylactically before IV calcium channel blockers to prevent hypotension **Precautions** • Do not use routinely in cardiac arrest • Do not mix with sodium bicarbonate
Cardioversion (Synchronized) • Administered via remote defibrillation electrodes or hand-held paddles from a defibrillator/monitor • Place defibrillator/monitor in synchronized (sync) mode • Sync mode delivers energy just after the R wave	**Technique** • Premedicate whenever possible • Engage sync mode before each attempt • Look for sync markers on the R wave • "Clear" the patient before each shock • Deliver monophasic shocks in the following sequence: f100 J, 200 J, 300 J, 360 J *Use this sequence for each of the following: —VT† —PSVT‡ —Atrial flutter‡ —Atrial fibrillation	**Indications** • All tachycardias (rate >150 beats/min) with serious signs and symptoms related to tachycardia • May give brief trial of medications based on specific arrhythmias **Precautions** • In critical conditions, go to immediate unsynchronized shocks • Urgent cardioversion is generally not needed if heart rate is £150 beats/min • Reactivation of sync mode is required after each attempted cardioversion (defibrillators/cardioverters default to unsynchronized mode)

Continued

TABLE B–1 **Advanced Cardiovascular Life Support Drugs and Electrical Therapy—cont'd**

Drug/Therapy	Adult Dosage	Indications/Precautions
Cardioversion (Synchronized) (cont'd)	Press "charge" button, "clear" the patient, and press both "shock" buttons simultaneously	• Prepare to defibrillate immediately if cardioversion causes VF • Synchronized cardioversion cannot be performed unless the patient is connected to monitor leads; lead select switch must be on lead I, II, or III and not on "paddles" • Contraindication: poison/drug induced tachycardia

Defibrillation Attempt	**Adult Monophasic Defibrillation Energy Levels****	
Use conventional monitor/defibrillator Use automated or shock advisory defibrillator Administer shocks via remote adhesive electrodes or hand-held paddles	• 200 J, first shock • 200–300 J, second shock • 360 J, third shock • If these shocks fail to convert VF/VT, continue at 360 J for future shocks • If VF recurs, shock again at the last successful energy level	**Indications** First intervention for VF or pulseless VT (class I) **Precautions** • Always "clear" the patient before discharging a defibrillation shock • Do not delay defibrillation for VF/VT • Asystole should not be routinely shocked • Treat VF/VT in hypothermic cardiac arrest with up to 3 shocks; repeat shocks for VF/VT only after core temperature rises above 30°C • If patient in VF/VT has an automatic implantable cardioverter defibrillator (AICD), perform external defibrillation per BLS guidelines; if AICD is delivering shocks, wait 30–60 sec for completion of cycle • If patient has implanted pacemaker, place paddles and pads several inches from the pacing generator

TABLE B–1 **Advanced Cardiovascular Life Support Drugs and Electrical Therapy—cont'd**

Drug/Therapy	Adult Dosage	Indications/Precautions
Digibind (Digoxin-Specific Antibody Therapy)	**Chronic Intoxication**	**Indications**
40-mg vial (each vial binds about 0.6 mg digoxin)	3–5 vials may be effective	Digoxin toxicity with the following:
	Acute Overdose	• Life-threatening arrhythmias
	• IV dose varies according to amount of digoxin ingested	• Shock or CHF
	• Average dose is 10 vials (400 mg); may require up to 20 vials (800 mg)	• Hyperkalemia (potassium level >5 mEq/L)
	• See package insert for details	• Steady-state serum levels >10–15 ng/mL for symptomatic patients
		Precautions
		Serum digoxin levels rise after digibind therapy and should not be used to guide continuing therapy
Digoxin	**IV Infusion**	**Indications**
0.25 mg/mL or 0.1 mg/mL supplied in 1- or 2-mL ampule (totals = 0.1–0.5 mg)	• Loading doses of 10–15 mg/kg lean body weight provide therapeutic effect with minimum risk of toxic effects	• To slow ventricular response in atrial fibrillation or atrial flutter
	• Maintenance dose is affected by body size and renal function	• Alternative drug for PSVT
		Precautions
		• Toxic effects are common and are frequently associated with serious arrhythmias
		Avoid electrical cardioversion if patient is receiving digoxin unless condition is life threatening; use lower current settings (10–20 J)
Diltiazem	**Acute Rate Control**	**Indications**
	• 15–20 mg (0.25 mg/kg) IV over 2 min	• To control ventricular rate in atrial fibrillation and atrial flutter; may terminate re-entrant arrhythmias that require AV nodal conduction for their continuation
	• May repeat in 15 min at 20–25 mg (0.35 mg/kg) over 2 min	• Use after adenosine to treat refractory PSVT in patients with narrow QRS complex and adequate BP

Continued

TABLE B–1 **Advanced Cardiovascular Life Support Drugs and Electrical Therapy—cont'd**

Drug/Therapy	Adult Dosage	Indications/Precautions
Diltiazem (cont'd)	**Maintenance Infusion** 5–15 mg/hr, titrated to HR	**Precautions** • Do not use calcium channel blockers for wide-QRS tachycardias of uncertain origin or for poison/drug-induced tachycardia • Avoid calcium channel blockers in patients with Wolff–Parkinson–White syndrome plus rapid atrial fibrillation or flutter, in patients with sick sinus syndrome, or in patients with AV block without a pacemaker • Expect BP drop resulting from peripheral vasodilatation (greater drop with verapamil than with diltiazem) • Avoid in patients receiving oral beta-blockers • Concurrent IV administration with IV beta-blockers can cause severe hypotension
Disopyramide (IV dose not approved for use in United States)	**IV Dose** 2 mg/kg over 10 min, followed by continuous infusion of 0.4 mg/kg/hr	**Indications** Useful for treatment of a wide variety of arrhythmias; prolongs the effective refractory period, similar to procainamide **Precautions/Contraindications** Must be infused relatively slowly; has potent anticholinergic, negative inotropic, and hypotensive effects that limit its use
Dobutamine IV infusion: dilute 250 mg (20 mL) in 250 mL NS or D5W	**IV Infusion** • Usual infusion rate is 2–20 mg/kg/min • Titrate so HR does not increase by >10% of baseline	**Indications** • Consider for pump problems (CHF, pulmonary congestion) with systolic BP of 70–100 mm Hg and no signs of shock

TABLE B–1 **Advanced Cardiovascular Life Support Drugs and Electrical Therapy—cont'd**

Drug/Therapy	Adult Dosage	Indications/Precautions
Dobutamine (cont'd)	• Hemodynamic monitoring is recommended for optimal use	**Precautions** • Avoid with systolic BP <100 mm Hg and signs of shock • May cause tachyarrhythmias, fluctuations in BP, headache, and nausea • Contraindication: suspected or known poison/drug-induced shock • Do not mix with sodium bicarbonate
Dofetilide (Not approved for use in United States)	**IV Infusion Dose** Single infusion of 8 mg/kg over 30 min	**Indications** Treatment of atrial fibrillation **Precautions/ Contraindications** • Adverse effects include QT prolongation, which can be associated with torsades de pointes; this complication is most likely to occur in patients with a history of CHF • Its use is limited by the need to infuse relatively slowly, which may be impractical under emergent conditions
Dopamine IV infusion: Mix 400–800 mg in 250 mL NS, lactated Ringer's solution, or D5W	**Continuous Infusions (Titrate to Patient Response)** **Low Dose:** 1–5 mg/kg/min **Moderate Dose:** 5–10 mg/kg/min ("cardiac doses") **High Dose:** 10–20 mg/kg/min ("vasopressor doses")	**Indications** • Second drug for symptomatic bradycardia (after atropine) • Use for hypotension (systolic BP £70–100 mm Hg) with signs and symptoms of shock **Precautions** • May use in patients with hypovolemia, but only after volume replacement

Continued

TABLE B–1 **Advanced Cardiovascular Life Support Drugs and Electrical Therapy—cont'd**

Drug/Therapy	Adult Dosage	Indications/Precautions
Dopamine (cont'd)		• Use with caution in cardiogenic shock with accompanying CHF • May cause tachyarrhythmias, excessive vasoconstriction • Taper slowly • Do not mix with sodium bicarbonate
Epinephrine Available in 1:10,000 and 1:1000 concentrations	**Cardiac Arrest** • **IV dose:** 1 mg (10 mL of 1:10,000 solution) administered of 3–5 min during resuscitation; follow each dose with 20 mL IV flush • **Higher dose:** higher doses (up to 0.2 mg/kg) may be used if 1 mg dose fails • **Continuous infusion:** add 30 mg epinephrine (30 mL of 1:1000 solution) to 250 mL NS or D5W; run at 100 mL/hr and titrate to response • **Tracheal route:** 2–2.5 mg diluted in 10 mL NS **Profound Bradycardia or Hypotension** 2–10 mg/min infusion (add 1 mg of 1:1000 to 500 mL NS; infuse at 1–5 mL/min)	**Indications** **Cardiac arrest:** VF, pulseless VT, asystole, pulseless electrical activity **Symptomatic bradycardia:** after atropine, dopamine, and transcutaneous pacing **Severe hypotension Anaphylaxis, severe allergic reactions:** combine with large fluid volumes, corticosteroids, antihistamines **Precautions** • Raising BP and increasing HR may cause myocardial ischemia, angina, and increased myocardial oxygen demand • High doses do not improve survival or neurologic outcome and may contribute to postresuscitation myocardial dysfunction • Higher doses may be required to treat poison/drug-induced shock
Fibrinolytic Agents For all agents, use 2 peripheral IV lines, one line exclusively for fibrinolytic administration		**Indications** For AMI in adults: • ST elevation (=1 mm in =2 contiguous leads) or new or presumably new LBBB; strongly suspicious for injury (BBB obscuring ST analysis)

TABLE B–1 **Advanced Cardiovascular Life Support Drugs and Electrical Therapy—cont'd**

Drug/Therapy	Adult Dosage	Indications/Precautions
Fibrinolytic Agents (cont'd) Alteplase, recombinant (Activase) Tissue plasminogen activator (tPA) 50- and 100-mg vials reconstituted with sterile water to 1 mg/mL Anistreplase (Eminase); Anisoylated Plasminogen Streptokinase Activator Complex (APSAC) Reconstitute 30 U in 50 mL sterile water or D5W	Recommended total dose is based on patient's weight. For AMI, the total dose should not exceed 100 mg; for acute ischemic stroke, the total dose should not exceed 90 mg. Note that there are 2 approved dose regimens for AMI patients and a different regimen for acute ischemic stroke. *For AMI:* • Accelerated infusion (1.5 hr) —Give 15-mg IV bolus —Then 0.75 mg/kg over next 30 min (not to exceed 50 mg) —Then 0.5 mg/kg over next 60 min (not to exceed 35 mg) • 3-hour infusion —Give 60 mg in first hour (initial 6–10 mg is given as a bolus) —Then 20 mg/hr for 2 additional hours *For acute ischemic stroke:* • Give 0.9 mg/kg (maximum 90 mg) infused over 60 min • Give 10% of the total dose as an initial IV bolus over 1 min • Give the remaining 90% over the next 60 min 30 IU IV over 2–5 min	• In context of signs and symptoms of AMI • Time from onset of symptoms <12 hr For acute ischemic stroke (alteplase is the only fibrinolytic agent approved for acute ischemic stroke): • Sudden onset of focal neurologic deficits or alterations in consciousness (e.g., language abnormality, motor arm, facial droop) • Absence of intracerebral or subarachnoid hemorrhage or mass effect on CT scan • Absence of variable or rapidly improving neurologic deficits • Alteplase can be started in <3 hr from symptom onset **Precautions** *Specific exclusion criteria* • Active internal bleeding (except menses) within 21 days • History of cerebrovascular, intracranial, or intraspinal event within 3 mo (stroke, arteriovenous malformation, neoplasm, aneurysm, recent trauma, recent surgery) • Major surgery or serious trauma within 14 days • Aortic dissection • Severe, uncontrolled hypertension • Known bleeding disorders • Prolonged CPR with evidence of thoracic trauma • Lumbar puncture within 7 days

Continued

TABLE B–1 **Advanced Cardiovascular Life Support Drugs and Electrical Therapy—cont'd**

Drug/Therapy	Adult Dosage	Indications/Precautions
Fibrinolytic Agents (cont'd)		• Recent arterial puncture at noncompressible site • During the first 24 hr of fibrinolytic therapy for ischemic stroke, do not administer aspirin or heparin
Reteplase, Recombinant (Retavase) 10-U vials reconstituted with sterile water to 1 U/mL **Streptokinase (Streptase)** Reconstitute to 1 mg/mL **Tenecteplase (TNKase)**	**Reteplase Recombinant** • Give first 10-U IV bolus over 2 min • 30 min later, give second 10-U IV bolus over 2 min (give NS flush before and after each bolus) • 1.5 million IU in a 1-hr infusion • Bolus: 30–50 mg	**Adjuvant Therapy for AM** • 160–325 mg aspirin chewed as soon as possible • Begin heparin immediately and continue for 48 hr if alteplase or reteplase is used
Flecainide (IV form not approved for use in United States)	**IV Dose** Administered at 2 mg/kg body weight at 10 mg/min; must be infused slowly	**Indications** • Treatment of ventricular arrhythmias • Treatment of supraventricular arrhythmias in patients without coronary artery disease • Effective for termination of atrial flutter and fibrillation, ectopic atrial tachycardia, AV nodal reentrant tachycardia, and SVTs associated with an accessory pathway **Precautions/Contraindications** • Should be avoided in patients with impaired LV function because it has significant negative inotropic effects • Must be infused slowly

TABLE B–1 **Advanced Cardiovascular Life Support Drugs and Electrical Therapy—cont'd**

Drug/Therapy	Adult Dosage	Indications/Precautions
Flecainide (cont'd)		• Adverse effects include bradycardia, hypotension, and neurologic symptoms such as oral paresthesias and visual blurring
Flumazenil	**First Dose** 0.2 mg IV over 15 sec **Second Dose** 0.3 mg IV over 30 sec; if no adequate response, give third dose **Third Dose** 0.5 mg IV over 30 sec; if no adequate response, repeat once every minute until adequate response or a total of 3 mg is given	Indications Reverse respiratory depression and sedative effects from pure benzodiazepine overdose Precautions • Effects may not outlast effect of benzodiazepines • Monitor for recurrent respiratory depression • Do not use in suspected tricyclic overdose • Do not use in seizure-prone patients • Do not use in unknown drug overdose or mixed drug overdose with drugs known to cause seizures (e.g., tricyclic antidepressants, cocaine, amphetamines)
Furosemide	IV Infusion • 0.5–1 mg/kg given over 1–2 min If no response, double dose to 2 mg/kg, slowly, over 1–2 min	Indications • For adjuvant therapy of acute pulmonary edema in patients with systolic BP >90–100 mm Hg (without signs and symptoms of shock) • Hypertensive emergencies • Increased intracranial pressure Precautions Dehydration, hypovolemia, hypotension, hypokalemia, or other electrolyte imbalance may occur

Continued

TABLE B–1 **Advanced Cardiovascular Life Support Drugs and Electrical Therapy—cont'd**

Drug/Therapy	Adult Dosage	Indications/Precautions
Glucagon Powdered in 1- and 10-mg vials Reconstitute with provided solution	**IV Infusion** 1–5 mg over 2–5 min	**Indications** Adjuvant treatment of toxic effects of calcium channel blocker or beta-blocker **Precautions** • Do not mix with saline • May cause vomiting, hyperglycemia
Glycoprotein IIb/IIIa inhibitors	Check package insert for current indications, doses, and duration of therapy; optimal duration of therapy has not been established	**Indications** These drugs inhibit the integrin glycoprotein IIb/IIIa receptor in the membrane of platelets, inhibiting platelet aggregation; indicated for acute coronary syndromes without ST segment elevation **Precautions/ Contraindications** Active internal bleeding or bleeding disorder in past 30 days, history of intracranial hemorrhage or other bleeding, surgical procedure or trauma within 1 mo, platelet count <150,000/mm^3, hypersensitivity and concomitant use of another GP IIb/IIIa inhibitor
Abciximab (ReoPro)	• Acute coronary syndromes with planned PCI within 24 hr: 0.25 mg/kg IV bolus (10–60 min before procedure), then 0.125 mg/kg/min IV infusion • Must use with heparin • PCI only: 0.25 mg/kg IV bolus, then 10 mg/kg/min IV infusion	**Indications** FDA-approved for patients with non-Q wave MI or unstable angina with planned PCI within 24 hr **Precautions/ Contraindications** • Binds irreversibly with platelets; platelet function recovery requires 48 hr (regeneration) • Readministration may cause hypersensitivity reaction

TABLE B–1 **Advanced Cardiovascular Life Support Drugs and Electrical Therapy—cont'd**

Drug/Therapy	Adult Dosage	Indications/Precautions
Eptifibatide (Integrilin)	• Acute coronary syndromes: 180 mg/kg IV bolus, then 2 mg/kg/min IV infusion • PCI: 135 mg/kg IV bolus, then begin 0.5 mg/kg/min IV infusion, then repeat bolus in 10 min	**Indications** Non-Q wave MI, unstable angina managed medically, and unstable angina/non-Q wave MI patients undergoing PCI **Actions/Precautions** Platelet function recovers within 4–8 hr after discontinuation
Tirofiban (Aggrastat)	Acute coronary syndromes or PCI: 0.4 mg/kg/min IV for 30 min, then 0.1 mg/min IV infusion	**Indications** Non-Q wave MI, unstable angina managed medically, and unstable angina/non-Q wave MI patients undergoing PCI **Actions/Precautions** Platelet function recovers within 4–8 hr after discontinuation
Heparin Unfractionated (UFH) Concentrations range from 1000 to 40,000 IU/mL	**IV Infusion** • Initial bolus 60 IU/kg (maximum bolus, 4000 IU) • Continue 12 IU/kg/hr (maximum, 1000 IU/hr for patients >70 kg) (round to the nearest 50 IU) • Adjust to maintain aPTT 1.5–2 times the control values for 48 hr or until angiography • Target range for aPTT after first 24 hr is between 50 and 70 sec (may vary with laboratory) • Check aPTT at 6,12, 18, and 24 hr • Follow institutional heparin protocol	**Indications** • Adjuvant therapy in AMI • Begin heparin with fibrin-specific lytics (e.g., alteplase) **Precautions** • Same contraindications as for fibrinolytic therapy: active bleeding, recent intracranial, intraspinal, or eye surgery; severe hypertension; bleeding disorders; GI bleeding • Doses and laboratory targets appropriate when used with fibrinolytic therapy

Continued

TABLE B–1 **Advanced Cardiovascular Life Support Drugs and Electrical Therapy—cont'd**

Drug/Therapy	Adult Dosage	Indications/Precautions
Heparin (cont'd) —Ultrasound		• Heparin reversal: protamine 25-mg IV infusion over 10 min or longer (calculate dose as 1 mg protamine per 100 IU of heparin remaining in patient; heparin plasma half-life is 60 min) • Do not use if platelet count is or falls below 100,000 or with history of heparin-induced thrombocytopenia; for these patients, consider direct antithrombins: —Desirudin: 0.1 mg/kg IV bolus, followed by infusion of 0.1 mg/kg/hr for 72 hr —Lepirudin: 0.4 mg/kg IV bolus, followed by infusion of 0.15 mg/kg/hr for 72 hr
Heparin —Low Molecular Weight (LMWH)		**Indications** For use in acute coronary syndromes, specifically patients with non–Q wave MI or unstable angina. These drugs inhibit thrombin generation by factor Xa inhibition and also inhibit thrombin indirectly by formation of a complex with antithrombin III. These drugs are not neutralized by heparin-binding proteins.
	Subcutaneous Dose	**Precautions**
Dalteparin (Fragmin)	1 mg/kg BID SC for 2–8 days, administered with aspirin	• Hemorrhage may complicate any therapy with LMWH
Enoxaparin (Lovenox)	1 mg/kg BID SC for 2–8 days, administered with aspirin	• Contraindicated in presence of hypersensitivity to heparin or pork products or history of sensitivity to drug
Nadroparin (Fraxiparine) (not available in in United States)		

TABLE B–1 **Advanced Cardiovascular Life Support Drugs and Electrical Therapy—cont'd**

Drug/Therapy	Adult Dosage	Indications/Precautions
Heparin (cont'd) —LMWH		• Use enoxaparin with extreme caution, if at all, in patients with heparin-induced thrombocytopenia • Contraindicated if platelet count <100,000; for these patients, consider direct antithrombins: —Desirudin: 0.1 mg/kg IV bolus, followed by infusion of 0.1 mg/kg/hr for 72 hr —Lepirudin: 0.4 mg/kg IV bolus, followed by infusion of 0.15 mg/kg/hr for 72 hr
Ibutilide	**Dose for Adults = 60 kg** 1 mg (10 mL) administered IV (diluted or undiluted) over 10 min; a second dose may be administered at the same rate 10 min later for the conversion of atrial fibrillation or **Dose for adults <60 kg** 0.01 mg/kg initial IV dose	**Indications** Treatment of supraventricular arrhythmias, including atrial fibrillation and atrial flutter. Because it has such a short duration of action, it is most effective flutter of relatively brief duration. **Precautions/ Contraindications** Ventricular arrhythmias develop in approximately 2% to 5% of patients (polymorphic ventricular tachycardia, including torsades de pointes, may be observed). Monitor ECG continuously for arrhythmias during administration and for 4–6 hr after administration, with defibrillator nearby. Patients with significantly impaired LV function are at highest risk for arrhythmias.

Continued

TABLE B–1 **Advanced Cardiovascular Life Support Drugs and Electrical Therapy—cont'd**

Drug/Therapy	Adult Dosage	Indications/Precautions
Isoproterenol *IV infusion:* mix mg in 250 mL NS, lactated Ringer's solution, D5W	**IV Infusion** • Infuse at 2–10 mg/min • Titrate to adequate HR • In torsades de pointes, titrate to increase HR until VT is suppressed	**Indications** • Use cautiously as temporizing measure if external 1 pacer is not available for treatment of symptomatic bradycardia • Refractory torsades de pointes unresponsive to magnesium sulfate • Temporary control of bradycardia in heart transplant patients (denervated heart unresponsive to atropine) • Poisoning from beta-adrenergic blockers **Precautions** • Do not use for treatment of cardiac arrest • Increases myocardial oxygen requirements, which may increase myocardial ischemia • Do not give with epinephrine; can cause VF/VT • Do not administer to patients with poison/drug-induced shock (exception: beta-adrenergic blocker poisoning) • Higher doses are class III (harmful) except for beta-adrenergic blocker poisoning
Lidocaine Can be given via tracheal tube	**Cardiac Arrest from VF/VT** • Initial dose: 1–1.5 mg/kg IV • For refractory VF, may give additional 0.5–0.75 mg/kg IV push, repeat in 5 to 10 min; maximum total dose, 3 mg/kg	**Indications** • Cardiac arrest from VF/VT (class IIb) • Stable VT, wide-complex tachycardias of uncertain type, wide-complex PSVT (class IIb) **Precautions** • Prophylactic use in AMI patients is not recommended

TABLE B–1 **Advanced Cardiovascular Life Support Drugs and Electrical Therapy—cont'd**

Drug/Therapy	Adult Dosage	Indications/Precautions
Lidocaine (cont'd)	• A single dose of 1.5 mg/kg IV in cardiac arrest is acceptable • Tracheal administration: 2–4 mg/kg **Perfusing Arrhythmia** For stable VT, wide-complex tachycardia of uncertain type, or significant ectopy, use as follows: • 1–1.5 mg/kg IV push • Repeat 0.5–0.75 mg/kg in 5–10 min; maximum total dose, 3 mg/kg **Maintenance Infusion** 1–4 mg/min (30–50 mg/kg/min)	• Reduce maintenance dose (not loading dose) in presence of impaired liver function or LV dysfunction • Discontinue infusion immediately if signs of toxicity develop
Magnesium Sulfate	**Cardiac arrest (for Hypomagnesemia or Torsades de Pointes** 1–2 g (2–4 mL of a 50% solution) diluted in 10 mL of D5W IV push **Torsades de Pointes (Not in Cardiac Arrest)** • Loading dose of 1–2 g mixed in 50–100 mL of D5W, over 5–60 min IV • Follow with 0.5–1 g/hr IV (titrate dose to control the torsades) **Acute Myocardial Infarction (if Indicated)** • Loading dose of 1–2 g, mixed in 50–100 mL of D5W, over 5–60 min IV • Follow with 0.5–1 g/hr IV for up to 24 hr	**Indications** • Recommended for use in cardiac arrest only if torsades de pointes of suspected hypomagnesemia is present • Refractory VF (after lidocaine) • Torsades de pointes with a pulse • Life-threatening ventricular arrhythmias due to digitalis • Toxicity • Prophylactic administration in hospitalized patients with AMI is not recommended **Precautions** • Occasional fall in BP with rapid administration • Use with caution if renal failure is present

Continued

TABLE B–1 **Advanced Cardiovascular Life Support Drugs and Electrical Therapy—cont'd**

Drug/Therapy	Adult Dosage	Indications/Precautions
Mannitol Strengths: 5%, 10%, 15%, 20%, and 25%	**IV Infusion** • Administer 0.5–1 g/kg over 5–10 min • Additional doses of 0.25–2 g/kg can be given q4–6 hr as needed • Use with support of oxygenation and ventilation	**Indications** Increased intracranial pressure in management of neurologic emergencies **Precautions** • Monitor fluid status and serum osmolality (not to exceed 310 mOsm/kg) • Use with caution in renal failure, because fluid overload may result
Morphine Sulfate	**IV Infusion** 2–4 mg IV (over 1–5 min) q 5–30 min	**Indications** • Chest pain with ACS unresponsive to nitrates • Acute cardiogenic pulmonary edema (if BP is adequate) **Precautions** • Administer slowly and titrate to effect • May compromise respiration; therefore, use with caution in the compromised respiratory state of acute pulmonary edema • Causes hypotension in volume-depleted patients • Reverse, if needed, with naloxone (0.4–2 mg IV)
Naloxone Hydrochloride	**IV Infusion** • 0.4–2 mg q2min • Use higher doses for complete narcotic reversal • Can administer up to 10 mg over short period (<10 min) • In suspected opiate addicted patients titrate dose until ventilations are adequate: begin with min ×3 doses, then 1.4 mg IV push	**Indications** Respiratory and neurologic depression due to opiate intoxication **Precautions** • May cause opiate withdrawal • Effects may not outlast effects of narcotics 0.2 mg q 2 • Monitor for recurrent respiratory depression • Rare anaphylactic reactions have been reported

TABLE B–1 **Advanced Cardiovascular Life Support Drugs and Electrical Therapy—cont'd**

Drug/Therapy	Adult Dosage	Indications/Precautions
Nitroglycerin Available in IV form, sublingual tablets, and aerosol spray	**IV Infusion** • IV bolus: 12.5–25 mg • Infuse at 10–20 mg/min • Route of choice for emergencies • Use appropriate IV sets provided by pharmaceutical companies • Titrate to effect **Sublingual Route** 1 tablet (0.3–0.4 mg); repeat every 5 min **Aerosol Spray** Spray for 0.5–1 sec at 5-min intervals (provides 0.4 mg/dose)	**Indications** • Initial antianginal for suspected ischemic pain • For initial 24–48 hr in patients with AMI and CHF, large anterior wall infarction, persistent or recurrent ischemia or hypertension • Continued use (beyond 48 hr) for patients with recurrent angina or persistent pulmonary congestion • Hypertensive urgency with ACS **Precautions/Contraindications** • With evidence of AMI, limit systolic BP drop to 10% if patient is normotensive, 30% drop if hypertensive, and avoid drop below 90 mm Hg • Do not mix with other drugs • Patient should sit or lie down when receiving this medication • Do not shake aerosol spray, because this affects metered dose • Contraindications —Hypotension —Severe bradycardia or severe tachycardia —RV infarction —Viagra within 24 hr
Nitroprusside (Sodium Nitroprusside) Mix 50 or 100 mg in 250 mL D5W only	**IV Infusion** • Begin at 0.1 mg/kg/min and titrate upward every 3–5 min to desired effect (up to 5.0 mg/kg/min) • Use with an infusion	**Indications** • Hypertensive crisis • To reduce afterload in heart failure and acute pulmonary edema • To reduce afterload in acute mitral or aortic valve regurgitation

Continued

TABLE B–1 **Advanced Cardiovascular Life Support Drugs and Electrical Therapy—cont'd**

Drug/Therapy	Adult Dosage	Indications/Precautions
Nitroprusside (Sodium Nitroprusside) (cont'd)	pump; use hemo-dynamic monitoring for optimal safety • Action occurs within 1–2 min • Cover drug reservoir and tubing with opaque material	**Precautions** • Light-sensitive; therefore, wrap drug reservoir in aluminum foil • May cause hypotension, thiocyanate toxicity, and CO_2 retention • May reverse hypoxic pulmonary vasoconstriction in patients with pulmonary disease, exacerbating intrapulmonary shunting, resulting in hypoxemia • Other side effects include headaches, nausea, vomiting, and abdominal cramps
Norepinephrine	**IV Infusion (Only Route)** Mix 4 mg in 250 mL of D5W or 5% dextrose in NS Avoid dilution in NS alone • 0.5–1 mg/min titrated to improve BP (up to 30 mg/min) • Do not administer in same IV line as alkaline solutions • Poison/drug-induced hypotension may require higher doses to achieve adequate perfusion	**Indications** • For severe cardiogenic shock and hemodynami-cally significant hypotension (systolic BP <70 mm Hg) with low total peripheral resistance • This is an agent of last resort for management of ischemic heart disease and shock **Precautions** • Increases myocardial oxygen requirements because it raises BP and HR • May induce arrhythmias; use with caution in patients with acute ischemia; monitor cardiac output • Extravasation causes tissue necrosis • If extravasation occurs, administer phentolamine 5–10 mg in 10–15 mL saline solution, infiltrated into area

TABLE B–1 **Advanced Cardiovascular Life Support Drugs and Electrical Therapy—cont'd**

Drug/Therapy	Adult Dosage			Indications/Precautions

Oxygen	**Device**	**Flow Rate**	**O$_2$ (%)**	**Indications**
Delivered from portable tanks or installed, wall-mounted sources through delivery devices	Nasal prongs	1–6 L/min	24–44	• Any suspected cardiopulmonary emergency, especially (but not limited to) complaints of shortness of breath and suspected ischemic chest pain
	Venturi mask	4–8 L/min	24–40	
	Partial re-breather mask			
	Bag-mask	15 L/min	Up to 100	• Note: Pulse oximetry provides a useful method of titrating oxygen administration to maintain physiologic oxygen saturation (see precautions)

Precautions
- Observe closely when using with pulmonary patients known to be dependent on hypoxic respiratory drive (very rare)
- Pulse oximetry inaccurate in low cardiac output states or with vasoconstriction

Procainamide	**Cardiac Arrest**	**Indications**

Cardiac Arrest
- 20 mg/min IV infusion (maximum total dose; 17 mg/kg)
- In refractory VF/VT, 100 mg IV push doses given q5min are acceptable

Other Indications
- 20 mg/min IV infusion until one of the following occurs:
  —Arrhythmia suppression
  —Hypotension
  —QRS widens by >50%
  —Total dose of 17 mg/kg is given

Indications
- Useful for treatment of a wide variety of arrhythmias
- May be used for treatment of PSVT uncontrolled by adenosine and vagal maneuvers if BP stable
- Stable wide-complex tachycardia of unknown origin
- Atrial fibrillation with rapid rate in Wolff–Parkinson–White syndrome

Precautions
- If cardiac or renal dysfunction is present, reduce maximum total dose to 12 mg/kg and maintenance infusion to 1–2 mg/min

Continued

TABLE B–1 **Advanced Cardiovascular Life Support Drugs and Electrical Therapy—cont'd**

Drug/Therapy	Adult Dosage	Indications/Precautions
Procainamide (cont'd)	**Maintenance Infusion** 1–4 mg/min	• Proarrhythmic, especially in setting of AMI, hypokalemia, or hypomagnesemia • May induce hypotension in patients with impaired LV function • Use with caution with other drugs that prolong QT interval (e.g., amiodarone, sotalol)
Propafenone IV form not approved for use in United States	**IV Dose** 1–2 mg/kg body weight at 10 mg/min ***Must be infused slowly***	**Indications** Antiarrhythmic agent used for treatment of ventricular and supraventricular arrhythmias **Precautions/ Contraindications** • Significant negative inotropic effects; must be infused slowly; may increase mortality in patients who have had MI, so should be avoided when coronary artery disease is suspected • Increased plasma concentrations can develop if taken with cimetidine; digoxin, and warfarin levels increase when these drugs are taken with propafenone • Reported side effects include bradycardia, hypotension, and GI upset
Sodium Bicarbonate	**IV Infusion** • 1 mEq/kg IV bolus • Repeat half this dose q10 min thereafter • If rapidly available, use ABG analysis to guide bicarbonate therapy (calculated base deficits or bicarbonate concentration)	**Indications** Specific indications for bicarbonate use are as follows: • Class I if known preexisting hyperkalemia • Class IIa if known pre-existing bicarbonate-responsive • acidosis (e.g., diabetic ketoacidosis) or overdose

TABLE B–1 **Advanced Cardiovascular Life Support Drugs and Electrical Therapy—cont'd**

Drug/Therapy	Adult Dosage	Indications/Precautions
Sodium Bicarbonate (cont'd)	**Blood Gas Interpretation** An acute change in $PaCO_2$ of 1 mm Hg is associated with an increase or decrease in pH of 0.008 U (relative to normal $PaCO_2$ of 40 mm Hg and normal pH of 7.4) (e.g., cardiac arrest and CPR without intubation)	(e.g., tricyclic antidepressant overdose, cocaine, diphenhydramine) to alkalinize urine in aspirin or other overdose • Class IIb if prolonged resuscitation with effective ventilation; upon return of spontaneous circulation after long arrest interval • Class III (not useful or effective) in hypercarbic acidosis
Sotalol IV form not approved for use in United States	**Dose** Administered at 1–1.5 mg/kg body weight, then infused at rate of 10 mg/min ***Must be infused slowly***	**Precautions** • Adequate ventilation and CPR, not bicarbonate, are the major "buffer agents" in cardiac arrest • Not recommended for routine use in cardiac arrest patients **Indications** In the United States, oral form is approved for treatment of ventricular and atrial arrhythmias. Outside the United States, used for treatment of supraventricular and ventricular arrhythmias in patients without structural heart disease **Precautions/ Contraindications** • Should be avoided in patients with poor perfusion because of significant negative inotropic effects; must be infused slowly

Continued

TABLE B–1 **Advanced Cardiovascular Life Support Drugs and Electrical Therapy—cont'd**

Drug/Therapy	Adult Dosage	Indications/Precautions
Sotalol (cont'd)		• Adverse effects include bradycardia, hypotension, and Arrhythmias (torsades de pointes) • Use with caution with other drugs that prolong QT interval (e.g., procainamide, amiodarone)
Thrombolytic Agents (See **Fibrinolytic Agents,** page 466)		
Transcutaneous Pacing External pacemakers have either fixed rates (non-demand or asynchronous mode) or demand rates (range, 30–180 beats/min) Current outputs range from 0 to 200 mA	**Technique** • Place pacing electrodes on chest per package instructions • Turn the pacer ON • Set demand rate to approximately 80 beats/min • Set current (mA) output as follows: —Bradycardia: Increase milliamperes from minimum setting until consistent capture is achieved (characterized by a widening QRS and a broad T wave after each pacer spike); then add 2 mA for safety margin —Asystole: Begin at full output (mA); if capture occurs, slowly decrease output until capture is lost (threshold); then add 2 mA for safety margin	**Indications** • Class I for hemodynamically unstable bradycardia (e.g., BP changes, altered mental status, angina, pulmonary edema) • Class I for pacing readiness in setting of AMI, as follows: —Symptomatic sinus node dysfunction —Type II second-degree heart block —Third-degree heart block —New left, right, or alternating BBB or bifascicular block • Class IIa for bradycardia with symptomatic ventricular escape rhythms • Class IIa for overdrive pacing of tachycardias refractory to drug therapy or electrical cardioversion **Precautions** • Contraindicated in severe hypothermia or prolonged bradyasystolic cardiac arrest

TABLE B–1 **Advanced Cardiovascular Life Support Drugs and Electrical Therapy—cont'd**

Drug/Therapy	Adult Dosage	Indications/Precautions
Transcutaneous Pacing (cont'd)	• Class IIb for bradyasystolic cardiac arrest. Not routinely recommended, but if used, use early	• Conscious patients may require analgesia for discomfort • Avoid using carotid pulse to confirm mechanical capture; electrical stimulation causes muscular jerking that may mimic carotid pulse
Vasopressin	**IV, IO, and ET Doses for Cardiac Arrest** 40 U IV push × 1	**Indications** • May be used as an alternative pressor to epinephrine in the treatment of adult shock-refractory VF (class IIb) • May be useful for hemodynamic support in vasodilatory shock (e.g., septic shock) **Precautions/Contraindications** • Potent peripheral vasoconstrictor; increased peripheral vascular resistance may provoke cardiac ischemia and angina • Not recommended for responsive patients with coronary artery disease
Verapamil	**IV Infusion** • 2.5–5 mg IV bolus over 2 min • Second dose: 5–10 mg, if needed, in 15–30 min; maximum dose, 20 mg • Alternative: 5-mg bolus q15min to total dose of 30 mg	**Indications** • Alternative drug (after adenosine) to terminate PSVT with narrow QRS complex and adequate BP and preserved LV function • May control ventricular response in patients with atrial fibrillation, flutter, or multifocal atrial tachycardia

Continued

TABLE B–1 **Advanced Cardiovascular Life Support Drugs and Electrical Therapy—cont'd**

Drug/Therapy	Adult Dosage	Indications/Precautions
Verapamil (cont'd)	• Older patients: administer over 3 min	**Precautions** • Give only to patients with narrow-complex PSVT or arrhythmias known to be of supraventricular origin; do not use calcium channel blockers for wide-QRS tachycardias of uncertain origin • Avoid calcium channel blockers in patients with Wolff–Parkinson–White syndrome and atrial fibrillation, sick sinus syndrome, or second- or third-degree AV block without pacemaker • Expect BP drop caused by peripheral vasodilation; IV calcium is an antagonist that may restore BP in toxic cases • May decrease myocardial contractility and may exacerbate CHF in patients with LV dysfunction • Concurrent IV administration with IV beta-blockers may produce severe hypotension • Use with extreme caution in patients receiving oral beta-blockers

*Biphasic waveforms using lower energy are acceptable if documented to be clinically equivalent or superior to reports of monophasic shock success.

**Biphasic devices shock at lower energy levels (approximately 150 J). In some clinical settings, initial and repeated shocks at these lower energy levels are acceptable.

†Treat polymorphic VT (irregular form and rate) with same currents used for VF:200 J, 200–300 J, 360 J.

‡PSVT and atrial flutter often respond to lower energy levels; start with 50 J.

Reproduced with permission, ACLS Provider Manual, 2002, Copyright American Heart Association.

TABLE B–2 **Emergency Treatment of Hyperkalemia**

Therapy	Dose	Onset of Effect	Duration of Effect
Antagonize			
Calcium chloride	5–10 mL IV of 10% solution (500–1000 mg)	1–3 min	30–60 min
Shift into cells			
Sodium bicarbonate	1 mEq/kg IV bolus	5–10 min	1–2 hr
Insulin plus glucose (use 1 U insulin/ 2.5 g glucose)	Regular insulin 10 U IV plus 50 mL D$_{50}$ (25 g glucose) IV bolus (1 50-mL prefilled syringe or vial or D$_{50}$)	30 min	4–6 hr
Nebulized albuterol	10–20 mg nebulized over 15 min	15 min	15–90 min
Remove from body			
Diuresis with furosemide	40–80 mg IV bolus	When diuresis starts, 1–2 hr	When diuresis ends, 4–6 hr
Cation-exchange resin (Kayexalate)	15–50 g PO or PR, plus sorbitol		
Peritoneal dialysis or hemodialysis	Per institution	As soon as started	Until dialysis completed

Reproduced with permission, ACLS Provider Manual, 2002, Copyright American Heart Association.

TABLE B–3 **Sympathomimetic, Inotropic, and Inodilator Drugs**

Drug	IV Infusion	Adrenergic		Arrhythmogenic Potential
		Alpha	Beta	
Epinephrine	2–10 mg/min	++	+++	+++
Norepinephrine	0.5–30 mg/min	+++	++	++
Dopamine	1–5 mg/kg/min	+	+*	+
	5–10 mg/kg/min	++	++*	++
	10–20 mg/kg/min	+++	++	+++
Dobutamine	2–20 mg/kg/min	+	+++	++
Isoproterenol	2–10 mg/min	0	+++	+++
Amrinone†	5–15 mg/kg/min (after loading dose)	0	0*	++

*Increases renal and splanchnic blood flow.
†Phosphodiesterase inhibitor.
Reproduced with permission, ACLS Provider Manual, 2002, Copyright American Heart Association.

Reading X-Rays, Reading ECGs

READING X-RAYS

1. Clavicles
2. Trachea
3. Right mainstem bronchus
4. Left mainstem bronchus
5. Aortic knuckle
6. Superior vena cava
7. Right pulmonary artery
8. Left pulmonary artery
9. Left atrium
10. Right atrium
11. Left ventricle
12. Aortic stripe
13. Costophrenic angles
14. Gastric bubble

Figure C–1 Posteroanterior chest x-ray. (Reprinted from Marshall SA, Ruedy J: On Call: Principles and Protocols, 2nd ed. Philadelphia, WB Saunders, 1993, p. 332.)

1. Trachea
2. Left mainstem bronchus
3. Right pulmonary artery
4. Left pulmonary artery
5. Aortic arch
6. Manubrium
7. Sternum
8. Breast shadow
9. Retrosternal space
10. Retrocardiac space
11. Left atrium
12. Right ventricle
13. Left ventricle
14. Inferior vena cava
15. Gastric air bubble
16. Left hemidiaphragm
17. Right hemidiaphragm
18. Costophrenic angle
19. Scapular shadows

Figure C–2 Lateral chest x-ray. (Reprinted from Marshall SA, Ruedy J: On Call: Principles and Protocols, 2nd ed. Philadelphia, WB Saunders, 1993, p. 333.)

READING ECGS

Rate

Multiply the number of QRS complexes in a 6-second period (30 large squares) (between the two large dots) by 10 = beats/minute (Fig. C–3).

    Normal = 60 to 100 beats/minute
    Tachycardia = >100 beats/minute
    Bradycardia = <60 beats/minute

Rhythm

Is the rhythm regular?

    Is there a P wave preceding every QRS complex? Is there a QRS complex following every P wave?

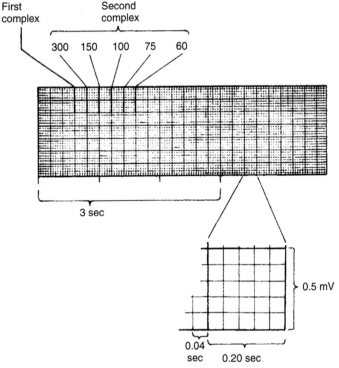

Figure C–3 Reading ECGs. Rate. (Reprinted from Marshall SA, Ruedy J: On Call: Principles and Protocols, 2nd ed. Philadelphia, WB Saunders, 1993, p. 328.)

1. Yes = sinus rhythm.
2. No P waves with irregular rhythm = atrial fibrillation.
3. No P waves with regular rhythm = junctional rhythm. Look for retrograde P waves in all leads.

Axis

See Figure C–4.

P Wave Configuration

Normal P wave. Look at all leads (Fig. C–5A).

Left Atrial Enlargement (Fig. C–5B)

Duration: 120 msec (three small squares in lead II). Often notched = P mitrale. Amplitude: Negative terminal P wave in lead V_1 >1 mm in depth *and* >40 msec (one small square).

Figure C–4 Axis. (Reprinted form Marshall SA, Ruedy J: On Call: Principles and Protocols, 2nd ed. Philadelphia, WB Saunders, 1993, p. 329.)

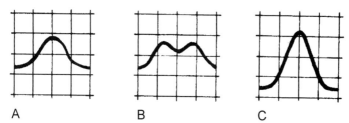

A   B   C

Figure C–5 Reading ECGs. P wave configuration in lead II. *A*, Normal P wave; *B*, Left atrial enlargement; *C*, Right atrial enlargement. (Reprinted from Marshall SA, Ruedy J: On Call: Principles and Protocols, 2nd ed. Philadelphia, WB Saunders, 1993, p. 329.)

Right Atrial Enlargement (Fig. C–5C)

Amplitude: 2.5 mm in leads II, III, or aVF (i.e., tall, peaked P wave of P pulmonale); 1.5 mm in the initial positive deflection of the P wave in lead V_1 or V_2.

QRS Configuration

Left Ventricular Hypertrophy

1. Increased QRS voltage (S in V_1 or V_2 plus R in V_5 >35 mm or R in aVL ≥11 mm)

2. Left atrial enlargement
3. ST segment depression and negative T wave in left lateral leads.

Right Ventricular Hypertrophy

1. $R > S$ in V_1
2. Right axis deviation (> +90 degrees)
3. ST segment depression and negative T wave in right precordial leads.

Conduction Abnormalities

First-Degree Block

PR interval >0.2 second (>1 large square)

Second-Degree Block

Occasional absence of QRS and T after a P of sinus origin.
1. Type I (Wenckebach): Progressive prolongation of the PR interval before the missed QRS complex
2. Type II: Absence of progressive prolongation of the PR interval before the missed QRS complex.

Third-Degree Block

Absence of any relationship between P waves of sinus origin and QRS complexes

Left Anterior Hemiblock Left axis deviation, Q in I and aVL; a small R in III, in the absence of left ventricular hypertrophy.

Left Posterior Hemiblock Right axis deviation, a small R in I and a small Q in III, in the absence of right ventricular hypertrophy.

Complete Right Bundle Branch Block. See Figure C–6A.

Complete Left Bundle Branch Block. See Figure C–6B.

V1 V6 V1 V6

A B

Figure C–6 Reading ECGs. QRS configuration. A, Complete right bundle branch block; B, complete left bundle branch block. (Reprinted from Marshall SA, Ruedy J: On Call: Principles and Protocols, 2nd ed. Philadelphia, WB Saunders, 1993, p. 331.)

Ventricular Preexcitation

1. PR interval <0.11 second with widened QRS (>0.12 second) due to a delta wave = Wolff–Parkinson–White syndrome.
2. PR interval <0.11 second with a normal QRS complex = Lown Ganong-Levine syndrome.

TABLE C–1 **Myocardial Infarction Patterns**

Type of Infarct	Patterns of Changes (Q Waves, ST Elevation or Depression, T Wave Inversion)*
Inferior	Q in II, III, aVF
Inferoposterior	Q in II, III, aVF, and V_6 $R > S$ and positive T in V_1
Anteroseptal	V_1 to V_4
Anterolateral to posterolateral	V_1 to V_5; Q in I, aVL, and V_6
Posterior	$R > S$ in V_1, positive T, and Q in V_6

*A significant Q wave is >40 msec wide or > one-third of the QRS height. ST segment or T wave changes in the absence of significant Q waves may represent a non-Q wave infarct.

Outlines of Common Surgical Notes

PREOP NOTE*

Date and time:
Preop diagnosis:
Procedure planned:
Staff surgeon:
Preop examination:
Preoperative laboratory studies:
List of routine medications/therapies:
Blood products available:
   (Confirm availability with a phone call to the blood bank the night before surgery)
Bowel preparation (if any):
"On call to OR" instructions:
Void:
Preop antibiotics:
SBE prophylaxis:
Steroid preparation:
Other special therapies needed:
   PAR statement (a brief statement that the procedure, alternatives, and risks have been discussed with the patient):
   For example, "Procedure, alternatives, benefits, complications, and risks, both foreseen and unforeseen, described in detail to the patient; questions were answered to his/her satisfaction. He/she elects to proceed as planned. Consent signed and witnessed. Surgical site confirmed."

BRIEF OP NOTE

Date and time:
Preop diagnosis:
Postop diagnosis:

---

*See also Chapter 24.

Procedure:
Staff surgeon:
Assistants:
Anesthesia:
Indications:
Findings:
   (Drawings are often useful to describe resultant anatomy)
Specimens:
   (including results of frozen sections, if any)
Drains:
Cultures:
Estimated blood loss:
Urine output:
Fluids received:
Complications:
("Returned to PAR/SICU in condition")

POSTOP CHECK

Date and time:
Date of procedure:
Procedure:
Staff surgeon:
Postop examination:
VS:
Mental status:
Cardiovascular:
Lungs:
Abdomen:
Extremities/skin:
Wound/dressing:
Specific surgical site:
Postop laboratory studies:
Urine output:
Drain output and character of fluid draining:
Pain control:
Patient status:
Time until reassessment:

ON CALL/CROSS-COVERAGE NOTE

Date and time:
Contacted by:
Patient identification:
Operation:
   (date and type of procedure, staff surgeon, complications)
Brief summary of course since the operation:

Current problem:
History of problem:
Examination (problem oriented):
VS:
Mental status:
Cardiovascular:
Lungs:
Abdomen:
Extremities/skin:
Wound/dressing:
Specific surgical site:
Specific problem site:
Recent laboratory studies:
Urine output:
Drain output and character of fluid draining:
Assessment:
Plans:
Persons contacted:
    (resident, attending, bedside care giver, family, consulting services, etc.)
Time until reassessment:

Antibiotic Standard Doses and Indications for Patients with Normal Renal Function

Drug	Dosage Range (g/day) IV/IM*	Usual Dosage (g/dosing interval) IV/IM*	Special Comments and Usage
Amikacin	5–7 mg/kg	5–7 mg/kg daily	Good coverage for Gram-negative rods. Useful for organisms resistant to gentamicin and tobramycin. Consider use in patients with Gram-negative infections with contraindication to aminoglycoside use
Amoxicillin	1–6	0.5–1 every 8 hr	Good for group B streptococcus, *Streptococcus viridans*, *S. pneumoniae*, and staphylococcus
Ampicillin	2–12	1 every 6 hr	Drug of choice for enterococcus, group B streptococcus, *Listeria*, and actinomycete. Useful for treatment of sepsis in combination with an aminoglycoside and either metronidazole or clindamycin

Continued

Drug	Dosage Range (g/ day) IV/IM*	Usual Dosage (g/dosing interval) IV/IM*	Special Comments and Usage
Aztreonam	1–8	0.5–2 every 8 hr	Good Gram-negative coverage. Consider use in patients with Gram-negative infections with renal insufficiency or contraindication to aminoglycoside use
Cefazolin	3–6	1 every 8 hr	Most common pre-operative antibiotic. Good *Staphylococcus aureus* and *Staphylococcus epidermidis* coverage. Moderate streptococcus groups A and B coverage. Does not cover enterococcus. Moderate coverage of streptococcus and staphylococcus, but does not cover enterococcus
Cefotaxime	3–8	1–2 every 6–8 hr	Useful in meningitis due to Gram-negative rods resistant to ampicillin
Cefoxitin	3–6	1–2 every 6–8 hr	Some staphylococcus and streptococcus coverage, and moderate anaerobic Gram-positive (*Clostridium*) and anaerobic Gram-negative coverage (*Bacteroides fragilis*) with a single agent
Ceftazidime	3–6	1 every 8 hr	Good *Pseudomonas* coverage. Consider use when Gram-negative infection and aminoglycosides are inappropriate

Drug	Dosage Range (g/day) IV/IM*	Usual Dosage (g/dosing interval) IV/IM*	Special Comments and Usage
Ceftriaxone	1–4	1–2 every 12–24 hr	Longer half-life than other cephalosporins. Moderate staphylococcus and streptococcus coverage. Useful in meningitis due to Gram-negative rods resistant to ampicillin
Cefuroxime	2–4.5	0.5–1 every 8 hr	Mixed lung infections in penicillin-allergic patients. *Haemophilus influenzae* resistant to ampicillin. Good coverage for streptococcus and staphylococcus except MRSA and enterococcus
Ciprofloxacin	0.4–0.8	200–400 mg every 12 hr	Broad-spectrum agent for urinary tract infections and as adjunct for complicated skin infection; also, good bone penetration. 500 mg PO every 12 hr has equal bioavailability as 400 mg IV every 12 hr
Clindamycin	0.6–2	0.6 every 8 hr	Good coverage for anaerobes "above the diaphragm". *B. fragilis* dosing
Erythromycin	1–4	0.5 every 6 hr	Drug of choice for *Legionella*, *Chlamydia*, *Mycoplasma*. Moderate *S. aureus* and streptococcus groups A and B coverage. Does not cover *S. epidermidis* or enterococcus

Continued

Drug	Dosage Range (g/ day) IV/IM*	Usual Dosage (g/dosing interval) IV/IM*	Special Comments and Usage
Gentamicin	5–7 mg/kg	5–7 mg/kg daily	Serious aerobic Gram-negative rod infections. Follow gentamicin levels and creatinine
Imipenem	1–2	0.5 every 6 hr	Good staphylococcus coverage, except MRSA. Good anaerobic and aerobic enteric coverage. Consider "big-gun agent"
Levofloxacin	0.25–0.5	0.25–0.5	Fluoroquinolone antibiotic used for community acquired pnuemoniae and some enterics. PO and IV form available
Meropenem	1.5–3	0.5–1 every 8 hr	Carbapenem antibiotic for multiply resistant Gram-negative enteric pathogens. May be combined with an amino-glycoside to cover *Psuedomonas sp*. A PO form is available
Metronidazole	1–2	0.5 every 8 hr	Good Gram-negative enteric coverage. Good for anaerobes "below the diaphragm". Well absorbed orally. Good for pseudomembranous colitis caused by *Clostridium difficile*
Penicillin	2–20 mu	1–4 mu every 4–6 hr	Drug of choice for streptococcal infec-tions. Good for oral infections, human bites, and anaerobic infections "above the diaphragm"

Drug	Dosage Range (g/day) IV/IM*	Usual Dosage (g/dosing interval) IV/IM*	Special Comments and Usage
Piperacillin	6–12	1.5–2 every 4 hr	Use for *Pseudomonas* infections. Moderate Gram-negative enteric coverage
Piperacillin and Tazobactam	13.5	3.375 g every 6 hr	Broad spectrum anti-*Pseudomonal* agent. Active against several gram-negative bacilli and is useful for empiric treatment of severe intra-abdominal infections, complex skin infections and nosocomial pneumoniae
Tetracycline	1–2	0.5 every 6 hr	Avoid use in children or pregnant patients, because bone and tooth development are affected
Tobramycin	5–7 mg/kg	5–7 mg/kg daily	More effective than gentamicin for *Pseudomonas* infection
Vancomycin	1–2	1 every 12 hr	Drug of choice for MRSA. Useful in multidrug-resistant Gram-positive infections

*Unless otherwise specified.

MRSA, methicillin-resistant *Staphylococcus aureus*; mu, million units.

Proprietary Names of Common Medications

Adalat	nifedipine
Aldactone	spironolactone
ALternaGEL	aluminum hydroxide gel
Alupent	metaproterenol sulfate
Amicar	aminocaproic acid
Amikin	amikacin
Amphojel	aluminum hydroxide gel
Anzemet	dolasetron
Apresoline	hydralazine hydrochloride
AquaMEPHYTON	phytonadione (vitamin K_1)
Aquasol A	retinol (vitamin A)
Asacol	mesalamine
Atarax	hydroxyzine hydrochloride
Ativan	lorazepam
Beclovent	beclomethasone dipropionate
Benadryl	diphenhydramine hydrochloride
Betaloc	metoprolol
Bumex	bumetanide
Calan	verapamil hydrochloride
Capoten	captopril
Carafate	sucralfate
Cardizem	diltiazem hydrochloride
Celebrex	celeloxib
Cipro	ciprofloxacin
Colace	docusate sodium
Compazine	prochlorperazine maleate
Coumadin	warfarin sodium
Cytotec	misoprostol
Demerol HCl	meperidine hydrochloride
Diabinese	chlorpropamide
Dialose	docusate
Diflucan	fluconazole
Dilacor XR	diltiazem hydrochloride
Dilantin	phenytoin sodium
Dulcolax	bisacodyl

Edecrin	ethacrynic acid
Esidrix	hydrochlorothiazide
Haldol	haloperidol
HydroDIURIL	hydrochlorothiazide
Imitrex	sumatriptan succinate
Imodium	loperamide
Inderal	propranolol hydrochloride
Indocin	indomethacin
Isoptin	verapamil hydrochloride
Isordil	isosorbide dinitrate
Kay Ciel	potassium chloride
Kayexalate	sodium polystyrene sulfonate
Lanoxin	digoxin
Lasix	furosemide
Levaquin	levofloxacin
Librium	chlordiazepoxide hydrochloride
Losec	omeprazole
Lomotil	diphenoxylate hydrochloride with atropine
Lopressor	metoprolol
Lotrimin	clotrimazole
Maalox	aluminum hydroxide; magnesium hydroxide
Maxeran	metoclopramide
Merrem	meropenim
Micro-K	potassium chloride
Motrin	ibuprofen
Mycelex	clotrimazole
Mycostatin	nystatin
Mylanta	aluminum hydroxide; magnesium hydroxide; simethicone
Naprosyn	naproxen
Narcan	naloxone hydrochloride
Nizoral	ketoconazole
Normodyne	labetalol hydrochloride
Osmitrol	mannitol
Pentam 300	pentamidine isoethionate
Pentasa	mesalamine
Pepcid	famotidine
Phenergan	promethazine hydrochloride
Phytonadione	vitamin K_1
Plavix	clopidourel
Prilosec	omeprazole
Primaxin	imipenem and cilastin
Prinivil	lisinopril
Procanbid	procainamide hydrochloride
Procardia	nifedipine
Protium	pantoprazole

Protonix	pantoprazole
Proventil	albuterol sulfate
Pyridium	phenazopyridine hydrochloride
Reglan	metoclopramide
Retinol	vitamin A
Romazicon	flumazenil
Serax	oxazepam
Sinemet	levodopa; carbidopa
Slow-K	potassium chloride
Sorbitrate	isosorbide dinitrate
Tagamet	cimetidine hydrochloride
Tazosyn	piperacillin and tazobactam
Thiamine	vitamin B_1
Thorazine	chlorpromazine
Trandate	labetalol hydrochloride
Tylenol	acetaminophen
Valium	diazepam
Vanceril	beclomethasone dipropionate
Vasotec	enalapril maleate
Ventolin	albuterol sulfate
Versed	midazolam hydrochloride
Vistaril	hydroxyzine pamoate
Vitamin A	retinol
Vitamin B1	thiamine hydrochloride
Vitamin K1	phytonadione
Xylocaine	lidocaine
Zantac	ranitidine hydrochloride
Zaroxolyn	metolazone
Zestril	lisinoprol
Zosyn	piperacillin and tazobactam
Zyloprim	allopurinol

On-Call Formulae

FLUIDS AND ELECTROLYTES

1. Determination of serum osmolality (mOsm)

Serum osmolality = 2[Na] + {[glucose]/[18]} + {[BUN]/[2.8]}

Na	Serum sodium concentration (in mEq/L)
Glucose	Serum glucose concentration (in mg/dL)
BUN	Blood urea nitrogen concentration (in mg/dL)
Normal range	280 to 295 mOsm

2. Determination of free water deficit (in L) in settings of hypernatremia

Water deficit = {[Na (observed) – Na (desired)] [0.6] [Wt]/ [Na (desired)]}

Na (observed)	Serum sodium concentration (in mEq/L)
Na (desired)	Assume 140 mEq/L
0.6	Volume of distribution of sodium
Wt	Weight (in kg)

3. Determination of actual serum sodium in settings of hyperglycemia

Na (corrected) = {[glucose (observed) – glucose (normal)] [1.4]/[glucose (normal)]} + Na (observed)

Na (corrected)	Actual serum concentration of sodium (in mEq/L)
Na (observed)	Serum sodium concentration (in mEq/L)
Glucose (observed)	Actual glucose concentration (in mg/dL)
Glucose (normal)	Assume 200 mg/dL
1.4	Correction factor, which considers the shift of water, that follows glucose into the interstitial space

4. Determination of sodium deficit in settings of hyponatremia

Na deficit = [Na (desired) − Na (observed)] [0.6] [Wt]

Na (desired)	Assume 135 mEq/L
Na (observed)	Serum sodium concentration (in mEq/L)
0.6	Volume of distribution of sodium
Wt	Weight (in kg)

5. Determination of bicarbonate (HCO_3) deficit (in mEq/L)

HCO_3 deficit = [Wt] [0.4] [HCO_3 (desired) − HCO_3 (actual)]

HCO_3 (desired)	Assume 15 to 20 mEq/L
HCO_3 (observed)	Serum concentration of bicarbonate (in mEq/L)
Wt	Weight (in kg)
0.4	Correction factor, which considers intracellular buffering of bicarbonate
Goal of therapy	Serum pH >7.2

6. Determination of bicarbonate (HCO_3) deficit (in mEq/L) by using base deficit

HCO_3 deficit = {[Base deficit] [Wt in kg] [0.4]/2}

7. Determination of anion gap (in mEq/L)

Anion gap = (Na + K) − (Cl + HCO_3)

Na	Serum sodium concentration (in mEq)
K	Serum potassium concentration (in mEq)
Cl	Serum chloride concentration (in mEq)
HCO_3	Serum bicarbonate ion concentration (in mEq)

8. Henderson–Hasselbach equation

pH = 6.1 + log {(HCO_3)/(0.03 × PCO_2)}

6.1	pH of the bicarbonate buffer system
HCO_3	Serum bicarbonate ion concentration (in mEq/L)
0.03	Solubility constant of CO_2 in arterial blood
PCO_2	Partial pressure of CO_2 in serum (in mm Hg)

9. Nitrogen balance (in g/day, may be a positive or a negative value)

N_2 balance = {24-hour protein intake/6.25} − [(24-hour UUN) + (4)]

24-hour UUN	Urinary urea nitrogen excretion (in g/day)
4	Obligatory loss (in g/day)

6.25   The number of grams of protein that yield 1 g N_2

Goal of therapy   +3 to 6 g/day balance

CARDIAC PHYSIOLOGY

1. Determination of cardiac output (CO)

$$CO = [HR] [SV]$$

CO	Cardiac output (in L/minute)
HR	Heart rate (in beats/minute)
SV	Stroke volume (in L/beat)
Normal	3.5 to 8.5 L/minute

Cardiac index (CI) = CO/patient surface area

2. Determination of cardiac index (CI)

$$CI = CO/body surface area$$

CO   Cardiac output (in L/minute)

3. Determination of blood pressure (BP)

$$BP = [CO] [SVR]$$

BP	Blood pressure (in mm Hg)
CO	Cardiac output (in L/minute)
SVR	Systemic vascular resistance in dyne-second/cm^5

4. Determination of mean arterial blood pressure (MAP)

$$MAP = \{DBP + [SBP-DBP]/[3]\}$$

MAP	Mean arterial pressure (in mm Hg)
DBP	Diastolic blood pressure (in mm Hg)
SBP	Systolic blood pressure (in mm Hg)

5. Determination of systemic vascular resistance (SVR)

$$SVR = \{[MAP-CVP] [80]/[CO]\}$$

SVR	Systemic vascular resistance in dyne-second/cm^5
MAP	Mean arterial pressure (in mm Hg)
CVP	Central venous pressure (in mm Hg)
CO	Cardiac output (in L/minute)

6. Conversion of pressure in millimeters of mercury (mm Hg) to pressure in centimeters of water (cm H_2O)

$$mm\ Hg = cm\ H_2O/1.36$$

7. Calculation of cerebral perfusion pressure (CPP)

$$CPP = MAP - ICP$$

CPP   Cerebral perfusion pressure (in mm Hg)
MAP   Mean arterial pressure (in mm Hg)
ICP   Intracranial pressure (in mm Hg)
Goal   65 mm Hg for adequate cerebral perfusion

8. Calculation of ankle-brachial index (ABI)

$$ABI = \{SBP\ (ankle)/SBP\ (arm)\}$$

ABI   Ankle-Brachial Index
SBP (ankle)   Systolic blood pressure taken at the ankle
SBP (arm)   Systolic blood pressure taken at the arm
Values: Normal: >0.95
               Claudication: 0.5–0.9
               Rest pain: 0.2–0.5
               Tissue necrosis: <0.3
               Notes: Noncompressible vessels (i.e., in diabetics)
                 can give falsely elevated values
               A Doppler is useful to perform this test at the
                 bedside.

RESPIRATORY PHYSIOLOGY

1. The Fick's law for transfer of gases

$$V_{gas} = \{(A)/0.5\}\ (k)\ (P_1 - P_2)$$

V_{gas} Rate of gas transfer across a membrane
A   Tissue area
0.5   Thickness of the pulmonary membrane (in µm)
k   Solubility coefficient of the gas
$P_1 - P_2$ Partial pressure gradient of the gas across the membrane
               (in mm Hg)
             (CO_2 diffuses 20 times faster than O_2 due to differences
               in their solubility coefficients)

2. Calculation of the alveolar oxygen partial pressure (PAO_2)

$$PAO_2 = (713)\ (FiO_2) - \{PaCO_2/0.8\}$$

PAO_2 Alveolar oxygen partial pressure (in mm Hg)
713   Sea level barometric pressure (760 mm Hg) minus the
             partial pressure of water vapor (pH_2O, 47 mm Hg)
FiO_2 Fractional concentration of inspired oxygen
$PaCO_2$ Partial pressure of CO_2 (in mm Hg, from arterial
             blood gas data)
0.8   Respiratory quotient

3. **Calculation of the alveolar-arterial oxygen gradient (P[A–a]O$_2$)**

$$P[A\text{–}a]O_2 = PAO_2 - PaO_2$$

P[A–a]O$_2$	Alveolar-arterial oxygen gradient (in mm Hg)
PAO$_2$	Alveolar oxygen partial pressure (in mm Hg)
PaO$_2$	Arterial oxygen partial pressure (in mm Hg, from arterial blood gas data)
	Normal ([A–a]O$_2$ is 12 mm Hg in young adults and increases to 20 mm Hg by the age of 70 years. In failure of ventilation, the P[A–a]O$_2$ will increase.

4. **Calculation of oxygen delivery (DO$_2$)**

$$DO_2 = CO \times 10 \times [(SaO_2 \times Hb \times 1.34 + (0.003 \times PaO_2)]$$

DO$_2$	Delivery of oxygen (in ml O$_2$ per minute)
CO	Cardiac output (in L/min)
SaO$_2$	Oxygen saturation of arterial blood (in %)
Hb	Hemoglobin concentration (in gm/dl)
1.34	O$_2$ binding capacity (in mL O$_2$/gm Hb)
0.003	Volume of O$_2$ dissolved in 100 mL of blood per mm Hg for each mm PaO$_2$
PaO$_2$	Partial pressure of O$_2$ in arterial blood (in mm Hg)
	Normal range is 800–1000 mL O$_2$ per minute. Note the relative importance of Hb in the equation.

RENAL PHYSIOLOGY

1. **Creatinine clearance (CrCl)**

$$CrCl = (140 - age)\,(wt)/(72)\,(Cr)$$

CrCl	Creatinine clearance (in mL/minute)
Age	Patient's age (in years)
Wt	Patient's weight (in kg)
Cr	Serum creatinine concentration (in mg/dL)
Normal	90 to 150 mL/minute

2. **Calculation of fractional excretion of Na (FENa)**

$$U_{Na} \times P_{Cr}/P_{Na} \times U_{Cr}$$

UNa	Urinary sodium concentration (in mEq)
PCr	Plasma creatinine concentration (in mg)
PNa	Plasma sodium concentration (in mEq)
UCr	Urinary creatinine concentration (in mg)
	As all units cancel, results are reported as percentage. May be performed on spot urine and plasma samples. A value lesser than 1% is indicative of prerenal causes of renal failure, a value greater than 1% is indicative of renal causes of failure.

On-Call Formulary

This formulary includes medications that are commonly used while on call. Dosages listed are for adults, and generic names are listed. Antibiotic dosages are listed in Appendix E. Always be mindful of the renal and hepatic function of the patient before administration of medications, and be aware that many patients require individualization of medications. Also, be aware that many medications require individualization of dose. For further information, consult the pharmacy or the medication insert instructions.

ACETAMINOPHEN

Proprietary name(s):	Tylenol and others
Therapeutic class:	Analgesic and antipyretic
Indications:	Pain and fever
Actions:	Diminishes pain response and has direct action on hypothalamus temperature regulation centers
Metabolism:	Hepatic
Excretion:	Renal
Side effects:	Uncommon; rash, drug fever, mucosal ulcerations, leukopenia, pancytopenia, and hepatic toxicity
Dose:	325–1000 mg PO/PR every 4 to 6 hours, as needed, to 4000 mg/24 hour.
Notes:	Little to no antiinflammatory action. Does not affect the aggregation of platelets.
	Does not interact with anticoagulants.
	Antidote for overdose is *N*-acetylcysteine.

ALBUTEROL

Proprietary name(s):	Proventil and Ventolin
Therapeutic class:	β_2-Adrenergic agonist
Indications:	Bronchospasm due to asthma, bronchitis, or chronic obstructive pulmonary disease (COPD)

Actions:	β_2-Adrenergic agonist
Metabolism:	Hepatic; less than 20% of the inhaled dose is absorbed systemically
Excretion:	Renal
Side effects:	Headache, tachycardia, lightheadedness, dizziness, tremor, palpitations, and nausea
Dose:	2.5 to 5 mg in 3 mL normal saline (NS) by nebulizer every 4 hours, as needed
	Severe acute bronchospasm may require doses every 3 to 5 minutes initially.
Notes:	May alternate with metaproterenol.

ALLOPURINOL

Proprietary name(s):	Zyloprim
Therapeutic class:	Xanthine oxidase inhibitor
Indications:	Symptomatic gout, uric acid nephropathy, and lysis of tumor
Actions:	Inhibits formation of uric acid
Metabolism:	Metabolite oxipurinol is also active
Excretion:	Renal
Side effects:	Rash, fever, gastrointestinal (GI) upset, cataracts, renal toxicity, and hepatotoxicity
Dose:	100 to 300 mg PO every day after meals. Severe cases may require doses up to 800 mg/day.
Notes:	Reduce the dose in renal or hepatic insufficiency. Acute gout episodes may follow initiation of therapy.
	Aminophylline, mercaptopurine, and azathioprine levels may be increased by allopurinol. Nonsteroidal anti-inflammatory drugs (NSAIDs) are the first-line therapy for acute gout.

ALUMINUM HYDROXIDE

Proprietary name(s):	Amphojel and ALternaGEL
Therapeutic class:	Antacid
Indications:	Epigastric pain due to peptic ulcer disease or gastritis. Prophylaxis for stress ulcers.
	Reduction of urinary phosphate in patients with phosphate-containing renal stones.

Actions: Buffers gastric acid; binds to phosphate in the GI tract

Side effects: Constipation, anorexia, nausea, hypophosphatemia and aluminum toxicity in patients with renal failure

Dose: For acute symptoms, 30 to 60 mL PO every 1 to 2 hours, as needed

For maintenance therapy, 30 to 60 mL PO every 1 to 3 hours when symptomatic and before bedtime, as needed

Notes: May bind to and reduce the absorption of tetracycline, thyroxine, and other medications.

ALUMINUM HYDROXIDE/MAGNESIUM HYDROXIDE

Proprietary name(s): Maalox and Mylanta

Therapeutic class: Antacid

Indications: Pain due to peptic ulcer disease, reflux esophagitis, and prophylaxis of stress ulcers

Actions: Buffers gastric acidity

Side effects: Diarrhea, hypermagnesemia, or aluminum toxicity in patients with renal failure

Dose: For acute symptoms, 30 to 60 mL PO every 1 to 2 hours, as needed

For maintenance therapy, 30 to 60 mL PO every 1 to 3 hours when symptomatic and before bedtime, as needed

Notes: Aluminum salts cause constipation. Magnesium salts cause diarrhea. The mixture of the salts tends to balance the effects. May bind to and reduce the absorption of tetracycline, thyroxine, and other medications.

AMIKACIN (SEE ANTIBIOTIC LISTING IN APPENDIX E)

AMINOCAPROIC ACID

Proprietary name(s): Amicar

Therapeutic class: Plasminogen activator inhibitor

Indications:	Hemorrhage due to fibrinolysis
Actions:	Inhibits plasminogen activator; also has antiplasmin activity
Metabolism:	65% of drug is excreted unchanged
Excretion:	Renal
Side effects:	Increased risk of deep venous thrombosis (DVT), cerebral embolism, and pulmonary embolism. Nausea, abdominal cramps, dizziness, rash, and headaches.
Dose:	Loading dose of 4 to 5 g IV over 1 hour, followed by maintenance infusion of 1 to 1.25 g/hour to achieve plasma levels of 0.13 mg/mL or until clinical bleeding stops.
	Maximum dose, 30 g/24 hours.
	Loading dose may be given PO.
Notes:	Rule out disseminated intravascular coagulation (DIC) before administration.

AMINOPHYLLINE

Therapeutic class:	Bronchodilator
Indications:	Bronchospasm due to asthma
Actions:	Methylxanthine; inhibits phosphodiesterase activity resulting in smooth muscle relaxation and bronchodilation. Also activates respiratory centers.
Metabolism:	Hepatic (90%)
Excretion:	Renal
Side effects:	Tachycardia, increased ventricular ectopy, nausea, vomiting, headaches, seizures, insomnia, and nightmares
Dose:	Loading dose of 6 mg/kg IV, followed by maintenance infusion of 0.5 to 0.7 mg/kg/hour. Use 0.5 loading dose if the patient is already taking theophylline.
Notes:	May follow plasma level, but patient side effects generally limit therapeutic usefulness. Decrease the dose in patients with congestive heart failure (CHF), liver disease and elderly patients.
	Aminophylline clearance is decreased by erythromycin, cimetidine, propranolol,

allopurinol, and a number of other medications.

AMIODARONE

Therapeutic class:	Antiarrhythmic
Indications:	Ventricular tachycardia
Actions:	The initial acute effects are predominantly due to an AV intranodal conduction delay and an increase in nodal refractoriness secondary to calcium channel blockade
Side effects:	Hypotension, bradycardia due to excess AV block, cardiac arrest, cardiogenic shock
Dose:	150 mg bolus in 100 mL 5% dextrose over 10 minutes, with a maintenance IV infusion of 540 mg over 18 hours (0.5 mg/minute)
Notes:	Use with extreme caution in patients known to be predisposed to bradycardia or AV block.

AMOXICILLIN (SEE ANTIBIOTIC LISTING IN APPENDIX E)

AMPHOTERICIN B

Proprietary name(s):	Fungizone
Therapeutic class:	Polyene antifungal
Indications:	Systemic fungal infections
Actions:	Disruption of fungal cell membrane
Excretion:	Renal
Side effects:	Fever, chills, nausea, vomiting, diarrhea, hypotension, nephrotoxicity, hypokalemia, hypomagnesemia, and thrombophlebitis
Dose:	Initial test dose: 0.1 mg/kg in 100 mL 50% dextrose in water IV over 2 hours
	If tolerated, further doses of 10 mg may be given on the first day.
	Daily dose then may be increased by 0.25 mg/kg/day until the desired dose of 0.5 to 1 mg/kg/day is achieved. Administer IV over 4 to 6 hours.

It is more important to administer a complete total course than it is to achieve the desirable daily dose. If the patient does not tolerate that high a concentration, simply lower the daily dose and extend the length of therapy.

Notes: Patients vary with respect to how well they tolerate amphotericin B therapy. Premedicate before each dose with antipyretics, antihistamines, antiemetics, and corticosteroids to reduce side effects. Follow serial potassium and magnesium levels during therapy and watch for renal insufficiency.

Liposomal-conjugated amphotericin B (Abelcet) may be given in doses of 5 mg/kg/day.

AMPICILLIN (SEE ANTIBIOTIC LISTING IN APPENDIX E)

ASPIRIN (ACETYLSALICYLIC ACID)

Therapeutic class: Analgesic, antipyretic, and anti-inflammatory

Indications: Pain due to inflammation, fever, and antiplatelet aggregation agent in coronary syndromes

Actions: Acts peripherally by interfering with the production of prostaglandins, thus reducing pain and inflammation

Acts centrally to reduce pain perception and reduce temperature by increasing heat loss

Side effects: Gastric erosion and bleeding, tinnitus, fever, thirst, and diaphoresis

Severe allergic reactions can occur, including asthma-like symptoms.

Dose: For mild pain or fever, 325 to 650 mg PO every 4 to 6 hours

For chest pain due to pericarditis, 650 mg PO 4 times per day

For angina and antiplatelet effects, 30 to 325 mg PO every day or every other day

For treatment of rheumatoid arthritis, 2.6 to 5.2 g/day in divided doses

AZTREONAM (SEE ANTIBIOTIC LISTING IN APPENDIX E)

BECLOMETHASONE

Proprietary name(s):	Beclovent and Vanceril
Therapeutic class:	Inhaled corticosteroid
Indications:	Bronchial asthma and long-term therapy
Actions:	Topical anti-inflammatory
Excretion:	Fecal
Side effects:	Oral and pharyngeal candidiasis, laryngeal myopathy
Dose:	2 inhalations 2 to 4 times per day. May be more effective if administered 3 to 5 minutes after a bronchodilator dose.
Notes:	Not indicated for acute bronchospasm.

BISACODYL

Proprietary name(s):	Dulcolax
Therapeutic class:	Laxative
Indications:	Constipation
Action:	Stimulates peristalsis
Metabolism:	Poorly absorbed
Side effects:	Abdominal cramping, nausea, rectal burning or bleeding
Dose:	10 to 15 mg PO every night, as needed
	10-mg suppository PR every night, as needed
Notes:	Avoid in pregnancy or after a myocardial infarction (MI). May worsen orthostatic hypotension, weakness, and incoordination in elderly patients.
	Avoid in acute abdomen, intestinal obstruction, or with recent intestinal anastomoses.
	Onset of action is 6 to 10 hours after PO dose, 15 to 60 minutes after a PR dose.

BUMETANIDE

Proprietary name(s):	Bumex
Therapeutic class:	Loop diuretic; rapid onset, short duration of action

Indications: Edema associated with CHF, cirrhosis, renal disease, or nephrotic syndrome

Actions: Inhibits the reabsorption of Na^+ and Cl^- in the ascending limb of the loop of Henle. Increases potassium excretion.

Excretion: Renal (80%)

Side effects: Electrolyte depletion, rash, hyperuricemia, and reversible deafness

Dose: 0.5 to 2 mg PO/IV per day in a single dose

                        May repeat every 20 minutes, if necessary, to a maximum of 3 mg.

Notes: 1 mg bumetanide is equivalent to 40 mg furosemide.

CALCIUM GLUCONATE

Therapeutic class: Calcium supplement

Indications: Symptomatic hypocalcemia and hyperkalemia. Adjunct therapy in cardiopulmonary resuscitation (CPR)

Actions: Replacement. Decreases cardiac automaticity and raises cardiac cell resting potential.

Side effects: Administration to patients concurrently on digoxin therapy may precipitate ventricular dysrhythmias due to combined effects of digoxin and Ca^{2+}.

Dose: For control of hypocalcemia, 1 to 15 g PO every day

                        For more rapid response, 5 to 10 mL of 10% solution IV

Notes: 500 mg of calcium gluconate = 2.3 mmol ionized Ca^{2+}.

                        10% solution contains 0.45 mmol ionized Ca^{2+}/mL.

CAPTOPRIL

Proprietary name(s):   Capoten

Therapeutic class: Angiotensin-converting enzyme (ACE) inhibitor

Indications: Hypertension, CHF, and prophylaxis against diabetic nephropathy

Actions: Inhibits the enzyme responsible for pulmonary conversion of angiotensin I to angiotensin II

Excretion:	Renal (59%)
Side effects:	Hypotension, impaired taste, cough, rash, angioedema, neutropenia, proteinuria, and renal insufficiency
Dose:	Begin with a test dose of 6.25 mg PO and monitor blood pressure (BP) for 4 hours.
	For hypertension, titrate to 25 to 50 mg PO 2 to 3 times per day
	For CHF, titrate to 25 to 50 mg PO 3 times per day
Notes:	May cause hyperkalemia if used in patients receiving potassium-sparing diuretics or receiving potassium supplementation.

CEFAZOLIN (SEE ANTIBIOTIC LISTING IN APPENDIX E)

CEFOTAXIME (SEE ANTIBIOTIC LISTING IN APPENDIX E)

CEFOXITIN (SEE ANTIBIOTIC LISTING IN APPENDIX E)

CEFTAZIDIME (SEE ANTIBIOTIC LISTING IN APPENDIX E)

CEFTRIAXONE (SEE ANTIBIOTIC LISTING IN APPENDIX E)

CEFUROXIME (SEE ANTIBIOTIC LISTING IN APPENDIX E)

CELECOXIB

Proprietary name(s):	Celebrex
Therapeutic class:	Selective COX-2 inhibitor
Indications:	Osteoarthritis, rheumatoid arthritis, familial adenomatous polyposis
Actions:	Inhibition of prostaglandin production via inhibition of cyclooxygenase-2
Metabolism:	Cytochrome P450 2C9
Excretion:	Hepatic metabolism
Side effects:	Rare, hepatic dysfunction, fluid retention, edema, GI bleeding

Dose: For arthritis pain relief, 100 to 200 mg PO two times per day

For familial adenomatous polyposis, 400 mg PO two times per day.

Notes: Not recommended in patients who have aspirin allergy. Not recommended in patients with sulfa allergy. Less GI upset reported than with nonselective NSAIDs. Probable adverse cardiovascular effects.

CHLORAL HYDRATE

Therapeutic class:	Alcohol hypnotic
Indications:	Insomnia
Actions:	Hypnotic
Side effects:	Gastric irritation, rash, paradoxical agitation
Dose:	0.5 to 1 g PO/PR every night, as needed
Notes:	Avoid in patients with liver or kidney disease.

CHLORDIAZEPOXIDE

Proprietary name(s):	Librium and others
Therapeutic class:	Benzodiazepine
Indications:	Anxiety and alcohol withdrawal
Actions:	Benzodiazepine sedative and anxiolytic agent
Metabolism:	Hepatic
Excretion:	Renal
Side effects:	Central nervous system (CNS) depression, drowsiness, ataxia, confusion, and pruritic rash
Dose:	For anxiety, 5 to 25 mg PO 3 to 4 times per day
	For alcohol withdrawal, 50 to 100 mg intramuscularly (IM)/IV every 2 to 6 hours as needed, maximum dose of 500 mg in the first 24 hours
Notes:	Dose must be individualized.
	Unpredictable absorption after IM injection.
	Antidote is flumazenil.

CHLORPROMAZINE

Proprietary name(s): Thorazine
Therapeutic class: Phenothiazine antipsychotic and anti-emetic
Indications: Agitation, nausea, vomiting, and hiccoughs
Actions: Antagonist of dopamine, histamine, muscarine, and α1-adrenergic responses
Side effects: CNS depression, hypotension, extrapyramidal effects, and jaundice
Dose: For mild agitation, 25 to 75 mg PO every day
For more severe cases, 150 mg PO or every day 25 to 50 mg IM with repeated doses every 3 to 4 hours, as needed
For hiccoughs, nausea, and vomiting, 10 to 15 mg PO/IM every 6 to 8 hours
Notes: For acute agitation, haloperidol may be a more appropriate choice as it has less effect on BP.

CHLORPROPAMIDE

Proprietary name(s): Diabinese and others
Therapeutic class: Oral hypoglycemic agent
Indications: Noninsulin-dependent diabetes mellitus (NIDDM)
Actions: Sulfonylurea. Stimulates insulin secretion and increases the effects of insulin on the liver to increase gluconeogenesis and on the muscle to increase glucose use.
Metabolism: Renal excretion
Side effects: Hypoglycemia, rash, blood dyscrasias, jaundice, hyponatremia, and edema
Dose: 100 to 500 mg PO every day in 1 or 2 doses
Notes: Has a long duration of action (20 to 60 hours). Hypoglycemic reactions may be prolonged in elderly patients and in those patients with renal impairment.
Drug associations causing hypoglycemia: NSAIDs, salicylates, sulfonamides, chloramphenicol, cimetidine, ranitidine, probenecid, warfarin, monoamine oxi-

dase (MAO) inhibitors, β-blockers, and metformin.

Drug associations causing hyperglycemia: Thiazides, diuretics, corticosteroids, phenothiazines, thyroid hormone replacement agents, oral contraceptive agents, phenytoin, sympathomimetics, calcium channel blockers, and isoniazid.

CIMETIDINE

Proprietary name(s):	Tagamet
Therapeutic class:	Histamine-2 antagonist
Indications:	Peptic ulcer disease and gastroesophageal reflux
Actions:	Inhibits histamine-induced secretion of gastric acid
Metabolism:	Hepatic
Excretion:	Renal
Side effects:	Gynecomastia, impotence, confusion, diarrhea, leukopenia, thrombocytopenia, and increased serum creatinine
Dose:	For peptic ulcer, 300 mg PO or IV every 6 to 8 hours, or 800 mg PO every night For reflux, 400 mg PO 2 times per day
Notes:	Reduces, microsomal enzyme metabolism of medications, including oral anticoagulants, phenytoin, and theophylline.

CIPROFLOXACIN (SEE ANTIBIOTIC LISTING IN APPENDIX E)

CLINDAMYCIN (SEE ANTIBIOTIC LISTING IN APPENDIX E)

CLOPIDOGREL

Proprietary name(s):	Plavix
Therapeutic class:	ADP-binding agent, inhibits platelet aggregation
Indications:	Atherosclerotic disease
Actions:	Inhibition of ADP-dependent platelet aggregation
Metabolism:	Hepatic

Excretion:	50% urine, 46% stool
Side effects:	Rare, GI bleeding, neutropenia, rash
Dose:	75 mg PO each day
Notes:	Risks of bleeding are similar to aspirin.

CODEINE

Therapeutic class:	Narcotic analgesic
Indications:	Pain, cough, and diarrhea
Actions:	Narcotic analgesic, depresses the medullary cough center, and decreases propulsive contractions of the small bowel
Metabolism:	Hepatic
Excretion:	Renal (90%)
Side effects:	Dysphoria, agitation, pruritus, constipation, lightheadedness, and sedation
Dose:	For analgesia, 30 to 60 mg PO/subcutaneously (SC)/IM every 4 to 6 hours, as needed
	For cough or diarrhea, 8 to 30 mg PO/SC/IM every 4 hours, as needed
Notes:	Useful for mild to moderate pain. May be habit forming.

CLOTRIMAZOLE

Proprietary name(s):	Lotrimin and Mycelex
Therapeutic class:	Antifungal
Indications:	Esophageal, vaginal, and intertrigonal candidiasis
Actions:	Damages fungal cell membranes
Side effects:	Local irritation
Dose:	For esophageal candidiasis, 10-mg troche PO 4 times per day
	For vaginal candidiasis, 100 mg intravaginally every night × 7 nights
	For intertrigonal candidiasis, 1% cream or solution applied 2 times per day

DIAZEPAM

Proprietary name(s):	Valium and others
Therapeutic class:	Enzodiazepine
Indications:	Anxiety, seizures, and alcohol withdrawal
Actions:	Benzodiazepine sedative and anxiolytic agent

Metabolism:	Hepatic (to active metabolites)
Excretion:	Renal
Side effects:	Sedation, hypotension, respiratory depression, and paradoxical agitation
Dose:	For anxiety, 2 to 10 mg PO/IM/IV 2 to 4 times per day
	For status epilepticus, 2 mg/minute IV until the seizure ceases or to a total dose of 20 mg
	For alcohol withdrawal, 5 to 10 mg IV at a rate of 2 to 5 mg/minute every 30 to 60 minute until the patient is sedated, then maintain on 10 to 20 mg PO 4 times per day
Notes:	Dose must be individualized.
	Unpredictable absorption after IM injection.
	Rectal and endotracheal tube (ET) administration possible in emergency situations.
	Antidote is flumazenil.

DIGOXIN

Proprietary name(s):	Lanoxin
Therapeutic class:	Digitalis glycoside
Indications:	Supraventricular tachycardia and CHF
Actions:	Slows atrioventricular (AV) conduction, increases the force of cardiac contraction, and Na^+/K^+-ATPase inhibitor
Metabolism:	Hepatic (<10%)
Excretion:	Renal (80%)
Side effects:	Dysrhythmias, nausea, vomiting, and neuropsychiatric disturbances
Dose:	Load with 0.125 to 0.5 mg IV every 6 hours to a total dose of 1 mg, or load with 0.125 to 0.5 mg PO every 6 hours to a total dose of 1.5 mg, then maintain on 0.125 to 0.25 mg PO/IV every day.
	Some supraventricular tachycardias may require higher doses.
Notes:	Reduce dose in elderly patients and in those patients with renal impairment. May cause arrhythmias in settings of hypokalemia or hypercalcemia.

DILTIAZEM

Proprietary name(s):	Cardizem
Therapeutic class:	Calcium channel blocker
Indications:	Angina pectoris, coronary spasm, and hypertension
Actions:	Calcium channel blocker and vasodilator
Metabolism:	Hepatic
Excretion:	Renal and biliary
Side effects:	First-degree AV block, bradycardia, flushing, dizziness, headache, peripheral edema, nausea, rash, and asthenia
Dose:	Initial dose, 30 mg PO 3 to 4 times per day, with titration to 180 to 360 mg/day administered in divided doses.
Notes:	Maximum antihypertensive effect is seen at 14 days. Sustained release forms are available.

DIPHENHYDRAMINE

Proprietary name(s):	Benadryl
Therapeutic class:	Antihistamine
Indications:	Allergic reactions
Actions:	Antihistamine and anticholinergic
Metabolism:	Hepatic
Excretion:	Renal
Side effects:	Drowsiness, dizziness, dry mouth, and urinary retention
Dose:	25 to 50 mg PO/IV/IM every 6 to 8 hours, as needed
Notes:	Anticholinergic effects may be additive to those noted with other medications such as tricyclic antidepressants.

DIPHENOXYLATE HCl WITH ATROPINE

Proprietary name(s):	Lomotil
Therapeutic class:	Antidiarrheal
Indications:	Control of noninfectious diarrheal symptoms
Actions:	Direct inhibition of GI peristalsis.
Side effects:	Abdominal cramping, distention, dry mouth, toxic megacolon
Dose:	2 tablets PO every 6 hours to control initial symptoms, decrease to 1 tablet every 12 hours for maintenance dose.
Notes:	Onset is in 1 to 2 hours.

DOCUSATE

Proprietary name(s):	Colace and Dialose
Therapeutic class:	Laxative
Indications:	Prevention of constipation
Actions:	Stool softener and lowers surface tension
Side effects:	Nausea and bitter taste
Dose:	100 mg PO 3 times per day
Notes:	Effects not immediate; may not be noticeable for 1 to 2 days.

DOLASETRON

Proprietary name(s):	Anzemet
Therapeutic class:	Antiemetic
Indications:	Prophylaxis and treatment of postoperative nausea and vomiting, and treatment of nausea associated with chemotherapy
Actions:	Selective serotonin 5-HT3 receptor antagonist
Metabolism:	To active metabolite hydrodolasetron
Excretion:	Renal (66%), stool (33%)
Side effects:	Headache, dizziness, hypotension
Dose:	12.5 mg IV, as needed
	Oral dose: 100 mg PO, as needed
Notes:	Use with caution in patients with prolonged cardiac intervals, especially QTc. Use with caution in patients with electrolyte abnormalities.

ENALAPRIL

Proprietary name(s):	Vasotec
Therapeutic class:	ACE inhibitor
Indications:	Hypertension and CHF
Actions:	Inhibits the enzyme responsible for conversion of angiotensin I to angiotensin II
Metabolism:	Hepatic (to active metabolite enalaprilat)
Excretion:	Renal
Side effects:	Hypotension, headache, nausea, and diarrhea
Dose:	Begin with a test dose of 2.5 mg PO and monitor BP for 4 hours. For hypertension, titrate to 2.5 to 40 mg PO every day For CHF, titrate to 10 to 40 mg PO every day

Notes: May cause hyperkalemia if used in patients receiving potassium-sparing diuretics or receiving potassium supplementation.

ERYTHROMYCIN (SEE ANTIBIOTIC LISTING IN APPENDIX E)

ETHACRYNIC ACID

Proprietary name(s):	Edecrin
Therapeutic class:	Loop diuretic
Indications:	CHF and edema
Actions:	Inhibition of the reabsorption of Na^+ and Cl^- in the ascending limb of the loop of Henle
Side effects:	Electrolyte depletion, hyperuricemia, hyperglycemia, anorexia, nausea, vomiting, diarrhea, and sensorineural hearing loss
Dose:	50 mg IV X 1 or 2 doses
Notes:	May have more side effects than other loop diuretics.
	Onset is rapid, within 30 minutes of a PO dose or within 5 minutes of an IV dose.

FAMOTIDINE

Proprietary name(s):	Pepcid
Therapeutic class:	Histamine-2 antagonist
Indications:	Peptic ulcer disease and gastroesophageal reflux
Actions:	Inhibits histamine-induced secretion of gastric acid
Metabolism:	Hepatic (to inactive metabolite)
Excretion:	Renal (70%)
Side effects:	Headache, dizziness, constipation, diarrhea, GI upset, and rash
Dose:	For acute disease, 40 mg PO every day or 20 mg IV 2 times per day
	For maintenance, 20 mg PO every night.
Notes:	Less affect on microsomal enzymes or androgen blocking than cimetidine.

FERROUS SULFATE

Therapeutic class:	Iron supplement
Indications:	Iron deficiency
Actions:	Replaces iron stores
Side effects:	Constipation, nausea, diarrhea, and abdominal cramping
Dose:	325 mg PO 3 times per day
Notes:	300 mg ferrous sulfate = 60 mg elemental iron.
	Stool may turn black.
	GI absorption enhanced on an empty stomach with concomitant vitamin C administration (200 mg vitamin C/30 mg iron).
	Iron stores will not be completely replaced for up to 4 to 6 months of therapy after normalization of the hematocrit.

FLUCONAZOLE

Proprietary name(s):	Diflucan
Therapeutic class:	Antifungal
Indications:	Oropharyngeal, esophageal, and systemic candidiasis; cryptococcal meningitis
Actions:	Inhibition of cell membranes of yeasts and fungi
Excretion:	Renal
Side effects:	Nausea, vomiting, headache, rash, abdominal pain, diarrhea, and hepatic necrosis
Dose:	For oral or esophageal disease, initial dose of 200 mg PO followed by 100 mg PO every day
	For systemic candidiasis and cryptococcal meningitis, 200 to 400 mg PO every day.
	Reduce the dose in those patients with renal impairment.
Notes:	Many drug interactions due to the microsomal enzyme inhibition, including sulfonylureas, phenytoin, warfarin, and cyclophosphamide.

FLUMAZENIL

Proprietary name(s):	Romazicon
Therapeutic class:	Benzodiazepine antagonist
Indications:	Reversal of benzodiazepine-induced sedation
Actions:	Benzodiazepine receptor antagonist
Metabolism:	Hepatic
Excretion:	Renal
Side effects:	Seizures, headache, vasodilation, nausea, vomiting, agitation, dizziness, abnormal vision, and paresthesias
Dose:	For reversal of sedation, 0.2 mg IV over 15 seconds
	Repeat as necessary in increments of 0.2 mg every 60 seconds, to a maximum dose of 1 mg.
	For treatment of benzodiazepine overdose, 0.2 mg IV over 30 seconds
	An additional 0.3 mg IV may be administered after 30 seconds, if necessary. Further doses of 0.5 mg may be given IV every 30 seconds, as needed, to a maximum of 3 mg.
Notes:	Avoid in patients with evidence of cyclic antidepressant overdose.
	Does not reverse benzodiazepine-induced respiratory depression.
	Monitor for return of benzodiazepine-related symptoms of sedation and respiratory depression.

FUROSEMIDE

Proprietary name(s):	Lasix
Therapeutic class:	Loop diuretic
Indications:	CHF, edema, hyperkalemia, and hypercalcemia
Actions:	Inhibition of the reabsorption of Na^+ and Cl^- in the ascending limb of the loop of Henle
Metabolism:	Hepatic
Excretion:	Renal
Side effects:	Electrolyte depletion, hyperuricemia, hyperglycemia, and reversible deafness
Dose:	For acute pulmonary edema, 20 to 40 mg PO/IV with repeat doses every 60 to

90 minutes, as needed, to a maximum of 600 mg/day

Higher doses may be required in patients with severe disease or renal failure.

Notes: Loop diuretics are well absorbed orally with rapid onset of action.

GENTAMICIN (SEE ANTIBIOTIC LISTING IN APPENDIX E)

HALOPERIDOL

Proprietary name(s):	Haldol
Therapeutic class:	Antipsychotic
Indications:	Psychotic disorders and acute agitation
Actions:	Antipsychotic neuroleptic butyrophenone
Side effects:	Extrapyramidal reactions, postural hypotension, sedation, galactorrhea, jaundice, blurred vision, bronchospasm, and neuroleptic malignant syndrome
Dose:	0.5 to 2 mg PO 3 times per day
	For acute psychotic crises, 2 to 10 mg IM every 1 hour, as needed
Notes:	Extrapyramidal side effects are more pronounced, but hypotension is less frequent than with phenothiazines.

HEPARIN SODIUM

Therapeutic class:	Anticoagulant
Indications:	Prophylaxis and treatment of DVT, pulmonary embolism, embolic cerebrovascular accident (CVA). Adjunct in treatment of unstable angina, and thrombolytic therapy.
Actions:	Acts in conjunction with antithrombin III, which neutralizes several activated clotting factors. Antithrombin effect.
Metabolism:	Hepatic
Excretion:	Renal
Side effects:	Hemorrhage and thrombocytopenia
Dose:	For DVT or pulmonary embolus, load IV with 5000 to 10,000 U followed by continuous infusion of 1000 to 2000 U/hour IV

Low-dose SC: 5000 U every 8 to 12 hours

High-dose SC: 10,000 to 12,500 U every 8 to 12 hours.

Titrate to desired partial thromboplastin time (PTT) (generally 1.5 to 2 X control).

Notes: Monitor PTT closely. Also prolongs prothrombin time (PT).

Overheparinization is treated with protamine sulfate. Usual dose is 1 mg protamine/100 U heparin given slowly IV.

HYDRALAZINE

Proprietary name(s):	Apresoline
Therapeutic class:	Arterial vasodilator
Indications:	Hypertension
Actions:	Arterial vasodilator
Metabolism:	Hepatic
Side effects:	Tachycardia, headache, blood dyscrasias, nausea, vomiting, diarrhea, systemic lupus erythematosus (SLE) reaction at higher doses (>200 mg/day)
Dose:	10 to 25 mg PO every 6 hours
	20 to 40 mg IV/IM every 3 to 6 hours, as needed
Notes:	Very limited effect on veins, so minimal postural hypotension.
	Monitor carefully in patients with coronary artery disease.

HYDROCHLOROTHIAZIDE

Proprietary name(s):	Esidrix and HydroDIURIL
Therapeutic class:	Thiazide diuretic
Indications:	Hypertension, CHF, and edema
Actions:	Blocks Na^+ and Cl^- reabsorption in the cortical diluting segment of the loop of Henle
Excretion:	Renal
Side effects:	Electrolyte depletion, hyperuricemia, hyperglycemia, hypercalcemia, pancreatitis, jaundice, nausea, vomiting, and diarrhea
Dose:	12.5 to 50 mg PO every day

Notes: Adequate potassium replacement necessary with long-term therapy

HYDROCORTISONE

Therapeutic class: Corticosteroid
Indications: Severe bronchospasm, anaphylaxis, hypercalcemia, and adrenal insufficiency
Actions: Anti-inflammatory
Side effects: Na^+ retention, hyperglycemia, K^+ loss, and behavioral disturbances
Dose: 250 mg IV followed by 100 mg IV every 6 hours.
Notes: Contraindicated in settings of systemic fungal infections.

HYDROXYZINE

Proprietary name(s):   Atarax and Vistaril
Therapeutic class: Antihistamine and antiemetic
Indications: Anxiety, pruritus, nausea, and vomiting
Actions: Suppression of activity in subcortical CNS sites
Metabolism: Hepatic
Side effects: Drowsiness, dry mouth, and tremor
Dose: For anxiety, 50 to 100 mg PO/IM 4 times per day
For pruritus or nausea, 25 to 100 mg PO/IM 3 to 4 times per day
Notes: May potentiate the sedation effects of other CNS depressants.

IBUPROFEN

Proprietary name(s):   Motrin and others
Therapeutic class: NSAID
Indications: Inflammation due to arthritis, soft-tissue injuries, and analgesia
Actions: Propionic acid derivative. Interferes with the production of prostaglandins.
Metabolism: Hepatic
Excretion: Renal
Side effects: Nausea, diarrhea, gastric pain, gastric erosions, dizziness, headache, tinnitus, and vision changes. May compromise

renal function in patients with renal impairment. Contraindicated in the syndrome of aspirin sensitivity, nasal polyps, and bronchospasm.

Dose:	For analgesia, 200 mg PO 3 to 4 times per day
	For anti-inflammatory effects, 200 to 400 mg PO 3 to 4 times per day
	Maximum dose: 3200 mg/day
Notes:	Available in many over-the-counter preparations.
	Should be used with caution in patients receiving anticoagulant medications.

IMIPENEM/CILASTIN (SEE ANTIBIOTIC LISTING IN APPENDIX E)

INDOMETHACIN

Proprietary name(s):	Indocin
Therapeutic class:	NSAID
Indications:	Inflammation due to arthritis, acute gout, soft-tissue injury, and pericarditis
Actions:	Indole acetic acid derivative. Interferes with the production of prostaglandins.
Metabolism:	Hepatic
Excretion:	Renal
Side effects:	Headache, dizziness and lightheadedness, and epigastric pain. May compromise renal function in patients with renal impairment.
	Contraindicated in the syndrome of aspirin sensitivity, nasal polyps, and bronchospasm.
Dose:	25 to 50 mg PO 3 times per day. Maximum daily dose: 150 to 200 mg/day
Notes:	May increase the risk of bleeding in patients receiving anticoagulants.
	Take with food to minimize GI upset.

INSULIN

Therapeutic class:	Hypoglycemic
Indications:	Diabetes mellitus
Actions:	Enhances hepatic glycogen storage, enhances entry of glucose and potas-

sium into cells, and inhibits the breakdown of protein and fat

Side effects:	Hypoglycemia, local skin reactions, and lipohypertrophy
Dose:	Must be individualized. See Chapter 14.
Notes:	Less immunogenicity is seen with recombinant human insulin than with insulins from animal sources.

ISOSORBIDE DINITRATE

Proprietary name(s):	Isordil and Sorbitrate
Therapeutic class:	Vasodilator
Indications:	Angina pectoris and CHF
Actions:	Venous, coronary, and arterial vasodilator
Side effects:	Headache, hypotension, and flushing
Dose:	5 to 30 mg PO 4 times per day
Notes:	Nitrate tolerance may develop with prolonged continuous administration.

KETOCONAZOLE

Proprietary name(s):	Nizoral
Therapeutic class:	Imidazole antifungal
Indications:	Esophageal candidiasis, pulmonary histoplasmosis
Actions:	Inhibition of yeast and fungal cell growth
Metabolism:	Hepatic
Excretion:	Biliary (>80%)
Side effects:	Nausea, anorexia, vomiting, rash, pruritus, gynecomastia, and impotence. Inhibits microsomal enzymes, so may interfere with the metabolism of warfarin, cyclophosphamide, and other medications.
Dose:	200 to 400 mg PO every day
Notes:	Absorption is impaired in patients receiving medications that reduce gastric acidity.

LABETALOL

Proprietary name(s):	Normodyne and Trandate
Therapeutic class:	α_1- and β-blocker
Indications:	Hypertensive emergencies

Actions:	α_1-Blocking action is predominant in acute use but is accompanied by non-specific β-blockade
Metabolism:	Hepatic
Excretion:	Renal
Side effects:	Postural hypotension, bronchospasm, jaundice, bradycardia, and negative inotropic effect. Avoid in patients with asthma or with severe bradycardia.
Dose:	20 mg IV every 10 to 15 minutes
	Increase the dose incrementally (e.g., 20 mg, 20 mg, 40 mg, 40 mg, . . .) every 10 minutes until the desired supine BP is achieved.
	Alternatively, a continuous drip may be started at 2 mg/minute with titration to desired BP response, with a maximum daily dose of 2400 mg.
Notes:	Contraindicated in patients in whom β-blockade is undesirable.

LEVODOPA-CARBIDOPA

Proprietary name(s):	Sinemet
Therapeutic class:	Dopamine agonist
Indications:	Parkinson's disease
Actions:	Levodopa is converted to dopamine in the basal ganglia.
	Carbidopa inhibits the peripheral destruction of levodopa.
Side effects:	Anorexia, nausea, vomiting, abdominal pain, dysrhythmias, behavioral changes, orthostatic hypotension, and involuntary motions
Dose:	Begin with 1 tablet (100 mg/10 mg) PO 2 times per day
	Increase the dose until the desired response is obtained, with a maximum daily dose of 8 tablets (800 mg/8 mg).
Notes:	Side effects are common.

LEVOFLOXACIN (SEE ANTIBIOTIC LISTING IN APPENDIX E)

LIDOCAINE

Proprietary name(s):	Xylocaine
Therapeutic class:	Class IB antiarrhythmic

Indications: Ventricular arrhythmias, prophylaxis, and treatment

Actions: Lengthens the effective refractory period in the ventricular conduction system. Decreases ventricular automaticity.

Metabolism: Hepatic

Excretion: Renal

Side effects: Nausea, vomiting, hypotension, confusion, seizures, perioral paresthesias, drowsiness, and dizziness

Dose: Load with 1 mg/kg IV over 2 to 3 minutes. Further doses of 50 mg IV may be given at 5- to 10-minute intervals to a total dose of 300 mg.

Maintain with 1 to 4 mg/minute continuous IV infusion.

For prophylaxis, a loading dose of 200 mg given in 50-mg increments every 5 minutes, followed by maintenance IV infusion of 3 mg/minute

Notes: Lower maintenance doses are required in elderly patients or in those with CHF, hepatic failure, or hypotension.

LISINOPRIL

Proprietary name(s):   Zestril, Prinivil

Therapeutic class: ACE inhibitor

Indications: Hypertension and CHF

Actions: Inhibits the enzyme responsible for conversion of angiotensin I to angiotensin II

Side effects: Hypotension, headache, nausea, and diarrhea

Dose: Begin with a test dose of 2.5 mg PO and monitor BP for 4 hours.

For hypertension, titrate to 2.5 to 20 mg PO every day.

For CHF, titrate to 5 to 20 mg PO every day

Notes: May cause hyperkalemia if used in patients receiving potassium-sparing diuretics or receiving potassium supplementation.

LOPERIMIDE

Proprietary name(s):   Imodium

Therapeutic class: Antidiarrheal

Indications:	Control of noninfectious diarrheal symptoms
Actions:	Direct inhibition of GI peristalsis.
Side effects:	Abdominal cramping, distention, dry mouth, toxic megacolon in ulcerative colitis
Dose:	4 mg PO every 4 hours up to a maximum of 16 mg in 24 hours
Notes:	Onset is in 2 to 4 hours. Less effective if given on a PRN basis.

LORAZEPAM

Proprietary name(s):	Ativan
Therapeutic class:	Benzodiazepine
Indications:	Insomnia and anxiety
Actions:	Benzodiazepine sedative-hypnotic
Metabolism:	Hepatic
Excretion:	Renal
Side effects:	Sedation and respiratory depression
Dose:	For sleep, 0.5 to 1 mg PO/IM every night. For anxiety, 1 mg PO/IM 2 times per day. Maximum dose: 4 mg/dose
Notes:	Peak effect in 1 to 6 hours. Antidote is flumazenil.

MANNITOL

Proprietary name(s):	Osmitrol
Therapeutic class:	Osmotic diuretic
Indications:	Peripheral edema, cerebral edema, and hemolytic transfusion reactions
Actions:	Osmotic diuresis
Excretion:	Renal
Side effects:	Volume overload, hyperosmolality, hyponatremia, nausea, and headache
Dose:	Test dose of 12.5 g over 3 to 5 minutes. Effects should be noted within 2 hours. 25 to 100 g IV over 15 to 30 minutes every 2 to 3 hours, as needed
Notes:	Requires functioning kidneys to work, contraindicated in renal failure. Monitor electrolytes.

MEPERIDINE

Proprietary name(s):	Demerol
Therapeutic class:	Narcotic analgesic

Indications:	Moderate to severe pain
Actions:	Narcotic analgesic
Metabolism:	Hepatic
Excretion:	Renal
Side effects:	Respiratory depression, hypotension, nausea, vomiting, constipation, agitation, and rash
Dose:	50 to 150 mg SC/IM/PO every 4 hours
Notes:	60 to 80 mg meperidine (SC/IM/PO) is equivalent to 10 mg morphine (SC/IV). Often administered with concomitant antinausea medication.
	Antidote is naloxone.
	May be habit forming.

MESALAMINE

Proprietary name(s):	Asacol, Pentasa
Therapeutic class:	Delayed release sulfasalazine, anti-inflammatory
Indications:	Inflammatory bowel disease
Actions:	Luminal anti-inflammatory, inhibition of prostaglandin synthesis
Metabolism:	Acetylated by gut mucosa
Excretion:	72% Stool (not absorbed), 28% kidney
Side effects:	Mild headache, GI upset, diarrhea, asthenia
Dose:	400 to 800 mg PO three time per day
Notes:	May cause aberrations in liver function tests.

METAPROTERENOL

Proprietary name(s):	Alupent
Therapeutic class:	β_2-Adrenergic agonist
Indications:	Bronchospasm due to asthma, bronchitis, or COPD
Actions:	β_2-Adrenergic agonist
Metabolism:	Hepatic. 3% of aerosol dose is systemically absorbed.
Side effects:	Headache, tachycardia, hypertension, lightheadedness, dizziness, tremor, palpitations, nausea, and vomiting
Dose:	0.2 to 0.3 mg in 3 mL NS by nebulizer every 4 hours, as needed
	Severe acute bronchospasm may require doses every 3 to 5 minutes initially.
Notes:	May alternate with albuterol.

METFORMIN

Proprietary name(s):	Glucophage
Therapeutic class:	Antihyperglycemic agent
Indications:	NIDDM as monotherapy or in conjunction with sulfonylureas
Actions:	Decreases hepatic glucose production, decreases intestinal absorption of glucose, and increases peripheral glucose uptake and utilization
Excretion:	Renal
Side effects:	Lactic acidosis, diarrhea, nausea, vomiting, abdominal bloating, flatulence, and anorexia
Dose:	Dose must be individualized.
	Start with 500 mg PO 2 times per day and increase to desired blood glucose effect, to a maximum daily dose of 2500 mg.
	Decrease dose in renal failure.
Notes:	Hypoglycemic reactions are not seen as with sulfonylureas.

METOCLOPRAMIDE

Proprietary names(s):	Reglan, Maxeran
Therapeutic class:	Antinausea agent
Indications:	Nausea, poor gastric motility
Actions:	Stimulates upper GI motility, increases gastric emptying. Increases lower esophageal sphincter tone.
Side effects:	Drowsiness, lethargy, tartive dyskinesia (rare)
Dose:	5 to 10 mg PO or 25 mg IM or IV every 4 to 6 hours PRN
Notes:	Reduce dosage with renal or hepatic impairment.

METOLAZONE

Proprietary name(s):	Zaroxolyn
Therapeutic class:	Quinazoline diuretic
Indications:	Hypertension, CHF, edema, and some types of renal failure
Actions:	Blocks Na^+ and Cl^+ reabsorption in the cortical diluting segment of the loop of Henle

Excretion:	Renal
Side effects:	Electrolyte depletion, hyperuricemia, hyperglycemia, and hypomagnesemia. Do not use in anuric patients.
Dose:	2.5 to 10 mg PO every day
Notes:	Similar properties to thiazide diuretics but longer acting than hydrochlorothiazide. Monitor electrolytes.
	Additive effects when administered with furosemide.

MEROPENEM (SEE ANTIBIOTIC LISTING IN APPENDIX E)

METOPROLOL

Proprietary name(s):	Lopressor, Betaloc
Therapeutic class:	Cardioselective beta-blocker
Indications:	Angina pectoris, post-MI, treatment of supraventricular tachycardia (SVT), hypertension, migraine and thyrotoxicosis
Metabolism:	Hepatic
Excretion:	Renal (<1%)
Side effects:	Fatigue, depression, confusion, nightmares, GI upset, headache, visual disturbances, hypotension, AV block, bronchospasm
Dose:	Hypertension, angina, post-MI or migraine prophylaxis: 50 to 200 mg PO BID
	1 to 2 mg/minute IV up to 5 mg IV push for hypertensive crisis, repeat PRN at 2 to 5 minute intervals up to a total of 15 mg
Notes:	Use care in patients at risk for bronchospasm, diabetes, or hepatic impairment.

METRONIDAZOLE (SEE ANTIBIOTIC LISTING IN APPENDIX E)

MIDAZOLAM

Proprietary name(s):	Versed
Therapeutic class:	Benzodiazepine

Indications: Sedation before surgery or diagnostic procedure

Actions: Benzodiazepine sedative-hypnotic

Side effects: Sedation, paradoxical agitation, respiratory depression

Dose: Induction dose, 0.2 to 0.35 mg/kg IV, as needed, over 20 to 30 seconds

Reduce dose in elderly patients and in those already receiving other sedative medications.

Notes: Inject slowly to avoid complications of respiratory depression and hypotension. Should be used with appropriate monitoring for respiratory complications.

Antidote is flumazenil.

MISOPROSTOL

Proprietary name(s): Cytotec

Therapeutic class: Synthetic prostaglandin E1 analog

Indications: Prophylaxis of NSAID-related gastric ulcers

Actions: Inhibits gastric acid secretion and protects mucosal cells

Excretion: Renal (80%)

Side effects: Diarrhea, abdominal pain, nausea, headache, flatulence, and dyspepsia

Dose: 0.1 to 0.2 mg PO 4 times per day with food

Notes: Do not administer to pregnant women.

MORPHINE SULFATE

Therapeutic class: Narcotic analgesic

Indications: Moderate to severe pain and pulmonary edema

Actions: Narcotic analgesic and splanchnic venodilation

Metabolism: Hepatic

Excretion: Renal (90%) and biliary (7% to 10%)

Side effects: Respiratory depression, hypotension, sedation, nausea, vomiting, and constipation

Dose: For pulmonary edema or chest pain due to coronary ischemia, 2 to 4 mg

IV every 5 to 10 minutes to a maximum dose of 10 to 12 mg

For pain, 2 to 15 mg IV/IM/SC every 4 hours, as needed

Notes: 10 mg morphine (IM/SC) is equivalent to 60 to 80 mg meperidine (IM/SC/PO). Often administered with concomitant antinausea medication.

May be habit forming.

Antidote is naloxone.

NALOXONE HYDROCHLORIDE

Proprietary name(s): Narcan
Therapeutic class: Narcotic antagonist
Indications: Reversal of narcotic-induced effects
Actions: Narcotic receptor antagonist metabolism

Hepatic
Excretion: Renal
Side effects: Nausea, vomiting, and may precipitate withdrawal in narcotic abusers
Dose: 0.2 to 2 mg IV/IM, SC every 5 minutes to a maximum dose of 10 mg
Notes: Effects are shorter than most narcotics. Monitor for return of narcotic-induced symptoms, and repeat naloxone dose as necessary.

May be administered via ET in emergency situations.

NAPROXEN

Proprietary name(s): Naprosyn
Therapeutic class: NSAID
Indications: Inflammation due to arthritis, soft-tissue injury, and pericarditis
Actions: Propionic acid derivative; interferes with production of prostaglandins
Metabolism: Hepatic
Excretion: Renal
Side effects: Headaches, dizziness and lightheadedness, and epigastric pain

May compromise renal function in patients with renal impairment.

Contraindicated in the syndrome of aspirin sensitivity, nasal polyps, and bronchospasm.

Dose: 250 mg PO 2 times per day. Maximum dose: 1250 mg/day

Notes: Should be used with caution in patients receiving anticoagulant medications.

NIFEDIPINE

Proprietary name(s): Adalat and Procardia
Therapeutic class: Calcium channel blocker
Indications: Angina pectoris, coronary spasm, and hypertension
Actions: Calcium channel blocker and vasodilator
Metabolism: Hepatic
Excretion: Renal (80%)
Side effects: Hypotension, flushing, dizziness, headache, and peripheral edema
Dose: 10 to 30 mg PO 3 times per day. Maximum dose: 180 mg/day.
Notes: The edema due to nifedipine is due to vasodilation and does not respond to diuretics.

Hypotension is often difficult to treat with fluids alone and may require vasopressor agent administration.

Nifedipine has a greater effect than verapamil and diltiazem in peripheral vasculature.

NITROGLYCERIN

Therapeutic class: Vasodilator
Indications: Angina pectoris and CHF
Actions: Venous, coronary, and arterial vasodilation
Metabolism: Hepatic
Excretion: Renal
Side effects: Headache, hypotension, and flushing
Dose: Sublingual (SL) 0.15 to 0.6 mg every 3 to 5 minutes

Lingual aerosol 1 to 2 sprays onto or under the tongue every 3 to 5 minutes to a maximum dose of 3 sprays/15 minutes

Transdermal patch 0.2 mg/hour, increasing to 0.4 mg/hour. Patch should be left on for 10 to 12 hours then removed for 12 to 14 hours to avoid tolerance.

Transdermal paste 0.5 to 4 inches every 4 to 8 hours. Rotate sites.

Oral (sustained-release) 2 to 9 mg PO 2 to 3 times per day

IV 0 to 3 mcg/kg/minute. Titrate to desired BP.

Notes: Nitrate tolerance may develop with prolonged continuous administration. Dose must be individualized.

NYSTATIN

Proprietary name(s):	Mycostatin
Therapeutic class:	Antifungal
Indications:	Oral and esophageal candidiasis
Actions:	Disruption of fungal cell membranes
Excretion:	Fecal for a PO dose
Side effects:	Minimal; nausea and vomiting
Dose:	400,000 to 600,000 U PO swish and swallow 4 times per day
Notes:	Not absorbed orally.

OMEPRAZOLE

Proprietary name(s):	Prilosec, Losec
Therapeutic class:	H^+/K^+-ATPase inhibitor
Indications:	Active peptic ulcer disease, gastro-esophageal reflux, severe erosive esophagitis, gastric acid hypersecretion
Actions:	Gastric acid pump inhibitor
Excretion:	Renal (77%), remainder biliary
Side effects:	Headache, diarrhea, abdominal pain, nausea, vomiting, rash, dizziness
Dose:	For ulcer, reflux, and esophagitis, 20 mg PO every day
	For hypersecretion syndromes, start with 60 mg PO every day, increase to 120 mg 3 times per day as required to achieve desired results
Notes:	Not recommended for long-term maintenance therapy.

OXAZEPAM

Proprietary name(s):	Serax
Therapeutic class:	Benzodiazepine
Indications:	Insomnia and anxiety

Actions:	Benzodiazepine sedative-hypnotic
Side effects:	Sedation, respiratory depression, and confusion
Dose:	For sleep, 10 to 30 mg PO every night, as needed
	For anxiety, 30 to 100 mg PO every day in divided doses
Notes:	Peak effect in 1 to 4 hours. Relatively short duration.
	Antidote is flumazenil.

PANTOPRAZOLE

Proprietary name(s):	Protonix, Protium
Therapeutic class:	H^+/K^+-ATPase inhibitor
Indications:	Active peptic ulcer disease, gastroesophageal reflux, severe erosive esophagitis, gastric acid hypersecretion
Actions:	Gastric acid pump inhibitor
Side effects:	Headache, diarrhea, abdominal pain, nausea, vomiting, rash, dizziness
Dose:	For ulcer, reflux, and esophagitis, 40 mg PO every day
Notes:	Not recommended for long-term maintenance therapy.

PENICILLIN (SEE ANTIBIOTIC LISTING IN APPENDIX E)

PENTAMIDINE ISETHIONATE

Proprietary name(s):	Pentam
Therapeutic class:	Anti-PCP agent
Indications:	Pneumocystis carinii pneumonia (PCP)
Actions:	Unknown
Excretion:	Renal
Side effects:	Hypotension, renal failure, cardiac arrhythmias, hypoglycemia, and pancreatitis
Dose:	4 mg/kg/day in 50 to 250 mL 5% dextrose in water IV over 2 hours
	Reduce dose in renal-impaired patients.

PHENAZOPYRIDINE

Proprietary name(s):	Pyridium
Therapeutic class:	Urinary analgesic
Indications:	Cystitis and urethritis

Actions:	Analgesic effect on inflamed urinary tract mucosa
Excretion:	Renal
Side effects:	Orange discoloration of secretions including urine, tears, and semen; nausea, headache, rash, and pruritus
Dose:	200 mg PO 3 times per day after meals, as needed
Notes:	No antibacterial effects. May stain contact lenses.

PHENYTOIN

Proprietary name(s):	Dilantin
Therapeutic class:	Anticonvulsant
Indications:	Seizure disorders, prophylaxis, and treatment
Actions:	Anticonvulsant and reduces Na^+ transport across cerebral cell membranes
Metabolism:	At therapeutic doses, phenytoin is metabolized by the liver in zero-order kinetics (a fixed amount of drug is metabolized per unit time).
	Relatively small changes in the dose can cause major changes in serum concentrations in the long term. Serum levels are greatly affected by medications altering microsomal enzyme activity.
Excretion:	Renal
Side effects:	Hypotension, cardiac dysrhythmias, ataxia, nystagmus, dysarthria, hepatotoxicity, gingival hypertrophy, hirsutism, megaloblastic anemia, lymphadenopathy, fever, and rash
Dose:	For status epilepticus, 18 mg/kg IV in NS loading dose at a rate of 25 to 50 mg/minute, followed by a maintenance dose of 300 mg PO/IV every day
Notes:	Dose must be individualized. Follow serum levels.
	IM administration is erratically absorbed.
	Abrupt withdrawal may precipitate seizure activity.

PHYTONADIONE (VITAMIN K1)

Proprietary name(s):	AquaMEPHYTON
Therapeutic class:	Vitamin replacement
Indications:	Replacement in vitamin K deficiency and reversal of warfarin effects
Actions:	Vitamin K is essential for hepatic synthesis of clotting factors II, VII, IX, and X
Side effects:	Hematoma formation with SC/IM administration
Dose:	For reversal of overcoumarinization: 2.5 to 5 mg PO/SC/IM
	For vitamin supplementation in total parenteral nutrition (TPN): 2.5 mg IM weekly
Notes:	Avoid IV administration because of hypotension and anaphylaxis.
	Severe hemorrhage due to warfarin therapy is best treated with fresh frozen plasma. The effects of vitamin K take several days to overcome with continuous warfarin therapy.

PIPERACILLIN (SEE ANTIBIOTIC LISTING IN APPENDIX E)

POTASSIUM

Proprietary name(s):	Slow K, Micro-K, and Kay Ciel
Therapeutic class:	Potassium supplement
Indications:	Hypokalemia
Actions:	Potassium supplement
Side effects:	Nausea, vomiting, diarrhea, abdominal discomfort, and hyperkalemia
Dose:	For prevention, 24 to 40 mEq/day
	For treatment, 60 to 120 mEq/day
Notes:	Danger of hyperkalemia in patients with renal impairment, patients receiving potassium-sparing diuretics, and in those on ACE inhibitors.

PROCAINAMIDE

Proprietary name(s):	Procanbid
Therapeutic class:	Class IA antiarrhythmic

Indications:	Atrial and ventricular arrhythmias
Actions:	Reduces the maximum rate of depolarization in atrial and ventricular conducting tissues
Metabolism:	Hepatic
Excretion:	Renal
Side effects:	Hypotension, anorexia, nausea, vomiting, heart block, proarrhythmia, rash, fever, SLE-like syndrome, and arthralgias
Dose:	Load with 1 g PO followed by 250 to 500 mg PO every 3 hours.
	Delayed-release formulations may be given every 12 hours.
	For life-threatening tachydysrhythmias, 100 mg IV over 2 minutes, repeating the dose until the arrhythmia abates or to a maximum dose of 1 g. Follow with a maintenance infusion of 2 to 4 mg/minute.
Notes:	Actions are similar to quinidine except no atropinic effect.
	Cross-allergic with procaine.

PROCHLORPERAZINE

Proprietary name(s):	Compazine
Therapeutic class:	Phenothiazine
Indications:	Agitation, nausea, and vomiting
Actions:	Antagonist of dopamine, histamine, muscarine, and α_1-adrenergic responses
Metabolism:	Hepatic, with enterohepatic recirculation
Excretion:	Renal
Side effects:	Drowsiness, dizziness, amenorrhea, blurred vision, skin reactions, hypotension, extrapyramidal effects, jaundice, tardive dyskinesia, and neuroleptic malignant syndrome
Dose:	For nausea, 5 to 10 mg PO/IM every 6 to 8 hours, as needed, or 2.5 to 10 mg IV every 6 to 8 hours, as needed
Notes:	Extrapyramidal symptoms may be treated with diphenhydramine.

PROMETHAZINE

| Proprietary name(s): | Phenergan |
| Therapeutic class: | Phenothiazine |

Indications:	Sedation, antianxiety, nausea, and vomiting
Actions:	Antihistamine and anticholinergic
Metabolism:	Hepatic excretion
	Renal and fecal
Side effects:	Extrapyramidal symptoms, drowsiness, dizziness, constipation, dry mouth, and urinary retention
Dose:	25 to 50 mg PO/PR/IM every 4 to 6 hours, as needed
	12.5 to 25 mg IV every 4 to 6 hours, as needed
Notes:	Anticholinergic effects are additive with those of other medications such as tricyclic antidepressants.

PROPRANOLOL

Proprietary name(s):	Inderal
Therapeutic class:	Nonspecific β-blocker
Indications:	Angina pectoris, post-MI treatment of supraventricular tachycardia (SVT), hypertension, and thyrotoxicosis
Actions:	Nonspecific β-blockade
Metabolism:	Hepatic
Excretion:	Renal (<1%)
Side effects:	Hypotension, bradycardia, bronchospasm, CHF, nausea, vomiting, fatigue, nightmares, and may mask symptoms of hypoglycemia
Dose:	10 to 80 mg PO 2 to 4 times per day
	Begin with a low dose and adjust to desired effect.
Notes:	Abrupt withdrawal may precipitate symptoms of angina in patients with coronary artery disease.
	Dose must be individualized.

PROTAMINE SULFATE

Therapeutic class:	Heparin antagonist
Indications:	Reversal of heparin-induced anticoagulation
Actions:	Binds to and inactivates heparin
Side effects:	Hypotension, bradycardia, and flushing
Dose:	1 mg/100 mg heparin. Administer by slow IV push, no more than 50 mg in a 10-minute period.

Notes: Overdosage may paradoxically worsen hemorrhage as protamine also possesses anticoagulant properties. Effects may be transient.

QUININE SULFATE

Therapeutic class: Antimalarial
Indications: Nocturnal leg cramps
Actions: Increases muscular refractory period, decreases motor endplate excitability, and affects the distribution of calcium within the muscle fiber
Side effects: Nausea, visual disturbances, hemolytic anemia, and thrombocytopenia
Dose: 300 mg PO every night, as needed
Notes: Side effects are unusual at this dose, which is 1/10th of that used to treat malaria.

RANITIDINE

Proprietary name(s): Zantac
Therapeutic class: Histamine-2 antagonist
Indications: Peptic ulcer disease and gastroesophageal reflux
Actions: Inhibits histamine-induced secretion of gastric acid
Metabolism: Hepatic
Excretion: Renal (30% of PO dose, 70% of IV dose)
Side effects: Jaundice, gynecomastia, headache, confusion, and leukopenia
Dose: For acute symptoms, 50 mg IV every 8 hours or 150 mg PO 2 times per day or 300 mg PO every night
For maintenance therapy, 150 mg PO every night
Notes: Generally well tolerated. Does not have the same effect as cimetidine on microsomal enzymes or androgen blocking.

RETINOL (VITAMIN A)

Proprietary name(s): Aquasol A
Therapeutic class: Vitamin replacement
Indications: Replacement in vitamin A deficiency

Actions:	Vitamin A is essential in the production of rhodopsin in the eye and preserves the integrity of epithelial cells.
Metabolism:	Fat-soluble vitamin, stored in liver and excreted in feces
Side effects:	Due to overdose; fatigue, malaise, lethargy, abdominal discomfort, anorexia, nausea, irritability, headache, and skin changes
Dose:	100,000 to 500,000 U every day × 3 days PO/IM, followed by 50,000 U PO/IM every day × 2 months
Notes:	May facilitate wound healing in steroid-dependent patients.

SODIUM POLYSTYRENE SULFONATE

Proprietary name(s):	Kayexalate
Therapeutic class:	Cation exchange resin
Indications:	Hyperkalemia
Actions:	Nonabsorbable cation exchange resin
Side effects:	Nausea, vomiting, gastric irritation, and sodium retention
Dose:	15 to 30 g in 50 to 100 mL NS, or 20% sorbitol PO every 3 to 4 hours, or 50 g in 200 mL 20% sorbitol of 20% dextrose in water PR by retention enema for 30 to 60 minutes
Notes:	20 mEq of Na^+ are exchanged for 20 mEq K^+ for each 15 g resin given PO. Mg^{2+} and Ca^{2+} may also be exchanged.
	Actual results are highly variable.

SPIRONOLACTONE

Proprietary name(s):	Aldactone
Therapeutic class:	Aldosterone antagonist and diuretic
Indications:	Ascites, edema, hypertension, and hyperaldosteronism
Actions:	Aldosterone antagonist
Metabolism:	Hepatic (into many active metabolites)
Excretion:	Renal > biliary
Side effects:	Hyponatremia, gynecomastia, confusion, and headache
Dose:	50 to 100 mg PO per day (may be divided into 4 doses per day, as desired)

Higher doses may be required in states of hyperaldosteronism.

Notes: Most effective in states of hyperaldosteronism; however, equipotent to thiazide diuretics in the treatment of hypertension.

SUCRALFATE

Proprietary name(s):	Carafate
Therapeutic class:	Sulfated disaccharide
Indications:	Peptic ulcer disease, prophylaxis, and treatment
Actions:	Formation of an ulcer-adherent complex that acts as a barrier to damage from gastric acid, bile salts, and pepsin; minimal antacid properties
Excretion:	Fecal, not absorbed
Side effects:	Side effects are rare: constipation, nausea, gastric discomfort, pruritus, rash, dizziness, headache, insomnia, and vertigo
Dose:	1 g PO 4 times per day
Notes:	May reduce the absorption and effects of many medications including cimetidine, ciprofloxacin, digoxin, ketoconazole, norfloxacin, phenytoin, ranitidine, tetracycline, and theophylline.
	Sucralfate binds and sequesters aluminum. Use with caution in renally impaired patients.

SUMATRIPTAN SUCCINATE

Proprietary name(s):	Imitrex
Indications:	Intermittent treatment of migraine
Actions:	Selective 5-hydroxytryptamine-like receptor agonist
	Causes vasoconstriction, particularly of the dilated carotid circulation in migraine disorder
Side effects:	May cause coronary artery spasm. Contraindicated in patients with coronary artery disease, concomitant use of ergot alkaloid medication, concomitant use of MAO inhibitors,

uncontrolled hypertension, or hemiplegic migraine disorder.

Flushing, dizziness, feelings of heat, pressure, malaise, fatigue, drowsiness, nausea, and vomiting

Dose: 6 mg SC or 100 mg PO

If initial dose is partially or completely successful, may repeat doses with an additional 6 mg SC or 100 mg.

Do not exceed a maximum daily PO dose of 300 mg.

Do not repeat if initial dose has no effect.

Notes: Peak effect in 15 minutes with SC dose, in 0.5 to 5 hours with PO dose. A nasal spray formulation is also available.

TETRACYCLINE (SEE ANTIBIOTIC LISTING IN APPENDIX E)

THIAMINE (VITAMIN B1)

Therapeutic class:	Vitamin replacement
Indications:	Thiamine deficiency and prophylaxis of Wernicke's encephalopathy
Actions:	Water-soluble vitamin B1 replacement
Side effects:	IV administration associated with hypotension or anaphylactic shock
Dose:	100 mg PO/IM/IV every day × 3 days
	If given IV, administer over 5 minutes
Notes:	Well absorbed orally. Consider the PO route, even in emergencies.

TOBRAMYCIN (SEE ANTIBIOTIC LISTING IN APPENDIX E)

VANCOMYCIN (SEE ANTIBIOTIC LISTING IN APPENDIX E)

VERAPAMIL

Proprietary name(s):	Isoptin and Calan
Therapeutic class:	Calcium channel blocker
Indications:	Angina pectoris, treatment of SVTs, hypertension, and left ventricular diastolic dysfunction

Actions:	Calcium channel blockade and depresses AV conduction
Metabolism:	Hepatic
Excretion:	Renal (70%) and fecal
Side effects:	CHF, bradycardia, hypotension, headache, dizziness, and constipation
Dose:	For angina and hypertension, 80 to 120 mg PO 3 times per day
	For SVT, 5 to 10 mg IV; IV administration should only occur in monitored patients.
Notes:	Calcium gluconate 1 to 2 g IV may reverse the negative inotropic and hypotensive effects, but not the AV block.

WARFARIN

Proprietary name(s):	Coumadin
Therapeutic class:	Oral anticoagulant
Indications:	Prophylaxis and treatment of DVT, pulmonary embolism, and embolic CVA
Actions:	Inhibits vitamin K-dependent clotting factors
Metabolism:	Hepatic and microsomal
Excretion:	Renal
Side effects:	Hemorrhage, nausea, vomiting, skin necrosis, fever, and rash
Dose:	10 mg PO every day × 2 days, then estimate maintenance dose at 5 to 7.5 mg every day PO based on PT
Notes:	Dosage must be individualized to maintain PT in the desired range.
	Many medications interact to increase or decrease the effects of warfarin. Always look up the interactions with warfarin of any newly prescribed medication. Fresh frozen plasma is the treatment of choice to reverse warfarin-associated hemorrhage. Vitamin K is used if further warfarin therapy is not desired.

Index

Note: Page numbers in *Italics* refer to illustrations. Page numbers followed by t refer to tables.